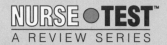

Medical-Surgical Nursing

SECOND EDITION

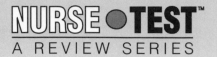

NURSE●TEST™
A REVIEW SERIES

Medical-Surgical Nursing

SECOND EDITION

Margaret M. Gingrich, RN, MSN

Associate Professor of Nursing

Harrisburg (Pa.) Area Community College

Janet H. Rhorer, RN, EdD, CS

Assistant Professor of Nursing

University of Texas at El Paso

SPRINGHOUSE CORPORATION ● SPRINGHOUSE, PENNSYLVANIA

STAFF

Vice President
Matthew Cahill

Editorial Director
Darlene Barela Cooke

Clinical Director
Judith Schilling McCann, RN, MSN

Art Director
John Hubbard

Managing Editor
David Moreau

Clinical Project Manager
Collette Bishop Hendler, RN, CCRN

Editor
Peter Johnson

Copy Editors
Brenna H. Mayer (manager), Virginia
Baskerville, Priscilla DeWitt, Stacey Ann
Follin, Barbara Long, Pamela Wingrod

Designers
Arlene Putterman (associate art director),
Linda Franklin (project manager), Donna
S. Morris, Stephanie Peters (cover design),
Jon Nelson (cover illustrator)

Manufacturing
Deborah Meiris (director), Patricia K.
Dorshaw (manager), Otto Mezei (book
production manager)

Editorial Assistants
Beverly Lane, Marcia Mills, Liz Schaeffer

℞ A member of the Reed Elsevier plc group

NTMS2 D N O S A J J M A
02 02 00   10 9 8 7 6 5 4 3 2

Library of Congress Cataloging-in-Publication Data
Medical-surgical nursing / [edited by] Margaret M. Gingrich, Janet H. Rhorer.
p. cm. — (Nurse test)
Includes bibliographical references and index.
1. Operating room nursing Examinations, questions, etc. 2. Surgical nursing Examinations, questions, etc. I. Gingrich, Margaret M. II. Rhorer, Janet H. III. Series: N.
[DNLM: 1. Perioperative Nursing Examination Questions. 2. Postoperative Care—nursing Examination Questions. WY 18.2 M4892 1999]
RD32.3M43 1999
610.73′677′076—dc21
DNLM/DLC   99-23705
ISBN 1-58255-003-4 (alk. paper)   CIP

CONTENTS

CONTRIBUTORS

Clare M. Brabson, RN, BSN
Staff Nurse
Fitzgerald Mercy Hospital
Darby, Pa.

Nancy M. Flynn, RN,C, MSN
Clinical Nurse Educator
Bryn Mawr (Pa.) Hospital

Linda B. Haas, RN, PhC, CDE
Endocrinology Clinical Nurse
  Specialist
Department of Veterans Affairs, Puget
Sound Health Care System
Seattle Division

Andrea R. Mann, RN, MSN
Instructor, Third Level Chairman
Frankford Hospital School of Nursing
Philadelphia
Adjunct Faculty
Pennsylvania State University
Abington

Jane V. McCloskey, RN, MSN
Faculty
Carolinas College of Health Science
Charlotte, N.C.

Gina Oliver, RN,C, PhD
Associate Professor
Deaconess College
St. Louis

Karin K. Roberts, RN, PhD
Associate Professor
Research College of Nursing
Kansas City, Mo.

INTRODUCTION

The commitment to a successful nursing career requires you to demonstrate that you have the knowledge to be a competent nurse. Passing rigorous challenge examinations and the NCLEX licensure examination shows your commitment to promoting high-quality nursing care.

NurseTest Medical-Surgical Nursing, Second Edition, is an in-depth question-and-answer review book that provides hundreds of multiple-choice questions to test your knowledge of the core nursing subject — medical-surgical nursing.

Organized by body system, each chapter contains questions related to that specific group of patients. Each question consists of a stem with four answer options. After answering the questions on the answer sheet, you can check your responses. The answers include rationales for both the correct and incorrect options. As an added feature, each question identifies the corresponding nursing process step, client needs category and subcategory, and taxonomic level.

Nursing process steps

When studying for a medical-surgical examination, keep in mind that the questions are designed to test your knowledge of the five nursing process steps: *assessment, analysis, planning, implementation, and evaluation.*

Client needs categories

The health needs of patients are organized by four major categories of client needs. These were identified during a 1996 job analysis study of newly licensed registered nurses. These four categories are further divided into 10 subcategories:

A. Safe, effective care environment
    1. *Management of care*
        Providing integrated, cost-effective care to patients by coordinating, supervising, or collaborating with members of the multidisciplinary health care team
    2. *Safety and infection control*
        Protecting patients and health care personnel from environmental hazards

B. Health promotion and maintenance
    1. *Growth and development through the life span*
        Assisting the patient and significant others through the normal, expected stages of growth and development from conception through advanced old age

2. *Prevention and early detection of disease*
Managing and providing care for patients in need of prevention and early detection of health problems

C. Psychosocial integrity
1. *Coping and adaptation*
Promoting patient's ability to cope, adapt, or troubleshoot situations related to illnesses or stressful events
2. *Psychosocial adaptation*
Managing and providing care for patients with acute or chronic mental illnesses

D. Physiological integrity
1. *Basic care and comfort*
Providing comfort and assistance in the performance of activities of daily living
2. *Pharmacological and parenteral therapies*
Managing and providing care related to the administration of medications and parenteral therapies
3. *Reduction of risk potential*
Reducing the likelihood that patients will develop complications or health problems related to existing conditions, treatments, or procedures
4. *Physiological adaptation*
Managing and providing care to patients with acute, chronic, or life-threatening physical health conditions

Taxonomic levels

The taxonomic or cognitive level of questions refers to the type of mental activity required to answer the question as defined in the cognitive domain. The NCLEX examination consists of multiple-choice questions at the cognitive levels of *knowledge, comprehension, application,* and *analysis.* Because the practice of nursing requires application of knowledge, skills, and abilities, most of the questions in the examination are written at the application or analysis level of cognitive ability.

Multiple-choice questions

Multiple-choice questions consist of an introductory statement, the stem, and four options. The introductory statement contains information about the clinical situation, and presents information about the patient, the disease, or interventions being done. The stem is the specific question you are to answer. The four options include, of course, the correct response and three distracters, which are options that are designed to resemble the correct answer but are incorrect. To successfully answer multiple-choice questions, you must separate what the question is telling you from what it is asking. Identify whether the stem is asking for a true response or false response.

True response stems ask you to identify appropriate nursing actions, prioritize nursing actions, or identify safe nursing judgments or therapeutic nursing responses. True response statements may also ask you to identify the action or statement that demonstrates success with teaching of the patient. Key words used with true response stems include *most, best, initially should, chief, immediate, indicative,* and *understands.*

False response stems are seeking wrong or negative information. Some key terms include *inappropriate, contraindicated, least important, lowest priority, required further instruction, unsafe,* and *least likely.*

Watch for such terms as *early, late, immediate, before, postoperative,* and *on admission.*

Thus, the first step in selecting the correct answer is identifying whether the stem is asking for a true or false response. Then read each option and identify whether it's a true or false response. Eliminate those that don't match what the stem is asking. Pay close attention to the timing indicated in each question. For example:

> Jon Walker, a 53-year-old patient with kidney stones, reports that he is allergic to shellfish. The nurse should anticipate administering which of the following agents before excretory urography?
>
> > **A.** Diphenhydramine (Benadryl)
> > **B.** Epinephrine
> > **C.** Albuterol (Proventil)
> > **D.** Interferon

Correct answer: **A**

Excretory urography requires contrast medium and radiography to visualize the urinary tract. Patients allergic to iodine or shellfish may react to the contrast medium because it contains iodine. Diphenhydramine, a histamine$_1$-receptor blocker is given to prevent an allergic response. Epinephrine and albuterol are bronchodilators used in the treatment of anaphylaxis and asthma; interferon is given to modulate immune responses to viruses.

> *Nursing process step:* Planning
> *Client needs category:* Physiological integrity
> *Client needs subcategory:* Pharmacological and parenteral therapies
> *Taxonomic level:* Application

Preparing for the test

Stress and anxiety are normal reactions to testing situations; however, uncontrollable anxiety will hurt your ability to do well. Proper study behaviors and a thorough preparation for an examination are the best ways to reduce the stress experienced before and during an examination. It doesn't matter if you start by reviewing lecture notes, textbooks, or various preparatory examinations, you must have a plan. Remember that the studying shouldn't just be for the exam, but to make you a better nurse as you start your career. Begin preparing early and don't try to cram all information into a few nights or hours of studying. The following is a suggested plan for scheduling your study time.

1. Set aside at least 2 to 3 hours for review per session. Review periods of 1 hour or less are often ineffective because of the time spent getting organized.
2. Take short breaks after an hour. Set a stopwatch so that you don't break your concentration by continuously thinking about the time and looking at your watch. When the timer goes off, get up and physically get away from the study area and materials. If you can't trust yourself to keep your break to about 10 minutes, use the timer again. Keep the television off, because there are no programs that short!
3. Start to review notes, texts, and other pertinent material.
4. Take a practice test that will diagnose your strengths and weaknesses.
5. One of the best ways to avoid the pitfalls of testing is to place yourself in the environment as often as possible. Practice with other tests as often as possible; compare results and identify your strengths and weaknesses.
6. Doing practice tests is a highly effective way to study and remember the material.

Day of the examination

1. Get up early.
2. Wear comfortable clothes, preferably layers that are easier to adjust to the environment.
3. Eat breakfast.
4. Leave early.
5. Arrive early.
6. Do NOT study while you wait for your examination.
7. Read, listen to music, relax.
8. Leave notes and books at home.
9. Listen carefully to the instructions given before entering the test room.

Test anxiety

Don't underestimate the power of positive thinking. If you tell yourself often enough "I'm going to fail this test," you just might do so. Therefore, if you keep convincing yourself that you're as prepared as anyone and are going to do well on the test, you're already ahead of the game.

If you find instant retrieval difficult and you feel as if facts and figures are just a jumble in your mind, you'll need to take a moment to relax. The simplest relaxation method is deep breathing. Just lean back in your chair, relax your muscles, and take three very deep breaths (count to 10 while you hold each one). That may be the only relaxing technique you need.

Other techniques involve focusing your mind on one thing and excluding everything else. While you're concentrating on one object, your mind can't be thinking of anything else.

Taking the test

You can improve your chances of performing well on multiple-choice tests by learning to choose between the best two options available and by following a set of proven guidelines.

Choosing between the two best options

The first step in choosing between the two best options is to be sure that you understand what the question is asking. Then eliminate the incorrect options. If you're having difficulty choosing between two seemingly correct responses, use the following strategies.

a. Eliminate similar distracters. If two options are essentially saying the same thing or include the same idea, then neither of them can be the answer. The answer has to be the option that is different.

b. Reread two seemingly correct options. If two options seem equally correct, reread them carefully; there must be some difference between them. Reread the stem; you may notice something you missed before.

c. Look for a global response. A more general statement may also include correct ideas from other options.

Guidelines to remember

- Budget your time. Although you may not know exactly how many questions you'll be asked to answer, you can estimate a little over 1 minute per question. Keep moving at a steady pace.
- Read each question thoroughly but quickly. In general, your first reaction to a question is the correct one. Remember that the examination is designed to determine if you're minimally competent and safe.
- Concentrate on one item at a time. Don't worry about how many questions you'll have to answer.

- Answer questions as if the situation were ideal. Assume the nurse had all the time and resources needed. You're only concerned about one patient, the one in the question.
- Focus on the key words in the stem.
- Identify whether the stem is seeking a true response or a false response. Those stems asking for false responses are easily misread.
- Reword a difficult stem.
- Try answering the question before you've read the options provided.
- Always read all options before selecting the best one.
- Relate each option to the stem.
- Use logic and common sense to figure out the correct response.
- Remember that the correct option will tend to have greater applicability and flexibility.
- Clueless? Look for clues in answer choices instead of in the stem of the question.
- Don't compare the situation to what your hospital does or to other experiences you may have had.

Judith Ann Driscoll, RN, MEd, MSN
Assistant Professor
Deaconess College of Nursing
St. Louis

CHAPTER 1

RESPIRATORY SYSTEM

QUESTIONS

1. A patient states that he has smoked a half a pack of cigarettes per day for 30 years. This should be documented as:

    A. 10 pack years.
    B. 15 pack years.
    C. 30 pack years.
    D. 40 pack years.

SITUATION: *Elisabeth Alexander, a 24-year-old factory worker with a history of asthma, presents to the emergency department with difficulty breathing.*

    Questions 2 to 4 refer to this situation.

2. When assessing Ms. Alexander, the nurse would expect to auscultate:

    A. diminished breath sounds and crackles in lung bases.
    B. moist crackles in lung bases.
    C. distant breath sounds and expiratory wheezes.
    D. bronchial breath sounds in lung bases.

3. A severe inflammatory response triggered Ms. Alexander's asthma attack. Which of the following drugs would the nurse expect to give to combat the inflammatory response?

    A. theophylline (Aminophylline)
    B. prednisone (Sterapred)
    C. metoprolol (Lopressor)
    D. albuterol (Proventil)

4. Ms. Alexander's condition worsens, requiring endotracheal intubation and mechanical ventilation. Her ventilator is set to respond with a positive pressure breath at a preset tidal volume every time she attempts to take a breath. If she fails to breathe, the machine automatically takes over ventilation at a preset rate and tidal volume. This ventilator mode is called the:

    A. pressure support mode.
    B. continuous positive airway pressure mode.
    C. synchronized intermittent mandatory ventilation mode.
    D. assist control mode.

SITUATION: *A 38-year old homeless man is brought to the emergency department by a police officer. The officer reports finding the man sitting on a street corner coughing up blood. After thorough assessment, the patient is thought to have tuberculosis.*

Questions 5 and 6 refer to this situation.

5. Which of the following diagnostic tests would confirm the diagnosis of tuberculosis (TB)?

    A. Chest X-ray
    B. Bronchoscopy
    C. Tuberculin skin test
    D. Sputum stains and cultures

6. Before giving the patient rifampin as prescribed, the nurse should warn the patient about which of the following possible adverse urinary reactions?

    A. Oliguria
    B. Reddish orange urine
    C. Polyuria
    D. Hematuria

SITUATION: *David Andrews, age 24, is admitted to the hospital following a motor vehicle accident. He wasn't wearing a seat belt. His blood pressure is 82/46 mm Hg; his heart rate, 118 beats/minute; and his respiratory rate, 32 breaths/minute.*

Questions 7 to 11 refer to this situation.

7. Mr. Andrews is restless and cyanotic. Based on this finding, the nurse should first:

    A. perform nasotracheal suctioning.
    B. inspect the patient's back for lacerations.
    C. observe the patient's chest for symmetry.
    D. palpate the patient's abdomen for tenderness.

8. While inspecting the patient's chest, the nurse notes that the chest wall contracts on inspiration and bulges on expiration. From this assessment, she suspects:

    A. hemothorax.
    B. flail chest.
    C. pneumothorax.
    D. tension pneumothorax.

9. Mr. Andrews's arterial blood gas (ABG) analysis reveals a pH of 7.20, a $Paco_2$ of 65 mm Hg, a Pao_2 of 45 mm Hg, and an HCO_3^- of 22 mEq/L. These laboratory values indicate:

    A. respiratory acidosis.
    B. metabolic acidosis.
    C. respiratory alkalosis.
    D. metabolic alkalosis.

10. Mr. Andrews's respiratory status continues to deteriorate. The nurse should prepare to assist with:

    A. chest decompression.
    B. chest tube insertion.
    C. pulmonary function tests.
    D. endotracheal intubation.

11. Mr. Andrews requires vecuronium bromide (Norcuron) to support mechanical ventilation. The patient's wife understands the nurse's teaching about the drug when she states:

    A. "I know he appears unconscious, but he's awake and can hear me."
    B. "I know he's unconscious and probably can't hear me."
    C. "I know he can see me but can't hear me."
    D. "I know he's unconscious and can't feel any pain."

SITUATION: *Anne Brown is a 45-year-old obese patient who had a colectomy for colon cancer 2 days ago. Her postoperative course has been uneventful, but she refuses to get out of bed.*

Questions 12 to 15 refer to this situation.

12. Which of the following interventions would help prevent complications of immobility?

    A. Performing passive range-of-motion exercises
    B. Administering I.V. fluids at a keep-vein-open rate
    C. Using the knee catch on the bed at all times
    D. Rubbing the patient's legs frequently to promote circulation

13. To assess Ms. Brown for possible Homans' sign, the nurse should:

    A. elevate the patient's leg and look for discoloration in the ankle area.
    B. squeeze the patient's calf and note any tenderness.
    C. dorsiflex the foot with the leg elevated, noting any calf pain.
    D. plantarflex the foot, noting any arch pain and discoloration.

14. Ms. Brown suddenly develops chest pain, shortness of breath, and air hunger. The nurse knows she must further assess Ms. Brown's chest pain to determine its origin. When determining whether the chest pain is cardiac or pleuritic in nature, the nurse knows that pleuritic chest pain typically:

   A. is described as crushing and substernal.
   B. worsens with deep inspiration.
   C. is relieved with nitroglycerin.
   D. is relieved when the patient leans forward.

15. Ms. Brown is diagnosed with a pulmonary embolus. Which of the following is the most appropriate nursing diagnosis for this patient?

   A. Ineffective airway clearance
   B. Risk for infection
   C. Impaired gas exchange
   D. Altered cardiopulmonary tissue perfusion

SITUATION: *Thomas Wood is a 19-year-old roofer who fell from a scaffold 20' (6 m) to the ground. He was admitted to the emergency department with multiple abrasions, complaining of shortness of breath.*

Questions 16 to 18 refer to this situation.

16. Mr. Wood's chest X-ray reveals a right pneumothorax. With this in mind, the nurse should first:

   A. help the patient turn, cough, and deep-breathe.
   B. prepare a chest drainage system.
   C. prepare the patient for a computed tomography (CT) scan of the chest.
   D. administer a sedative.

17. As the nurse helps Mr. Wood out of bed, his chest tube becomes dislodged and falls to the floor. Which of the following must be done first?

   A. Positioning the patient on the side where the chest tube was placed
   B. Reinserting the chest tube
   C. Sealing off the insertion site
   D. Having the patient perform Valsalva's maneuver

18. Assessment of Mr. Wood after chest tube insertion should include:

   A. noting bubbling within the drainage chamber.
   B. measuring chest drainage every 24 hours.
   C. auscultating breath sounds every 4 hours and as needed.
   D. percussing for subcutaneous emphysema every 8 hours.

SITUATION: *John Corinth, age 68, has been hospitalized repeatedly for chronic obstructive pulmonary disease (COPD). He's now being admitted to the medical-surgical floor for an exacerbation of COPD.*

Questions 19 to 23 refer to this situation.

19. The nurse is performing Mr. Corinth's admission assessment. She should obtain subjective data by:

    A. speaking to the patient's family.
    B. assessing the patient's respiratory rate.
    C. asking the patient to describe his symptoms.
    D. assessing the patient's breathing pattern.

20. During assessment, Mr. Corinth is having difficulty breathing. When interviewing him about his health history, the nurse should:

    A. ask him as few questions as possible.
    B. quickly ask as many questions as possible.
    C. postpone asking questions.
    D. ignore his breathing difficulty to avoid embarrassing him.

21. The doctor orders pulmonary function tests for Mr. Corinth. Which of the following instructions should be given to him before testing?

    A. "Don't take bronchodilators for 4 hours before testing."
    B. "These tests measure your breathing at rest."
    C. "You may eat a clear liquid breakfast the morning of the testing."
    D. "A blood sample will be drawn during testing."

22. Mr. Corinth returns to his room after pulmonary function testing and develops an acute episode of respiratory distress. How is oxygen most accurately administered for this condition?

    A. Simple mask
    B. Partial rebreather mask
    C. Venturi mask
    D. Bag-valve mask

23. Mr. Corinth refuses to participate in his self-care. Every time the nurse approaches him he states, "I just want to die. I'm no good to anyone anymore." The nurse realizes that he's experiencing:

    A. self-actualization.
    B. confabulation.
    C. reaction formation.
    D. grief.

SITUATION: *Brittany Evans, age 52, is admitted to the medical-surgical floor with a 2-week history of hemoptysis. The doctor suspects lung cancer and has ordered the appropriate diagnostic tests.*

Questions 24 to 27 refer to this situation.

24. While preparing Ms. Evans for a diagnostic test, the nurse explains, "The doctor will insert a tube down your throat to visualize your trachea and lung passages." The nurse has explained which of the following diagnostic tests?

    A. Bronchoscopy
    B. Ventilation and perfusion scan
    C. Pulmonary angiography
    D. Oral endoscopy

25. The nurse is caring for Ms. Evans immediately following her bronchoscopy. Which of the following nursing diagnoses should receive priority?

    A. Pain related to throat irritation
    B. Risk for aspiration related to gag reflex suppression
    C. Risk for injury related to restraint use during the procedure
    D. Anxiety related to possible diagnosis

26. Ms. Evans undergoes a right pneumonectomy for lung cancer. Which of the following positions shouldn't be used when repositioning her immediately following the procedure?

    A. Semi-Fowler's position
    B. Left side-lying position
    C. Right side-lying position
    D. High Fowler's position

27. Ms. Evans should be assessed closely for which of the following complications of a pneumonectomy?

    A. Pulmonary edema
    B. Transposition of the great vessels
    C. Pleurisy
    D. Pericarditis

SITUATION: *Wayne Dale is a 46-year-old patient brought to the emergency department after a tonic-clonic seizure. His blood pressure is 159/88 mm Hg; his heart rate, 111 beats/minute; and his respiratory rate, 22 breaths/minute.*

Questions 28 to 30 refer to this situation.

28. Following the tonic-clonic seizure, Mr. Dale has snoring respirations. The doctor orders a nasopharyngeal airway inserted to protect Mr. Dale's airway. The nurse is inserting the airway correctly when she:

    A. depresses the tongue as the airway is inserted.
    B. lubricates the airway with petroleum jelly.
    C. inserts the airway with the tip upward.
    D. gently pushes the airway along the floor of the nostril.

29. Mr. Dale experiences additional seizure activity after admission to the medical-surgical floor and is given lorazepam (Ativan). Later, his respirations become shallow and drop to a rate of 6 breaths/minute. What is the most appropriate oxygen delivery system for this patient?

    A. Nasal cannula
    B. Simple face mask
    C. Venturi mask
    D. Bag-valve mask

30. Mr. Dale requires endotracheal intubation and mechanical ventilation. Disconnecting the ventilator and vigorously suctioning Mr. Dale for a prolonged period could lead to which of the following complications?

    A. Hypoxemia
    B. Hypovolemia
    C. Hyperthermia
    D. Septicemia

SITUATION: *Priscilla Graver, age 57, went to her doctor complaining of difficulty breathing and pain in the left side of her chest. She states she has had shaking chills and a productive cough. The doctor advises Mrs. Graver's husband to take her to the hospital for admission.*

Questions 31 to 34 refer to this situation.

31. The doctor orders a sputum culture for Mrs. Graver. When collecting a sputum specimen, the nurse should:

    A. tell the patient to cough deeply and expectorate into the specimen container.
    B. place the patient in the semi-Fowler position and tell her to cough shallowly.
    C. place the patient in the high Fowler position and tell her to expectorate saliva into the specimen container.
    D. tell the patient to breathe deeply, cough shallowly, and expectorate into the specimen container.

32. Mrs. Graver is admitted to the medical-surgical floor with a diagnosis of bacterial pneumonia. The most common causative organism of bacterial pneumonia is:

   A. *Streptococcus pneumoniae.*
   B. *Proteus* species.
   C. *Haemophilus influenzae.*
   D. *Escherichia coli.*

33. Aggressive chest physiotherapy is instituted but isn't successful in removing Mrs. Graver's secretions. Which type of drug would the nurse expect the doctor to prescribe following physiotherapy?

   A. Anticholinergic
   B. Mucolytic
   C. Antibiotic
   D. Diuretic

34. Which is the most appropriate nursing diagnosis for the patient with pneumonia?

   A. Fluid volume deficit
   B. Decreased cardiac output
   C. Impaired gas exchange
   D. Risk for infection

SITUATION: *Kelsey Killian is a 43-year-old unrestrained driver admitted to the hospital after a motor vehicle crash. She sustained fractured ribs on the left side, a pelvic fracture, and a left femur fracture. She has a history of type 1 diabetes and breast cancer and is presently using birth control pills.*

Questions 35 to 38 refer to this situation.

35. Which of the following factors places Ms. Killian at risk for developing adult respiratory distress syndrome (ARDS)?

   A. Traumatic injury
   B. History of diabetes
   C. History of breast cancer
   D. Use of birth control pills

36. A classic finding in the patient with acute respiratory distress syndrome (ARDS) is:

   A. sudden hypocalcemia with tetany.
   B. severe hyperkalemia.
   C. hypoxia resistant to oxygen therapy.
   D. hypercapnia.

37. What pathologic change is responsible for the development of pulmonary edema in the patient with acute respiratory distress syndrome (ARDS)?

  A. Right-sided heart failure
  B. Alveolocapillary membrane damage
  C. Extravascular fluid volume excess
  D. Pulmonary artery infarct

38. Ms. Killian continues to show signs of hypoxemia. The nurse knows that the patient's treatment plan is appropriate when the doctor:

  A. prescribes mechanical ventilation.
  B. prescribes chest physiotherapy.
  C. prescribes low FIO_2 concentrations.
  D. inserts a chest tube.

SITUATION: *Debbie James, a 24-year-old patient, comes to the emergency department hyperventilating and complaining of numbness and tingling in her hands. She states she had an argument with her boyfriend about 45 minutes ago.*

Questions 39 and 40 refer to this situation.

39. The doctor prescribes an arterial blood gas analysis, which reveals a pH of 7.64, a $Paco_2$ of 26 mm Hg, a Pao_2 of 100 mm Hg, and an HCO_3^- of 28 mEq/L. After analyzing the results, the nurse determines that the patient is experiencing:

  A. respiratory acidosis.
  B. metabolic acidosis.
  C. respiratory alkalosis.
  D. metabolic acidosis.

40. The nurse should tell Ms. James to do which of the following to arrest the hyperventilation?

  A. Take frequent shallow breaths.
  B. Breathe into a paper bag.
  C. Take frequent deep breaths.
  D. Sit quietly and forget about the argument.

SITUATION: *Lynne Jones is a 21-year-old patient with a history of type 1 diabetes. She presents to the emergency department with nausea, which she has had for 2 days. Her serum glucose level is 556 mg/dl and her urine is positive for ketones.*

Questions 41 and 42 refer to this situation.

41. Ms. Jones has abnormally deep, gasping respirations. This breathing pattern is known as:

  A. bradypnea.
  B. Cheyne-Stokes respirations.
  C. Biot's respirations.
  D. Kussmaul's respirations.

42. Ms. Jones's arterial blood gas analysis reveals a pH of 7.25, a $Paco_2$ of 33 mm Hg, a Pao_2 of 102 mm Hg, and an HCO_3^- of 19 mEq/L. After analyzing these values, the nurse determines that the patient is experiencing:

  A. respiratory acidosis.
  B. metabolic acidosis.
  C. respiratory alkalosis.
  D. metabolic alkalosis.

SITUATION: *Ronald Emerson is returned to the medical-surgical floor after tracheostomy insertion. His respirations are regular and unlabored but his tracheostomy is producing large amounts of sputum.*

  Questions 43 to 45 refer to this situation.

43. During the immediate postoperative period, the priority nursing diagnosis for Mr. Emerson would be:

  A. ineffective airway clearance related to bronchial secretions.
  B. risk for infection related to new surgical incision.
  C. risk for injury related to confusion from anesthesia.
  D. body image disturbance related to tracheostomy insertion.

44. Mr. Emerson requires tracheostomy care at each shift. When providing tracheostomy care, the nurse should:

  A. wash the suction catheter with soap and water.
  B. suction the patient first using low wall suction.
  C. replace the disposable inner cannula daily.
  D. clean the stoma with equal parts saline solution and hydrogen peroxide.

45. The next day, Mr. Emerson has coughing episodes while taking clear liquids by mouth. The nurse should immediately:

  A. check to see if the tracheostomy cuff is inflated.
  B. check to see if the tracheostomy cuff is deflated.
  C. consult speech therapy for swallowing studies.
  D. place the patient in Trendelenburg's position.

SITUATION: *Terrance Rex is a 53-year-old mine worker admitted to the hospital after his doctor detects a lesion on his chest X-ray during an annual physical examination. A lung biopsy confirms a diagnosis of sarcoidosis.*

Questions 46 to 48 refer to this situation.

46. The nurse should describe sarcoidosis to Mr. Rex as:

    A. a disease characterized by multiple body organ masses.
    B. an occupational disease caused by air pollution.
    C. a contagious disease that affects mostly blacks.
    D. a highly infectious disease of the respiratory tract.

47. The doctor prescribes a corticosteroid for Mr. Rex. To assess him for adverse effects of the corticosteroid the nurse should do which of the following?

    A. Observe for signs of hyperglycemia.
    B. Check for signs of hyponatremia.
    C. Weigh the patient weekly.
    D. Monitor for hypotension.

48. Mr. Rex shows that he understands the discharge instructions he's received about corticosteroid administration when he states:

    A. "I shouldn't eat 1 hour before or 2 hours after taking the drug."
    B. "I'm glad I don't have to watch my salt intake."
    C. "I know I shouldn't suddenly stop taking the drug."
    D. "I'm so glad I can still visit my granddaughter even though she has a bad cold."

SITUATION: *Jason Miller, a 19-year-old college student, is on the varsity football team. During the game, he's tackled and sustains fractured ribs on the right side of the chest. He's taken to the emergency department of a local hospital.*

Questions 49 to 55 refer to this situation.

49. Which initial clinical manifestation would the nurse expect Jason to exhibit?

    A. Paradoxical respiration
    B. Crackles heard in the right lung base
    C. A clicking sensation during inspiration
    D. Shallow, painful breathing

50. Jason becomes increasingly irritable and short of breath. A chest X-ray shows 30% of his right lung has collapsed. He's given oxygen via nasal cannula while awaiting chest tube insertion. At this point, the nurse should assess for which early sign of hypoxia?

A. Bradycardia
B. Restlessness
C. Hypotension
D. Glycosuria

51. Jason asks the nurse, "What if I stop breathing when the doctor inserts the chest tube?" The most appropriate response would be to:

A. explain how the tubes function.
B. assure him that the nurse and doctor will be present.
C. ask the doctor to postpone the procedure.
D. ask the chaplain to talk to the patient about the procedure.

52. The doctor orders diazepam (Valium) I.V. before chest tube insertion primarily to:

A. alleviate pain.
B. increase respiratory rate.
C. relieve anxiety and tension.
D. increase muscle activity.

53. While Jason is connected to the chest drainage device, the nurse should immediately report:

A. excessive bubbling in the water-seal chamber.
B. fluctuation of fluid in the water-seal chamber.
C. dark red drainage in the collection chamber.
D. a fluid level of 20 cm in the suction control chamber.

54. Which observation would most likely indicate that Jason's chest tube should be removed?

A. 120 ml of chest tube drainage in 24 hours
B. Cessation of pain and dyspnea
C. Absence of fluid fluctuation in the water-seal chamber
D. Lung reexpansion on chest X-ray

55. Which method would best prevent air from entering the pleural cavity when Jason's chest tube is removed?

A. Breathing through pursed lips
B. Inhaling quickly and shallowly
C. Breathing with an opened mouth
D. Performing Valsalva's maneuver

SITUATION: *Henry Chung, age 48, has a persistent cough from a cold. His doctor prescribes guaifenesin (Breonesin) every 4 hours.*

Questions 56 to 58 refer to this situation.

56. Which of the following conditions requires cautious use of guaifenesin?

    A. Hypertension
    B. Acute angle-closure glaucoma
    C. Respiratory insufficiency
    D. Prostatic hyperplasia

57. How soon after taking the first dose of guaifenesin should Mr. Chung experience relief from coughing?

    A. Within 30 minutes
    B. In 45 to 60 minutes
    C. In 1½ to 2 hours
    D. In 2½ to 3 hours

58. During a teaching session, the nurse double-checks Mr. Chung's current medication usage. Which of the following drugs could interact with guaifenesin?

    A. Anticonvulsants
    B. Antiarrhythmics
    C. Antihypertensives
    D. Anticoagulants

SITUATION: *Nicholas Minucci, a 55-year-old patient with respiratory failure, is complaining of shortness of breath. His blood pressure is 176/90 mm Hg; his heart rate, 126 beats/minute; and his respiratory rate, 34 breaths/minute.*

Questions 59 and 60 refer to this situation.

59. The nurse notices that Mr. Minucci's chest is covered with hair. To accurately assess his breath sounds with the stethoscope, the nurse should:

    A. shave his chest first.
    B. use the diaphragm instead of the bell of the stethoscope.
    C. place her stethoscope on the patient's gown.
    D. lightly wet the hair.

60. Mr. Minucci's condition deteriorates, requiring endotracheal intubation. During intubation, he experiences cardiac arrest and his I.V. catheter becomes dislodged. Which of the following drugs can be administered down an endotracheal tube as an alternative route?

A. Naloxone, atropine, diazepam, epinephrine, and lidocaine
B. Naloxone, amrinone, diazepam, epinephrine, and lidocaine
C. Norepinephrine, atropine, diazepam, epinephrine, and lidocaine
D. Naloxone, atropine, digoxin, epinephrine, and lidocaine

SITUATION: *Michael Horowitz has had a persistent cough for about 4 months. One week ago, he noted blood in his sputum. He was admitted to the hospital where diagnostic testing confirmed lung cancer.*

Questions 61 to 63 refer to this situation.

61. After a lobectomy, Mr. Horowitz is returned to his room with chest tubes in place. The nurse assigns a nursing diagnosis of impaired gas exchange related to lung surgery. With this diagnosis, the expected outcome is that the patient will:

A. report loss of chest pain.
B. assume the semi-Fowler position.
C. request pain medication frequently.
D. exhibit a pulse oximetry of 94% or above.

62. Mr. Horowitz requires radiation therapy on an outpatient basis to treat the cancer. When teaching Mr. Horowitz about skin care, the nurse should encourage him to:

A. use skin lotions and powders on the irradiated area.
B. avoid washing off the marks placed on his skin to guide radiation therapy.
C. wear constrictive clothing.
D. massage the irradiated area to increase circulation.

63. Mr. Horowitz's wife is concerned about his poor appetite and weight loss. The nurse explains to her that radiation treatment, anxiety, and the disease itself can cause anorexia in cancer patients. The nurse should encourage Mr. Horowitz to:

A. limit his activities before and after meals.
B. force fluids.
C. eat high-calorie foods.
D. eat hot meat dishes with special sauces.

ANSWER SHEET

	A B C D		A B C D		A B C D
1	○ ○ ○ ○	22	○ ○ ○ ○	43	○ ○ ○ ○
2	○ ○ ○ ○	23	○ ○ ○ ○	44	○ ○ ○ ○
3	○ ○ ○ ○	24	○ ○ ○ ○	45	○ ○ ○ ○
4	○ ○ ○ ○	25	○ ○ ○ ○	46	○ ○ ○ ○
5	○ ○ ○ ○	26	○ ○ ○ ○	47	○ ○ ○ ○
6	○ ○ ○ ○	27	○ ○ ○ ○	48	○ ○ ○ ○
7	○ ○ ○ ○	28	○ ○ ○ ○	49	○ ○ ○ ○
8	○ ○ ○ ○	29	○ ○ ○ ○	50	○ ○ ○ ○
9	○ ○ ○ ○	30	○ ○ ○ ○	51	○ ○ ○ ○
10	○ ○ ○ ○	31	○ ○ ○ ○	52	○ ○ ○ ○
11	○ ○ ○ ○	32	○ ○ ○ ○	53	○ ○ ○ ○
12	○ ○ ○ ○	33	○ ○ ○ ○	54	○ ○ ○ ○
13	○ ○ ○ ○	34	○ ○ ○ ○	55	○ ○ ○ ○
14	○ ○ ○ ○	35	○ ○ ○ ○	56	○ ○ ○ ○
15	○ ○ ○ ○	36	○ ○ ○ ○	57	○ ○ ○ ○
16	○ ○ ○ ○	37	○ ○ ○ ○	58	○ ○ ○ ○
17	○ ○ ○ ○	38	○ ○ ○ ○	59	○ ○ ○ ○
18	○ ○ ○ ○	39	○ ○ ○ ○	60	○ ○ ○ ○
19	○ ○ ○ ○	40	○ ○ ○ ○	61	○ ○ ○ ○
20	○ ○ ○ ○	41	○ ○ ○ ○	62	○ ○ ○ ○
21	○ ○ ○ ○	42	○ ○ ○ ○	63	○ ○ ○ ○

ANSWERS AND RATIONALES

1. *Correct answer:* **B**

The formula for determining pack years is the number of years the patient smoked multiplied by the number of packs of cigarettes smoked per day. Thus: 30 years × one-half pack/day = 15 pack years.

> *Nursing process step:* Assessment
> *Client needs category:* Health promotion and maintenance
> *Client needs subcategory:* Prevention and early detection of disease
> *Taxonomic level:* Comprehension

2. *Correct answer:* **C**

During an asthma attack, breath sounds are distant. Expiration is prolonged with high-pitched wheezes throughout the lungs. Diminished breath sounds and crackles at lung bases may be a sign of atelectasis, a complication that is common with immobility. Moist crackles in lung bases may indicate left-sided heart failure. Bronchial breath sounds in lung bases may indicate bilateral lower-lobe pneumonia.

> *Nursing process step:* Assessment
> *Client needs category:* Physiological integrity
> *Client needs subcategory:* Reduction of risk potential
> *Taxonomic level:* Application

3. *Correct answer:* **B**

Prednisone, a corticosteroid, is a potent anti-inflammatory agent used in the acute management of asthma. Theophylline is a smooth-muscle relaxant that is used also to treat asthma. Metoprolol is a beta-adrenergic blocking agent that is contraindicated in patients with asthma. Albuterol is a selective $beta_2$-adrenergic bronchodilator used to prevent and treat bronchospasm in patients with asthma.

> *Nursing process step:* Planning
> *Client needs category:* Physiological integrity
> *Client needs subcategory:* Pharmacological and parenteral therapies
> *Taxonomic level:* Application

4. *Correct answer:* **D**

In assist control mode, the ventilator responds with a positive pressure breath at the preset tidal volume to every patient effort, and if the patient stops breathing, it automatically takes over ventilation at a preset rate and tidal volume. In pressure support mode, the ventilator supplements the patient's spontaneous breath with a preset positive pressure. It doesn't provide the entire volume, and the patient determines the respiratory rate. In continuous positive airway pressure mode, the intubated patient breathes spontaneously while the machine maintains airway pressure above atmospheric pressure. In synchronized intermittent mandatory ventilation mode, the ventilator allows the patient to breathe spontaneously but also delivers a synchronized positive-pressure breath at a predetermined rate.

Nursing process step: Implementation
Client needs category: Physiological integrity
Client needs subcategory: Physiological adaptation
Taxonomic level: Knowledge

5. *Correct answer:* **D**

Sputum stains and cultures that reveal tubercle bacilli confirm the diagnosis of TB. Chest X-rays can help diagnose TB by revealing nodular lesions, patchy infiltrates (mainly in the upper lobes), cavity formation, scar tissue, and calcium deposits, but they don't confirm the diagnosis. Bronchoscopy shows inflammation and altered lung tissue. It may also aid diagnosis by obtaining a sputum specimen if the patient is unable to produce one but bronchoscopy alone doesn't confirm the diagnosis. Tuberculin skin test reveals infection has occurred at some point but doesn't indicate active disease.

Nursing process step: Assessment
Client needs category: Health promotion and maintenance
Client needs subcategory: Prevention and early detection of disease
Taxonomic level: Knowledge

6. *Correct answer:* **B**

Rifampin may cause urine, tears, sweat, and feces to turn reddish orange. Oliguria, polyuria, and hematuria aren't adverse effects of rifampin.

Nursing process step: Planning
Client needs category: Physiological integrity
Client needs subcategory: Pharmacological and parenteral therapies
Taxonomic level: Comprehension

7. *Correct answer:* **C**

The patient is exhibiting signs of hypoxia; therefore, the first priority is to inspect his chest for symmetry. Unequal chest expansion indicates a possible pneumothorax and paradoxical chest movement indicates a flail chest. Nasotracheal suctioning would further deprive him of oxygen and wouldn't help diagnose the cause of his cyanosis. The patient's back and abdomen can be assessed after the cyanosis is addressed.

Nursing process step: Implementation
Client needs category: Physiological integrity
Client needs subcategory: Reduction of risk potential
Taxonomic level: Application

8. *Correct answer:* **B**

Flail chest occurs when two or more adjacent ribs are fractured at two or more sites resulting in a free-floating segment. This loss of chest wall stability causes respiratory impairment and notable paradoxical chest wall movement. Hemothorax or pneumothorax both decrease chest wall excursion on the affected side. A tension pneumothorax causes a mediastinal shift and tracheal deviation toward the unaffected side.

Nursing process step: Assessment
Client needs category: Physiological integrity
Client needs subcategory: Reduction of risk potential
Taxonomic level: Comprehension

9. *Correct answer:* **A**

Normal ABG values are: pH, 7.35 to 7.45; $Paco_2$, 35 to 45 mm Hg; Pao_2, 75 to 100 mm Hg; and HCO_3^-, 22 to 26 mEq/L. Mr. Andrews's ABG analysis shows a low pH and an elevated $Paco_2$, indicating respiratory acidosis. The kidneys haven't begun to compensate for the acidosis because the HCO_3^- is normal. With metabolic acidosis, the pH and HCO_3^- are low and the $Paco_2$ is normal. In the patient with respiratory alkalosis, the pH is elevated and the $Paco_2$ is low. In metabolic alkalosis, both pH and HCO_3^- are elevated.

Nursing process step: Assessment
Client needs category: Physiological integrity
Client needs subcategory: Physiological adaptation
Taxonomic level: Analysis

10. *Correct answer:* **D**

The treatment of choice for a patient with flail chest in respiratory distress is endotracheal intubation and mechanical ventilation. A chest tube or decompression would only be indicated for a flail chest if a pneumothorax were present. Pulmonary function tests aren't indicated for the unstable patient who has a flail chest.

Nursing process step: Planning
Client needs category: Physiological integrity
Client needs subcategory: Physiological adaptation
Taxonomic level: Application

11. *Correct answer:* **A**

When a neuromuscular blocking agent such as vecuronium bromide is used to support mechanical ventilation, the patient loses motor function and can't move. However, sensation remains intact, so the patient can still hear, see, taste, and smell. A sedative must be administered simultaneously to alleviate anxiety and provide comfort to the patient.

> *Nursing process step:* Evaluation
> *Client needs category:* Physiological integrity
> *Client needs subcategory:* Pharmacological and parenteral therapies
> *Taxonomic level:* Comprehension

12. *Correct answer:* **A**

Passive range-of-motion prevents venous pooling of blood in the extremities, reducing the risk of clot formation. Decreasing I.V. fluids to a keep-vein-open rate increases blood viscosity, increasing the risk of clot formation. Using the knee catch on the bed causes blood to pool in the lower leg. Rubbing the legs vigorously can displace any thrombi that might be present.

> *Nursing process step:* Implementation
> *Client needs category:* Physiological integrity
> *Client needs subcategory:* Reduction of risk potential
> *Taxonomic level:* Application

13. *Correct answer:* **C**

To assess for Homans' sign, the nurse should elevate the patient's leg and dorsiflex the foot, noting any calf tenderness or pain. Squeezing the calf could dislodge any thrombi that might be present. Elevating the patient's leg while looking for discoloration in the ankle area and plantarflexing the foot and noting arch pain and discoloration aren't steps to assessing for Homans' sign.

> *Nursing process step:* Assessment
> *Client needs category:* Physiological integrity
> *Client needs subcategory:* Reduction of risk potential
> *Taxonomic level:* Comprehension

14. *Correct answer:* **B**

Pleuritic chest pain is typically described as intermittent, sharp, and very painful and is aggravated with deep inspiration or movement. Crushing, substernal chest pain that is relieved by nitroglycerin is usually of cardiac origin. Leaning forward typically relieves pain associated with endocarditis.

> *Nursing process step:* Assessment
> *Client needs category:* Physiological integrity
> *Client needs subcategory:* Physiological adaptation
> *Taxonomic level:* Application

15. *Correct answer:* **D**

Pulmonary embolus occurs when a thrombus lodges in a branch of the pulmonary artery, partially or totally occluding it. The lung is adequately ventilated but can't be perfused, so there is altered cardiopulmonary tissue perfusion. There is no increase in secretions with a pulmonary embolus, so ineffective airway clearance wouldn't be appropriate. The patient isn't at risk for infection.

> *Nursing process step:* Analysis
> *Client needs category:* Physiological integrity
> *Client needs subcategory:* Physiological adaptation
> *Taxonomic level:* Application

16. *Correct answer:* **B**

When a pneumothorax is diagnosed, a chest tube must be inserted to evacuate air from the pleural space. The nurse must prepare the chest drainage system so that it can be attached to the chest tube immediately after insertion. A CT scan of the chest isn't used to diagnose a pneumothorax. Turning, coughing, and deep breathing can be encouraged after the chest tube is inserted. Sedation may be administered immediately prior to chest tube insertion, but the nurse should prepare the chest drainage system first.

> *Nursing process step:* Implementation
> *Client needs category:* Physiological integrity
> *Client needs subcategory:* Physiological adaptation
> *Taxonomic level:* Application

17. *Correct answer:* **C**

Sealing off the insertion site with an occlusive dressing takes top priority when a chest tube becomes dislodged. This prevents air from reentering the pleural space through the opening in the chest wall. After the insertion site is sealed off, the doctor should be notified so that a new chest tube can be inserted. Placing the patient on his side wouldn't help him at this time. The patient should perform Valsalva's maneuver to prevent air embolus when a central venous catheter cap is replaced.

> *Nursing process step:* Implementation
> *Client needs category:* Physiological integrity
> *Client needs subcategory:* Reduction of risk potential
> *Taxonomic level:* Application

18. *Correct answer:* **C**

In a patient with a chest tube, the nurse should auscultate for breath sounds every 4 hours and as needed to ensure that the tube is patent, expansion is achieved and maintained, and the patient's pulmonary status isn't deteriorating. Chest tube drainage should be assessed at least every 4 hours for patients whose condition is stable and more frequently for those who have just had a chest tube placed or who have had significant drainage. Subcutaneous emphysema is best evaluated by palpation or auscultation and should be assessed at least every 4 hours. Bubbling shouldn't occur in the drainage chamber of the chest tube drainage system.

> *Nursing process step:* Assessment
> *Client needs category:* Physiological integrity
> *Client needs subcategory:* Reduction of risk potential
> *Taxonomic level:* Application

19. *Correct answer:* **C**

The patient's perspective on his physical problem is subjective data. Assessing the patient's respiratory rate and breathing pattern are examples of objective data collection; objective data are information collected by the nurse about the patient's condition. Speaking to the patient's family can add insight into the patient's condition but isn't considered subjective data.

> *Nursing process step:* Assessment
> *Client needs category:* Physiological integrity
> *Client needs subcategory:* Reduction of risk potential
> *Taxonomic level:* Comprehension

20. *Correct answer:* **A**

To avoid worsening his dyspnea, the nurse should ask the patient as few questions as possible. Asking many questions quickly will exacerbate the patient's dyspnea by forcing him to answer quickly. Postponing the patient history at this time risks missing important information needed to adequately plan his care. The patient may feel the nurse is minimizing his problem if she ignores it.

> *Nursing process step:* Assessment
> *Client needs category:* Physiological integrity
> *Client needs subcategory:* Reduction of risk potential
> *Taxonomic level:* Application

21. *Correct answer:* **A**

Because pulmonary function tests evaluate ventilatory function through spirometric measurements, bronchodilators shouldn't be used for 4 hours before testing. The patient should have nothing by mouth after midnight the evening before the test. Pulmonary function testing doesn't require blood samples.

> *Nursing process step:* Planning
> *Client needs category:* Physiological integrity
> *Client needs subcategory:* Reduction of risk potential
> *Taxonomic level:* Application

22. *Correct answer:* **C**

A Venturi mask is used when accuracy of oxygen administration is essential; it delivers consistent FIO_2, regardless of the patient's breathing pattern. Accurate administration is especially important for the patient with chronic obstructive pulmonary disease because too much oxygen could stop his respiratory drive, driven by a low PaO_2. A simple mask delivers oxygen in a range of 40% to 60% but can't be set to deliver a specific amount of oxygen. A partial rebreathing mask delivers oxygen in higher concentrations than a simple mask but delivers it in a range and not a specific amount. A bag-valve mask is used as a temporary measure to deliver high concentrations of oxygen until the patient can be intubated and mechanically ventilated.

> *Nursing process step:* Implementation
> *Client needs category:* Physiological integrity
> *Client needs subcategory:* Physiological adaptation
> *Taxonomic level:* Application

23. *Correct answer:* **D**

The patient with a chronic illness goes through a grieving process related to the loss of his previous level of function. Grief is commonly manifested as loss of motivation and refusal to perform functions of which the patient is fully capable. Self-actualization is the process of fulfilling one's potential. Confabulation is a behavioral reaction in which the patient creates stories or invents answers to fill in memory gaps in an unconscious attempt to maintain self-esteem. In reaction formation, the patient uses behaviors that are the opposite of what he would like to do.

> *Nursing process step:* Evaluation
> *Client needs category:* Psychosocial integrity
> *Client needs subcategory:* Coping and adaptation
> *Taxonomic level:* Analysis

24. *Correct answer:* **A**

During a bronchoscopy the doctor uses a flexible fiber-optic bronchoscope to visualize the trachea, the mainstem bronchus, and the major subdivisions of the bronchial tubes. Ventilation and perfusion scans use a radioisotope tracer and a scanning machine. Ventilation scans visualize patterns of air movement and air distribution in the lungs, and perfusion scans visualize patterns of blood flow through the lungs. Pulmonary angiography requires the administration of a contrast medium to visualize the pulmonary vasculature by X-ray. Oral endoscopy is the visual examination of the lining of the esophagus, the stomach, and the upper duodenum, using a flexible fiber-optic endoscope.

Nursing process step: Implementation
Client needs category: Physiological integrity
Client needs subcategory: Reduction of risk potential
Taxonomic level: Comprehension

25. *Correct answer:* **B**

During bronchoscopy, the gag and cough reflexes are suppressed by an anesthetic agent to allow passage of the bronchoscope. This leaves the patient at risk for aspiration until these reflexes return. The patient may also be anxious, experience pain, or be at risk for injury, but airway maintenance must always take top priority.

Nursing process step: Analysis
Client needs category: Physiological integrity
Client needs subcategory: Reduction of risk potential
Taxonomic level: Application

26. *Correct answer:* **B**

When the patient isn't lying on her back in a semi-Fowler's or high-Fowler's position, she should be placed with the affected side down immediately following a pneumonectomy. This allows optimal expansion of the remaining lung and promotes oxygenation; it also helps keep fluid that accumulates in the pleural space below the level of the bronchial stump.

Nursing process step: Implementation
Client needs category: Physiological integrity
Client needs subcategory: Reduction of risk potential
Taxonomic level: Application

27. *Correct answer:* **A**

Possible complications of a pneumonectomy include pulmonary edema, mediastinal shift, and atrial arrhythmias. Transposition of the great vessels is a congenital cardiac anomaly, pleurisy is an inflammation of the membrane that lines the chest and covers the lung, and pericarditis is an inflammation of the pericardium; none of these are complications of pneumonectomy.

Nursing process step: Assessment
Client needs category: Physiological integrity
Client needs subcategory: Reduction of risk potential
Taxonomic level: Analysis

28. *Correct answer:* **D**

The nurse is inserting the nasopharyngeal airway correctly when she places the patient in a supine position, pushes the tip of the patient's nose upward, and inserts the airway along the floor of the nostril into the posterior pharynx. The airway should be inserted to a predetermined length (measuring from the tip of the nose to the ear lobe and marking the distance on the tube) or until the flange is flush with the nostril. An oropharyngeal (not nasopharyngeal) airway should be inserted by pointing the tip upward toward the roof of the mouth. Only water-based lubricant, not petroleum jelly, should be used. Because the airway is inserted nasally, the patient's tongue is bypassed and doesn't need to be depressed.

> *Nursing process step:* Evaluation
> *Client needs category:* Safe, effective care management
> *Client needs subcategory:* Management of care
> *Taxonomic level:* Application

29. *Correct answer:* **D**

A bag-valve mask is the most appropriate oxygen delivery system for a patient who can't exert adequate respiratory effort. This mask should be used until the respiratory effects of lorazepam are reversed or the patient is endotracheally intubated and mechanically ventilated. A nasal cannula, simple face mask, and Venturi mask require the patient to have an adequate spontaneous respiratory effort, so they wouldn't be appropriate for this patient.

> *Nursing process step:* Implementation
> *Client needs category:* Physiological integrity
> *Client needs subcategory:* Physiological adaptation
> *Taxonomic level:* Analysis

30. *Correct answer:* **A**

Hypoxemia, cardiac arrhythmias, and hypotension can result from prolonged vigorous suctioning. When a suction catheter is placed in the airway and suction applied, oxygen-enriched air is removed and replaced by room air, resulting in moderate to severe hypoxemia. This can cause cardiac arrhythmias and hypotension. Therefore, suctioning should be performed after oxygenating the patient and then only intermittently for no longer than 10 seconds. Hypovolemia, hyperthermia, and septicemia don't result from prolonged suctioning.

> *Nursing process step:* Evaluation
> *Client needs category:* Physiological integrity
> *Client needs subcategory:* Reduction of risk potential
> *Taxonomic level:* Application

31. *Correct answer:* **A**

To successfully collect a sputum specimen, the nurse should place the patient in the high Fowler position. Ask the patient to rinse her mouth with water to reduce specimen contamination by oral bacteria or food particles. Then tell her to cough deeply and expectorate directly into the specimen container. Ask her to produce at least 15 ml of sputum, if possible.

Nursing process step: Implementation
Client needs category: Physiological integrity
Client needs subcategory: Reduction of risk potential
Taxonomic level: Knowledge

32. *Correct answer:* **A**

Streptococcus pneumoniae is the most common cause of bacterial pneumonia. It's most prevalent during the winter and spring. *Proteus* bacteria are found in fecal material. *Haemophilus influenzae* causes viral pneumonia. *Escherichia coli* normally occurs in the intestinal tract.

Nursing process step: Assessment
Client needs category: Health promotion and maintenance
Client needs subcategory: Prevention and early detection of disease
Taxonomic level: Knowledge

33. *Correct answer:* **B**

The doctor would prescribe a mucolytic to thin the secretions. An anticholinergic or a diuretic would thicken the secretions; an antibiotic would have already been ordered to treat the pneumonia but it won't help thin the secretions.

Nursing process step: Planning
Client needs category: Physiological integrity
Client needs subcategory: Pharmacological and parenteral therapies
Taxonomic level: Comprehension

34. *Correct answer:* **C**

Impaired gas exchange is the most appropriate nursing diagnosis for a patient with pneumonia. The patient is prone to fluid volume excess because I.V. fluids are needed to hydrate the patient. Decreased cardiac output is unlikely in a patient with pneumonia unless there is some preexisting cardiac disease. The patient with pneumonia already has an infection.

Nursing process step: Analysis
Client needs category: Physiological integrity
Client needs subcategory: Reduction of risk potential
Taxonomic level: Analysis

35. *Correct answer:* **A**

Trauma is the most common cause of ARDS. ARDS is a form of pulmonary edema that can quickly lead to acute respiratory failure. Also known as shock, stiff, white, wet, or Da Nang lung, ARDS may follow a direct or indirect lung injury. It can prove fatal within 48 hours of onset if not promptly diagnosed and treated. The patient's history of type 1 diabetes may slow her healing process but it doesn't put her at risk for developing ARDS. Her history of breast cancer and use of birth control pills don't increase her risk of developing ARDS.

> *Nursing process step:* Evaluation
> *Client needs category:* Physiological integrity
> *Client needs subcategory:* Reduction of risk potential
> *Taxonomic level:* Analysis

36. *Correct answer:* **C**

A decreasing Pao_2 level despite administration of higher oxygen concentrations is a classic sign of ARDS. Electrolyte imbalance isn't a classic finding in the patient with ARDS. Hypercapnia may be present in later stages of ARDS but isn't a classic sign.

> *Nursing process step:* Assessment
> *Client needs category:* Physiological integrity
> *Client needs subcategory:* Reduction of risk potential
> *Taxonomic level:* Comprehension

37. *Correct answer:* **B**

Injury reduces normal blood flow to the lungs. Platelets aggregate and release histamine, serotonin, and bradykinin. Those substances, especially histamine, inflame and damage the alveolocapillary membrane, increasing capillary permeability. Fluids then shift into the interstitial space. As capillary permeability increases, proteins and fluids leak out, increasing interstitial osmotic pressure and causing pulmonary edema. Pulmonary edema associated with ARDS doesn't occur as a result of right-sided heart failure, extravascular fluid volume excess, or pulmonary artery infarct.

> *Nursing process step:* Evaluation
> *Client needs category:* Physiological integrity
> *Client needs subcategory:* Physiological adaptation
> *Taxonomic level:* Analysis

38. *Correct answer:* **A**

Appropriate treatment for the patient with acute respiratory distress syndrome who continues to show signs of hypoxemia is mechanical ventilation with positive end–expiratory pressure (PEEP). Chest physiotherapy may be prescribed after the patient is intubated and mechanically ventilated. A chest tube isn't indicated unless the patient develops a pneumothorax as a result of PEEP. High Fio_2 concentrations are administered to combat hypoxemia.

> *Nursing process step:* Evaluation
> *Client needs category:* Physiological integrity
> *Client needs category:* Physiological adaptation
> *Taxonomic level:* Analysis

39. *Correct answer:* **C**

The pH is greater than 7.45, which indicates alkalosis. The $Paco_2$ is less than 35 mm Hg, indicating that the alkalosis originated from a respiratory source. Hyperventilation caused by anxiety associated with arguing was the cause of respiratory alkalosis in this patient. The HCO_3^- is normal, so there is no metabolic source for the alkalosis.

> *Nursing process step:* Assessment
> *Client needs category:* Physiological integrity
> *Client needs subcategory:* Reduction of risk potential
> *Taxonomic level:* Analysis

40. *Correct answer:* **B**

The nurse should tell the patient to blow into a paper bag and reinhale CO_2 to stop the hyperventilation. The patient should also be encouraged to take slow even breaths when feeling anxious. Encourage the patient to express her feelings and help her work through her anxiety. If the patient is extremely anxious, a sedative may be needed.

> *Nursing process step:* Implementation
> *Client needs category:* Physiological integrity
> *Client needs subcategory:* Reduction of risk potential
> *Taxonomic level:* Application

41. *Correct answer:* **D**

Kussmaul's respirations are abnormally deep, gasping respirations that result from air hunger and are associated with severe diabetic acidosis and coma. Bradypnea is regular but abnormally slow respirations. Cheyne-Stokes respirations are a respiratory pattern marked by alternating periods of apnea and deep, rapid breathing. Typically, the cycle starts with slow, shallow breaths, which slowly increase to abnormal depth and rapidity. Respiration then becomes slow and shallow, ending in a 10- to 20-second apneic episode before the cycle begins again. Biot's respirations are an abnormal breathing pattern characterized by irregular periods of apnea alternating with periods of 4 or 5 breaths having the same depth.

> *Nursing process step:* Assessment
> *Client needs category:* Physiological integrity
> *Client needs subcategory:* Physiological adaptation
> *Taxonomic level:* Application

42. *Correct answer:* **B**

The pH is less than 7.35, which indicates acidosis. The $Paco_2$ isn't elevated, so the acidosis doesn't originate from a respiratory source. The HCO_3^- is less than 22 mEq/L, indicating metabolic acidosis.

Nursing process step: Evaluation
Client needs category: Physiological integrity
Client needs subcategory: Physiological adaptation
Taxonomic level: Analysis

43. *Correct answer:* **A**

Airway patency always takes priority, so ineffective airway clearance would be the most important nursing diagnosis for this patient. The patient is at risk for infection and he'll have a disturbance of body image, but these don't take priority over airway clearance. The patient shouldn't be at risk for injury because he shouldn't be confused as a result of anesthesia.

Nursing process step: Analysis
Client needs category: Physiological integrity
Client needs subcategory: Reduction of risk potential
Taxonomic level: Analysis

44. *Correct answer:* **D**

The stoma should be cleaned with a solution of equal parts saline solution and hydrogen peroxide. If the patient requires suctioning before tracheostomy care, a new sterile suction catheter must be used with wall suction set on "high." The inner cannula should be replaced every time tracheostomy care is given.

Nursing process step: Implementation
Client needs category: Physiological integrity
Client needs subcategory: Reduction of risk potential
Taxonomic level: Application

45. *Correct answer:* **A**

Mr. Emerson's coughing episodes may be caused by aspiration of liquids taken by mouth. The nurse should check to see that the tracheostomy cuff is inflated to decrease the risk of aspiration. Swallowing studies aren't indicated at this time. The patient should be positioned with his head elevated to prevent aspiration.

Nursing process step: Implementation
Client needs category: Physiological integrity
Client needs subcategory: Reduction of risk potential
Taxonomic level: Application

46. *Correct answer:* **A**

Sarcoidosis, a systemic disease with multiple masses (granulomas) characteristically produces lymphadenopathy, pulmonary infiltration, and skeletal, liver, eye, or skin lesions. The cause of the disease is unknown, but it may result from a hypersensitivity response — possibly T-cell imbalance — to such agents as atypical mycobacteria, fungi, and pine pollen. The disease is probably airborne; it isn't caused by air pollution associated with certain occupations. Although a high percentage of people with sarcoidosis are black, it isn't a contagious disease, and it isn't a highly infectious disease of the respiratory tract.

Nursing process step: Implementation
Client needs category: Health promotion and maintenance
Client needs subcategory: Prevention and early detection of disease
Taxonomic level: Knowledge

47. *Correct answer:* **A**

The nurse should observe for adverse effects, such as hyperglycemia, hypernatremia, fluid retention, elevated blood pressure, changes in emotional state and, in women, menstrual irregularities. The nurse should also check fingerstick blood glucose levels before meals and at bedtime to assess for hyperglycemia, weigh the patient daily to assess for fluid retention, and observe for mood swings. Corticosteroids don't cause hyponatremia or hypotension.

Nursing process step: Implementation
Client needs category: Physiological integrity
Client needs subcategory: Pharmacological and parenteral therapies
Taxonomic level: Application

48. *Correct answer:* **C**

Mr. Rex understands his discharge instructions when he verbalizes that he shouldn't stop taking the drug suddenly. He should also decrease his sodium intake, take the drug with food, and protect himself against infection.

Nursing process step: Evaluation
Client needs category: Physiological integrity
Client needs subcategory: Pharmacological and parenteral therapies
Taxonomic level: Analysis

49. *Correct answer:* **D**

Initial assessment of the patient with fractured ribs would reveal shallow breathing to minimize the pain accompanying any movement. Paradoxical respiration, in which the chest expands on expiration and contracts on inspiration, would be present only if the ribs sustained multiple fractures. Crackles auscultated over the right lung base would indicate atelectasis or heart failure. Diminished breath sounds on the affected side would present only if the patient had a pneumothorax. A clicking sensation during inspiration would be present only with costochondral separation.

Nursing process step: Assessment
Client needs category: Physiological integrity
Client needs subcategory: Physiological adaptation
Taxonomic level: Application

50. *Correct answer:* **B**

Hypoxia — insufficient oxygenation of the tissues — is characterized by restlessness, dyspnea, and tachycardia. Bradycardia, hypotension, and glycosuria aren't signs of hypoxia.

Nursing process step: Assessment
Client needs category: Physiological integrity
Client needs subcategory: Physiological adaptation
Taxonomic level: Comprehension

51. *Correct answer:* **A**

Explaining that the tube helps the collapsed portion of the lung reinflate, thereby making breathing easier, should decrease the patient's fear of death. Assuring him that the nurse and doctor will be present may reduce his anxiety but not as much as a detailed explanation will. Asking the doctor to postpone the procedure is inappropriate because the chest tube must be inserted immediately. Asking the chaplain to talk to the patient before the procedure may reduce the patient's anxiety and fears but would delay the procedure.

Nursing process step: Implementation
Client needs category: Physiological integrity
Client needs subcategory: Reduction of risk potential
Taxonomic level: Application

52. *Correct answer:* **C**

Diazepam relieves anxiety and tension related to organic or functional conditions. This drug has no analgesic effect. Because diazepam enhances muscle relaxation, it decreases muscle activity and respiratory rate.

Nursing process step: Evaluation
Client needs category: Physiological integrity
Client needs subcategory: Pharmacological and parenteral therapies
Taxonomic level: Comprehension

53. *Correct answer:* **A**

Bubbling in the water-seal chamber may indicate an air leak in the system, which predisposes the patient to tension pneumothorax. Fluid fluctuation in the water-seal chamber is normal unless the lung has reexpanded, the suction isn't working, or the tube is obstructed. Dark red drainage, indicating previous bleeding, is expected, but bright red drainage, indicating fresh bleeding, should be reported immediately. The drainage device was set at 20 cm of suction, so a fluid level of 20 cm in the suction control chamber is normal.

> *Nursing process step:* Implementation
> *Client needs category:* Physiological integrity
> *Client needs subcategory:* Physiological adaptation
> *Taxonomic level:* Application

54. *Correct answer:* **D**

A chest X-ray must confirm lung reexpansion before the chest tube can be removed. The amount of chest tube drainage and the cessation of pain and dyspnea aren't indications for removal. The chest tube may be irritating and painful, increasing the patient's dyspnea. Absence of fluid fluctuation in the water-seal chamber may indicate that the lung has reexpanded, but it also could mean that the chest tube is obstructed or the drainage device isn't working.

> *Nursing process step:* Evaluation
> *Client needs category:* Physiological integrity
> *Client needs subcategory:* Physiological adaptation
> *Taxonomic level:* Application

55. *Correct answer:* **D**

Valsalva's maneuver causes a bearing-down effect, increasing pressure throughout the body and preventing air from entering the pleural cavity. Breathing through pursed lips, quickly and shallowly, or with an open mouth won't prevent air from entering the pleural cavity when chest tubes are removed.

> *Nursing process step:* Implementation
> *Client needs category:* Physiological integrity
> *Client needs subcategory:* Reduction of risk potential
> *Taxonomic level:* Analysis

56. *Correct answer:* **C**

Guaifenesin requires cautious use in a patient with respiratory insufficiency, one with an ineffective cough reflex, or one who is pregnant or breast-feeding.

> *Nursing process step:* Evaluation
> *Client needs category:* Physiological integrity
> *Client needs subcategory:* Pharmacological and parenteral therapies
> *Taxonomic level:* Knowledge

57. *Correct answer:* **A**

The onset of action for expectorants such as guaifenesin is immediate to 30 minutes.

> *Nursing process step:* Evaluation
> *Client needs category:* Physiological integrity
> *Client needs subcategory:* Pharmacological and parenteral therapies
> *Taxonomic level:* Knowledge

58. *Correct answer:* **D**

Concomitant use of guaifenesin and an anticoagulant may increase the risk of bleeding. Guiafenesin doesn't interact significantly with the other drug classes.

> *Nursing process step:* Evaluation
> *Client needs category:* Physiological integrity
> *Client needs subcategory:* Pharmacological and parenteral therapies
> *Taxonomic level:* Knowledge

59. *Correct answer:* **D**

The nurse should lightly wet the chest hair to prevent friction on the endpiece of the stethoscope, which can mimic abnormal breath sounds. Shaving the patient's chest would alter his body image and provide unnecessary discomfort. When auscultating breath sounds, the nurse should hold the diaphragm tightly against the patient's skin (not against any covering fabric), just enough to form a seal.

> *Nursing process step:* Assessment
> *Client needs category:* Health promotion and maintenance
> *Client needs subcategory:* Prevention and early detection of disease
> *Taxonomic level:* Comprehension

60. *Correct answer:* **A**

If I.V. access isn't available, naloxone, atropine, diazepam, epinephrine, and lidocaine can be administered down the endotracheal tube. Norepinephrine, amrinone, and digoxin can't be administered via an endotracheal tube.

> *Nursing process step:* Implementation
> *Client needs category:* Physiological integrity
> *Client needs subcategory:* Pharmacological and parenteral therapies
> *Taxonomic level:* Knowledge

61. *Correct answer:* **D**

Pulse oximetry of 94% or above and a normal respiratory rate (less than 20 breaths/minute) without dyspnea indicates probable lung expansion and effective chest tube functioning. Reporting less chest pain or requesting more pain medication would be more appropriate patient outcomes for a nursing diagnosis of pain related to lung impairment and chest surgery. Assuming the semi-Fowler position, which facilitates breathing, may indicate that gas exchange is still impaired.

Nursing process step: Evaluation
Client needs category: Physiological integrity
Client needs subcategory: Reduction of risk potential
Taxonomic level: Analysis

62. *Correct answer:* B

The patient should be instructed to avoid washing off the marks placed on his skin to guide radiation therapy. If the marks are washed off, the patient must be reassessed and the marks reapplied—a time-consuming task. Skin lotions and powders are contraindicated because they may irritate the skin in the irradiated area. The patient should avoid wearing constrictive clothing, which decreases circulation. Massaging an area already tender from radiation can cause irritation and pain.

Nursing process step: Planning
Client needs category: Physiological integrity
Client needs subcategory: Reduction of risk potential
Taxonomic level: Application

63. *Correct answer:* C

Because Mr. Horowitz's loss of appetite causes him to eat less than normal, he should make every mouthful count by eating high-calorie foods. Moderate activity increases a person's appetite. Forcing fluids typically causes a feeling of fullness, further reducing the patient's appetite and nutritional intake. He should avoid hot meat dishes, which commonly cause a metallic taste in patients receiving radiation therapy.

Nursing process step: Implementation
Client needs category: Physiological integrity
Client needs subcategory: Basic care and comfort
Taxonomic level: Knowledge

CHAPTER 2

CARDIOVASCULAR SYSTEM

QUESTIONS

1. The nurse is performing her admission assessment of a patient. When grading arterial pulses, a 1+ pulse indicates:

    A. above normal perfusion.
    B. absent perfusion.
    C. normal perfusion.
    D. diminished perfusion.

2. Murmurs that indicate heart disease are often accompanied by other symptoms such as:

    A. dyspnea on exertion.
    B. subcutaneous emphysema.
    C. thoracic petechiae.
    D. periorbital edema.

3. Which pregnancy-related physiologic change would place the patient with a history of cardiac disease at the greatest risk of developing severe cardiac problems?

    A. Decreased heart rate
    B. Decreased cardiac output
    C. Increased plasma volume
    D. Increased blood pressure

4. The priority nursing diagnosis for the patient with cardiomyopathy is:

    A. anxiety related to risk of declining health status.
    B. ineffective individual coping related to fear of debilitating illness.
    C. fluid volume excess related to altered compensatory mechanisms.
    D. decreased cardiac output related to reduced myocardial contractility.

5. A patient with thrombophlebitis reached her expected outcomes of care. Her affected leg appears pink and warm. Her pedal pulse is palpable and there is no edema present. Which step in the nursing process is described above?

    A. Planning
    B. Implementation
    C. Analysis
    D. Evaluation

SITUATION: *For 4 years, David Sawyer, age 57, has had episodes of paroxysmal supraventricular tachycardia one or two times a month, usually following heavy exercise or caffeine intake. About 2 months ago, the episodes increased to every 1 to 2 days, with symptoms including dyspnea, dizziness, and palpitations.*

Questions 6 to 9 refer to this situation.

6. The doctor orders preliminary tests to help assess Mr. Sawyer's condition. The diagnostic test that depicts a graphical representation of the heart's electrical activity is called:

   A. a Holter monitor.
   B. a cardiac catheterization.
   C. an echocardiogram.
   D. an electrocardiogram (ECG).

7. Tachycardia may result from:

   A. vagal stimulation.
   B. fear, anger, or pain.
   C. stress, pain, or vomiting.
   D. vomiting or suctioning.

8. Diltiazem (Cardizem) is ordered to control the patient's paroxysmal supraventricular tachycardia (PSVT). This drug is classified as:

   A. a calcium channel blocker.
   B. a beta-adrenergic blocker.
   C. an angiotensin-converting enzyme inhibitor.
   D. an inotropic agent.

9. Mr. Sawyer shows no improvement with drug therapy, so radio frequency catheter ablation is performed. Discharge instructions should include:

   A. resuming antiarrhythmic drug therapy after discharge.
   B. calling the doctor if his heart rate increases with exercise.
   C. telling Mr. Sawyer that he may feel palpitations for a few weeks.
   D. returning for a weekly follow-up ECG for 2 months.

SITUATION: *Mary Walker, age 72, came to the clinic at the request of her daughter. She has a history of type 2 diabetes mellitus and her blood pressure is 172/94 mm Hg.*

Questions 10 to 12 refer to this situation.

10. Diagnosis of Mrs. Walker's hypertension is based on:

    A. symptoms such as headache and visual changes.
    B. serial elevation of diastolic blood pressure.
    C. a family history of atherosclerosis.
    D. a history of renal disease.

11. Mrs. Walker is prescribed captopril (Capoten) to treat her hypertension. This drug is classified as:

    A. an angiotensin-converting enzyme (ACE) inhibitor.
    B. a beta-adrenergic blocker.
    C. a calcium channel blocker.
    D. a vasodilator.

12. According to the National Institutes of Health stepped-care approach to treating primary hypertension, the first step involves:

    A. correcting the underlying cause.
    B. modifying lifestyle.
    C. using drug monotherapy.
    D. using combination drug therapy.

SITUATION: *Robert Williams, age 65, is standing at the bus stop with his daughter when he suddenly groans and collapses.*

Questions 13 and 14 refer to this situation.

13. The nurse is walking down the street when she hears Mr. William's daughter screaming for help. How should the nurse intervene?

    A. She should determine if the victim is unresponsive, summon emergency medical services (EMS), and initiate cardiopulmonary resuscitation (CPR) in the interim.
    B. She should provide rescue efforts for 1 minute, then activate the EMS system.
    C. She should assess the victim's pulse and breathing, open his airway, and activate the EMS.
    D. She should open the victim's airway, assess his breathing, provide rescue breathing, assess his pulse, then activate EMS.

14. Which of the following statements is true concerning endotracheal intubation following cardiac arrest?

A. It shouldn't be delayed so that ventilations can be delivered by another device.
B. It increases the risk of gastric content aspiration.
C. It should only be performed by persons proficient at the procedure.
D. It should precede defibrillation in patients with ventricular defibrillation or pulseless ventricular tachycardia.

SITUATION: *Bill Knowles, a 74-year-old smoker with advanced coronary artery disease, is scheduled for surgical revascularization of the coronary arteries to bypass plaque obstructions.*

Questions 15 to 19 refer to this situation.

15. Revascularization of the coronary arteries is also known as:

A. percutaneous transluminal coronary angioplasty.
B. coronary artery bypass graft.
C. percutaneous transluminal valvuloplasty.
D. valvular annuloplasty.

16. Which of Mr. Knowles's medications should be stopped before surgery?

A. Furosemide (Lasix)
B. Isosorbide dinitrate (Isordil)
C. Aspirin
D. Heparin sodium (Liquaemin)

17. When giving discharge instructions to Mr. Knowles following his coronary artery bypass graft (CABG) surgery, the nurse should include information about all of the following symptoms, the most common of which is:

A. confusion.
B. syncope.
C. ankle edema.
D. depression.

18. Which of the following would be the most appropriate nursing diagnosis for a patient with coronary artery disease?

A. Ineffective thermoregulation
B. Impaired gas exchange
C. Risk for injury
D. Decreased cardiac output

19. Which of the following would be the best expected outcome for a patient with decreased cardiac output?

A. The patient will exhibit no evidence of confusion.
B. The patient will have normal blood urea nitrogen (BUN) and creatinine levels.
C. The patient's blood pressure and pulse will be within normal limits.
D. The patient will exhibit no evidence of skin breakdown.

SITUATION: *A nurse is watching her son's baseball game when a pitch hits the batter, a 19-year-old, in the middle of his chest and he collapses.*

Questions 20 to 24 refer to this situation.

20. The nurse tells someone to call for an ambulance and report a cardiac arrest while she begins cardiopulmonary resuscitation. How deeply should the nurse apply compressions to the lower sternum on this patient?

   A. 1″ to 2″ (2.5 to 5 cm)
   B. 1½″ to 3″ (3.5 to 7.5 cm)
   C. 2½″ to 3″ (6 to 7.5 cm)
   D. 1½″ to 2″ (3.5 to 5 cm)

21. Paramedics prepare the injured player for defibrillation. The portable defibrillator's quick-look mode displays the rhythm as ventricular fibrillation. How many joules should the paramedic administer with the first shock?

   A. 100 joules
   B. 200 joules
   C. 300 joules
   D. 360 joules

22. The first three shocks are unsuccessful. Which medication should be administered next?

   A. Sodium bicarbonate
   B. Lidocaine (Xylocaine)
   C. Epinephrine
   D. Bretylium (Bretylol)

23. After the patient is successfully intubated and his heart rhythm is stabilized, the ambulance brings him to the emergency department. What other complications could arise from the baseball hitting his chest?

   A. Spinal cord injury
   B. Abdominal injury
   C. Blunt cardiac injury
   D. Renal-pelvic injury

24. The young man's condition is stabilized in the hospital and he's ready for discharge. What discharge instructions should the parents be given?

    A. They would benefit from taking a CPR course.
    B. They should discourage their son from playing contact sports.
    C. They should be told about the long-term effects of a cardiac contusion.
    D. They should be warned about drug-to-drug interactions associated with his cardiac medications.

SITUATION: *Bill Filano, age 54, comes to the emergency department complaining of sharp, substernal chest pain that increases with deep inspiration. He had a myocardial infarction (MI) 2 months prior to admission.*

Questions 25 to 28 refer to this situation.

25. Mr. Filano says the pain radiates to his neck, shoulders, back, and arms, and it decreases when he sits up and leans forward. Based on this assessment, you suspect that he has:

    A. developed another MI.
    B. endocarditis.
    C. pericarditis.
    D. myocarditis.

26. When auscultating Mr. Filano's heart sounds, the nurse would expect to hear:

    A. a grating sound.
    B. a murmur.
    C. a loud snap.
    D. a click.

27. Mr. Filano begins showing signs of heart failure (dyspnea, orthopnea, and tachycardia) and complains of generalized substernal chest pain and fullness in his chest. He's at risk for developing which of the following complications of pericarditis?

    A. Neoplasms
    B. Cardiac tamponade
    C. Infiltrates
    D. Myalgia

28. The nurse should prepare Mr. Filano for which of the following emergency treatments for cardiac tamponade?

A. Pericardiorrhaphy
B. Pericardiolysis
C. Pericardectomy
D. Pericardiocentesis

SITUATION: *John Harkins was admitted to the coronary care unit 1 day ago with an acute myocardial infarction (MI). His vital signs and heart rhythm stabilized during the night, but this morning the nurse has found him cold, pale, diaphoretic, and confused.*

Questions 29 to 32 refer to this situation.

29. Mr. Harkins's blood pressure has fallen to 80/60 mm Hg; pulse is thready at 118 beats/minute; and respirations are rapid and shallow at 36 breaths/minute. Auscultation reveals distant heart sounds and bibasilar crackles in the lung fields. Based on these findings, what is the most probable diagnosis?

A. Cardiogenic shock
B. Thromboembolism
C. Cardiomyopathy
D. Cardiac tamponade

30. Blood is pumped out into the systemic circulation during contraction of the:

A. right atrium.
B. left ventricle.
C. coronary arteries.
D. sinoatrial (SA) node.

31. Mr. Harkins' s severe left-sided heart failure will lead to a decrease in the total amount of blood ejected per minute. This quantity is known as:

A. stroke volume.
B. ejection fraction.
C. cardiac output.
D. heart rate.

32. The doctor prescribes dopamine (Intropin) to improve Mr. Harkins's hemodynamic status. The nurse knows that this drug is prescribed to:

A. decrease the oxygen demand of the heart.
B. increase cardiac output and stroke volume.
C. decrease the heart's workload.
D. decrease the circulating blood volume.

SITUATION: *Angela Riccardi, age 68, comes to the emergency department complaining of severe right-sided chest pain that radiates to the back. electrocardiography, echocardiography, and computed tomography rule out a myocardial infarction but confirm a thoracic aortic aneurysm.*

Questions 33 and 34 refer to this situation.

33. Which of the following is the most common cause of thoracic aortic aneurysm in Mrs. Riccardi's history?

    A. Atherosclerosis
    B. Hepatomegaly
    C. Diabetes mellitus
    D. Dermatophytosis

34. Mrs. Riccardi should be monitored for which of the following major complications associated with thoracic aortic aneurysm?

    A. Hypertension
    B. Aortic dissection
    C. Coarctation of the aorta
    D. Polyphagia

SITUATION: *Margaret Driver, age 48, has a medical history of rheumatic fever, type 1 diabetes mellitus, hypertension, pernicious anemia, and appendectomy. She's admitted to the hospital and undergoes mitral valve replacement surgery.*

Questions 35 and 36 refer to this situation.

35. After discharge, Mrs. Driver is scheduled for a tooth extraction. Which history finding is a major risk factor for infective endocarditis?

    A. Appendectomy
    B. Pernicious anemia
    C. Diabetes mellitus
    D. Valve replacement

36. What medication should be given as a precaution prior to Mrs. Driver's tooth extraction?

    A. Antianginal
    B. Antibiotic
    C. Antiemetic
    D. Antidiuretic

SITUATION: *Mr. Wolf has a history of chronic obstructive pulmonary disease. He comes to the clinic for evaluation because he hasn't been feeling well lately and his daughter thinks he may have a heart problem.*

Questions 37 to 39 refer to this situation.

37. To find out more information about Mr. Wolf's condition, the nurse should begin her interview by questioning him about:

    A. his educational background.
    B. his medical insurance.
    C. the duration of his problem.
    D. his support systems.

38. What cardiac complication might be expected as a result of chronic obstructive pulmonary disease (COPD)?

    A. Right ventricular hypertrophy
    B. Right ventricular atrophy
    C. Left ventricular hypertrophy
    D. Left ventricular atrophy

39. Mr. Wolf develops right-sided heart failure. Which of the following symptoms are common in this disorder?

    A. Respiratory acidosis
    B. Hypertension
    C. Dyspnea
    D. Jugular vein distention

SITUATION: *Mrs. Kelly, age 72, comes to the emergency department complaining of palpitations and dizziness. An electrocardiogram shows atrial fibrillation.*

Questions 40 and 41 refer to this situation.

40. An electrocardiogram (ECG) for the patient with atrial fibrillation will show:

    A. inverted P waves.
    B. multifocal QRS complexes.
    C. erratic P waves.
    D. a regular rhythm.

41. The doctor prescribes digoxin (Lanoxin) twice a day until a therapeutic drug level is attained. When the nurse takes Mrs. Kelly's apical pulse on the 3rd day, her pulse is 52 beats/minute, and she complains of nausea. The nurse should:

A. withhold the digoxin and notify the doctor.
B. withhold the digoxin and obtain a serum digoxin level.
C. administer the digoxin and medicate for nausea.
D. administer the digoxin and notify the doctor.

SITUATION: *Brad O'Reilly, age 42, was admitted to the emergency department with substernal chest pain. He received nitroglycerin (Nitrostat) in the ambulance on his way to the hospital. Cardiac enzyme levels were drawn and results are pending.*

Questions 42 to 45 refer to this situation.

42. Laboratory results show the creatine kinase (CK) level is elevated. The nurse should anticipate planning care for a patient with:

A. a pulmonary embolism.
B. a ventricular arrhythmia.
C. a myocardial infarction.
D. a cerebrovascular accident.

43. After Mr. O'Reilly's condition has been stabilized in the emergency department, he's admitted to the coronary care unit with a suspected diagnosis of an acute myocardial infarction. Increased serum levels of the isoenzyme CK-MB can be detected how soon after the onset of chest pain?

A. 30 minutes to 1 hour
B. 2 to 3 hours
C. 4 to 6 hours
D. 12 to 18 hours

44. When providing care for Mr. O'Reilly, the nurse should avoid which route when taking a temperature?

A. Oral
B. Rectal
C. Axillary
D. Tympanic

45. A primary nursing care goal for Mr. O'Reilly is to recognize the life-threatening complications of a myocardial infarction (MI). The major cause of death after an MI is:

A. cardiogenic shock.
B. heart failure.
C. pulmonary embolism.
D. cardiac arrhythmia.

SITUATION: *Marie Depitro, age 54, is admitted to the hospital for treatment of Prinzmetal's angina. Her blood pressure is 146/88 mm Hg; her heart rate, 90 beats/minute; and her respiratory rate, 22 breaths/minute.*

Questions 46 to 48 refer to this situation.

46. When developing Mrs. Depitro's plan of care, the nurse should remember that this type of angina is triggered by:

    A. coronary artery spasm.
    B. an unpredictable amount of activity.
    C. activities that increase oxygen demand.
    D. an unknown source.

47. Mrs. Depitro should receive which of the following agents to reduce the incidence of coronary artery spasm?

    A. Coronary artery blockers
    B. Calcium channel blockers
    C. Alpha-adrenergic blockers
    D. Angiotensin-converting enzyme (ACE) inhibitors

48. Mrs. Depitro has a blockage in the proximal portion of a coronary artery. She decides to undergo percutaneous transluminal coronary angioplasty (PTCA). During this procedure, the nurse expects to administer:

    A. an antibiotic.
    B. an anticonvulsant.
    C. an anticoagulant.
    D. an antihypertensive agent.

SITUATION: *Anna Krane, age 89, was brought to the emergency department by a neighbor who found her dyspneic and unable to remember when she last took her medication.*

Questions 49 to 51 refer to this situation.

49. Mrs. Krane reports a new onset of chest pain that occurs sporadically and with exertion. She complains of fatigue and mild ankle swelling, which worsens at the end of the day. The nurse should question Mrs. Krane to determine if she has which of the following common cardiac symptoms?

    A. Irritability and confusion
    B. Shortness of breath
    C. Difficulty sleeping
    D. Lower abdominal pain

50. Mrs. Krane's blood pressure is 168/108 mm Hg; which stage of hypertension is this?

    A. Stage 1 (mild)
    B. Stage 2 (moderate)
    C. Stage 3 (severe)
    D. Stage 4 (very severc)

51. Mrs. Krane's daughter arrived at the hospital and stated that her mother takes a "water pill" for high blood pressure. The doctor orders furosemide (Lasix) for Mrs. Krane. Her daughter asks the nurse how furosemide lowers blood pressure. The nurse's best response would be that furosemide reduces the heart's workload by:

    A. reducing the circulating blood volume.
    B. blocking the sympathetic nervous system.
    C. acting as a peripheral vasodilator.
    D. blocking renin angiotensin conversion.

SITUATION: *Jim Jennings comes to the emergency department complaining of visual changes and a severe headache. He has no significant past medical history and his blood pressure is 220/108 mm Hg.*

Questions 52 to 56 refer to this situation.

52. Mr. Jennings is diagnosed with malignant hypertension. What is the most common cause of this disorder?

    A. Pheochromocytoma
    B. Pyelonephritis
    C. Dissecting aneurysm
    D. Untreated hypertension

53. When teaching Mr. Jennings about the pathophysiology of hypertension, the nurse states that arterial baroreceptors are found in the carotid sinus and aorta. Arterial baroreceptors are also found in the:

    A. left ventricular wall.
    B. right ventricular wall.
    C. dorsalis pedis artery.
    D. common iliac artery.

54. The nurse knows that antihypertensive drugs commonly cause dizziness when the patient rises. Mr. Jenning's teaching plan should include which instruction to minimize postural hypotension?

A. "Avoid drinking alcoholic beverages and straining at stool; eat lots of fruits and fiber."

B. "Flex your calf muscles, avoid alcoholic beverages, and change positions slowly."

C. "Rest between demanding activities and drink 6 to 8 cups of fluid daily."

D. "Change positions quickly, and hold onto a stationary object when rising."

55. Mr. Jennings should be taught about complications of untreated hypertension, such as:

A. viral meningitis.

B. myoclonic seizure.

C. cerebrovascular accident.

D. status epilepticus.

56. Mr. Jennings must adhere to his antihypertensive drug regimen and modify which of the following risk factors associated with hypertension?

A. Serum lipid levels

B. Family history

C. Coronary artery disease

D. Diabetes mellitus

SITUATION: *Jim McCarthy, age 63, is admitted to the medical-surgical floor preoperatively and is scheduled for a left carotid endarterectomy. The nurse needs to complete an admission assessment.*

Questions 57 to 61 refer to this situation.

57. How should the nurse position Mr. McCarthy to assess his carotid pulse?

A. In a supine position with legs elevated on pillows

B. With the neck hyperextended away from the nurse

C. With the head elevated and facing the nurse

D. In Trendelenburg's position

58. What preexisting condition might you expect to find with Mr. McCarthy?

A. Renal disease

B. Atherosclerosis

C. Crohn's disease

D. Cervical dysplasia

59. As the nurse interviews Mr. McCarthy, he complains of another symptom associated with peripheral artery occlusion, namely:

A. burning.
B. redness.
C. pain.
D. warmth.

60. The nurse is teaching Mr. McCarthy about his upcoming surgery. Which of the following statements best describes carotid endarterectomy?

A. "A balloon-tipped catheter is inserted into the artery and emboli are removed."
B. "A mesh of wires is surgically implanted to prevent carotid artery re-occlusion."
C. "The thrombosed carotid artery segment is replaced by a graft."
D. "The carotid artery is incised and plaque is removed."

61. When caring for Mr. McCarthy after surgery, which assessment should take top priority?

A. Level of consciousness
B. Skin temperature and color
C. Intake and output
D. Dressing drainage

SITUATION: *Jane Egan, age 34, is admitted with systemic lupus erythematosus. She tells the nurse during a routine examination that her fingers become cyanotic and numb when it's cold outside.*

Questions 62 and 63 refer to this situation.

62. Mrs. Egan is most likely to be suffering from which of the following disorders?

A. Buerger's disease
B. Raynaud's disease
C. Thrombophlebitis
D. Ménière's disease

63. Before discharge, Mrs. Egan should be taught to monitor her:

A. heart rate.
B. skin condition.
C. blood pressure.
D. temperature.

SITUATION: *Despite lifestyle modifications and metoprolol (Aldomet) therapy, Richard Barrone's blood pressure remains elevated. He's admitted to the medical-surgical floor for blood pressure management.*

Questions 64 to 66 refer to this situation.

64. Mr. Barrone's doctor prescribes hydralazine (Apresoline) as adjunct therapy. What type of drug is hydralazine?

    A. Sympatholytic
    B. Vasodilator
    C. Diuretic
    D. Angiotensin-converting enzyme (ACE) inhibitor

65. While teaching Mr. Barrone about hydralazine therapy, the nurse explains the regimen. When should he take his daily dose of hydralazine?

    A. Upon arising in the morning
    B. Just before bedtime
    C. On an empty stomach
    D. With a meal

66. The nurse teaches Mr. Barrone about possible adverse reactions to hydralazine. Which of these adverse reactions is most likely to occur?

    A. Dry eye syndrome
    B. Pharyngitis
    C. Orthostatic hypotension
    D. Somnolence

ANSWER SHEET

	A B C D		A B C D		A B C D
1	○ ○ ○ ○	23	○ ○ ○ ○	45	○ ○ ○ ○
2	○ ○ ○ ○	24	○ ○ ○ ○	46	○ ○ ○ ○
3	○ ○ ○ ○	25	○ ○ ○ ○	47	○ ○ ○ ○
4	○ ○ ○ ○	26	○ ○ ○ ○	48	○ ○ ○ ○
5	○ ○ ○ ○	27	○ ○ ○ ○	49	○ ○ ○ ○
6	○ ○ ○ ○	28	○ ○ ○ ○	50	○ ○ ○ ○
7	○ ○ ○ ○	29	○ ○ ○ ○	51	○ ○ ○ ○
8	○ ○ ○ ○	30	○ ○ ○ ○	52	○ ○ ○ ○
9	○ ○ ○ ○	31	○ ○ ○ ○	53	○ ○ ○ ○
10	○ ○ ○ ○	32	○ ○ ○ ○	54	○ ○ ○ ○
11	○ ○ ○ ○	33	○ ○ ○ ○	55	○ ○ ○ ○
12	○ ○ ○ ○	34	○ ○ ○ ○	56	○ ○ ○ ○
13	○ ○ ○ ○	35	○ ○ ○ ○	57	○ ○ ○ ○
14	○ ○ ○ ○	36	○ ○ ○ ○	58	○ ○ ○ ○
15	○ ○ ○ ○	37	○ ○ ○ ○	59	○ ○ ○ ○
16	○ ○ ○ ○	38	○ ○ ○ ○	60	○ ○ ○ ○
17	○ ○ ○ ○	39	○ ○ ○ ○	61	○ ○ ○ ○
18	○ ○ ○ ○	40	○ ○ ○ ○	62	○ ○ ○ ○
19	○ ○ ○ ○	41	○ ○ ○ ○	63	○ ○ ○ ○
20	○ ○ ○ ○	42	○ ○ ○ ○	64	○ ○ ○ ○
21	○ ○ ○ ○	43	○ ○ ○ ○	65	○ ○ ○ ○
22	○ ○ ○ ○	44	○ ○ ○ ○	66	○ ○ ○ ○

ANSWERS AND RATIONALES

1. *Correct answer:* **D**

A 1+ pulse indicates weak pulses and is associated with diminished perfusion. A 4+ pulse is bounding perfusion, a 3+ is increased perfusion, a 2+ is normal perfusion, and 0 is absent perfusion.

> *Nursing process step:* Assessment
> *Client needs category:* Physiological integrity
> *Client needs subcategory:* Reduction of risk potential
> *Taxonomic level:* Comprehension

2. *Correct answer:* **A**

A murmur that indicates heart disease is often accompanied by dyspnea on exertion, which is a hallmark of heart failure. Other indicators are tachycardia, syncope, and chest pain. Subcutaneous emphysema, thoracic petechiae, and periorbital edema aren't associated with murmurs and heart disease.

> *Nursing process step:* Assessment
> *Client needs category:* Health promotion and maintenance
> *Client needs subcategory:* Prevention and early detection of disease
> *Taxonomic level:* Comprehension

3. *Correct answer:* **C**

Pregnancy increases plasma volume and expands the uterine vascular bed, possibly increasing both the heart rate and cardiac output. These changes may cause cardiac stress, especially during the second trimester. Blood pressure during early pregnancy may decrease, but it gradually returns to prepregnancy levels.

> *Nursing process step:* Assessment
> *Client needs category:* Health promotion and maintenance
> *Client needs subcategory:* Growth and development through the life span
> *Taxonomic level:* Application

4. *Correct answer:* **D**

Decreased cardiac output related to reduced myocardial contractility is the greatest threat to the survival of a patient with cardiomyopathy. The other options can be addressed once cardiac output and myocardial contractility have been restored.

> *Nursing process step:* Analysis
> *Client needs category:* Physiological integrity
> *Client needs subcategory:* Physiological adaptation
> *Taxonomic level:* Comprehension

5. *Correct answer:* **D**

Evaluation assesses the effectiveness of the treatment plan by determining if the patient has met the expected treatment outcome. Planning refers to designing a plan of action that will help the nurse deliver quality patient care. Implementation refers to all of the nursing interventions directed toward solving the patient's nursing problems. Analysis is the process of identifying the patient's nursing problems.

> *Nursing process step:* Evaluation
> *Client needs category:* Physiological integrity
> *Client needs subcategory:* Physiological adaptation
> *Taxonomic level:* Comprehension

6. *Correct answer:* **D**

An ECG is a noninvasive test that detects normal and abnormal heart rhythms. A Holter monitor continuously records the heart's electrical activity for 24 hours. Cardiac catheterization is a fluoroscopic examination of intracardiac structures. An echocardiogram is a test that uses echoes from sound waves to visualize intracardiac structures.

> *Nursing process step:* Assessment
> *Client needs category:* Health promotion and maintenance
> *Client needs subcategory:* Prevention and early detection of disease
> *Taxonomic level:* Knowledge

7. *Correct answer:* **B**

Tachycardia—overly rapid heart rate—may occur as a result of fear, anger, or pain. Bradycardia—slowed heart rate—can result from vomiting, suctioning (causing vagal nerve stimulation), and certain medications.

> *Nursing process step:* Assessment
> *Client needs category:* Health promotion and maintenance
> *Client needs subcategory:* Prevention and early detection of disease
> *Taxonomic level:* Comprehension

8. *Correct answer:* **A**

Diltiazem is a calcium channel blocker that inhibits calcium ion influx across cardiac and smooth-muscle cell membranes. When given to the patient with PSVT it slows conduction through the atrioventricular node, decreasing myocardial contractility and oxygen demand.

> *Nursing process step:* Implementation
> *Client needs category:* Physiological integrity
> *Client needs subcategory:* Pharmacological and parenteral therapies
> *Taxonomic level:* Knowledge

9. *Correct answer:* **C**

In radio frequency catheter ablation, radio frequency energy is delivered through an intracardiac electrode catheter that selectively destroys or modifies cardiac tissue. Beats that triggered the PSVT will no longer do so because the reentrant circuit has been destroyed; the palpitations will subside after 2 to 3 weeks. Antiarrhythmic drugs will no longer be needed following radio frequency ablation. An increase in heart rate is a normal response to exercise. A follow-up ECG is usually done in 1 to 3 months.

> *Nursing process step:* Planning
> *Client needs category:* Physiological integrity
> *Client needs subcategory:* Reduction of risk potential
> *Taxonomic level:* Application

10. *Correct answer:* **B**

Serial elevation of diastolic pressure (greater than 90 mm Hg) confirms the diagnosis of hypertension. Symptoms, such as headache and visual changes, and a history of renal disease and atherosclerosis help determine whether hypertension has a primary (idiopathic) or secondary cause. The etiology of primary hypertension is complex, involving several interacting homeostatic mechanisms. Hypertension is classified as secondary if it's related to a systemic disease that raises peripheral vascular resistance or cardiac output.

> *Nursing process step:* Assessment
> *Client needs category:* Physiological integrity
> *Client needs subcategory:* Reduction of risk potential
> *Taxonomic level:* Knowledge

11. *Correct answer:* **A**

Captopril is an ACE inhibitor that works by blocking the conversion of angiotensin I to angiotensin II, which reduces sodium and water retention and lowers blood pressure. ACE inhibitors may also slow the progression of diabetic renal disease in clients with associated renal insufficiency.

> *Nursing process step:* Implementation
> *Client needs category:* Physiological integrity
> *Client needs subcategory:* Pharmacological and parenteral therapies
> *Taxonomic level:* Knowledge

12. *Correct answer:* **B**

Modifying lifestyle (diet, exercise, weight-reduction, smoking and alcohol cessation) is the first step in treating primary hypertension. If the patient fails to achieve the desired blood pressure or make significant progress, he or she would continue lifestyle modifications and begin drug therapy with one drug (monotherapy). The next step would be to increase the drug dosage, substitute a drug in the same class, or add a drug from a different class (combination therapy). Correction of the underlying cause is the first step in treating secondary hypertension, which results from renal disease or another identifiable cause.

Nursing process step: Planning
Client needs category: Health promotion and maintenance
Client needs subcategory: Prevention and early detection of disease
Taxonomic level: Knowledge

13. *Correct answer:* A

Ventricular fibrillation is the cause of cardiac arrest in 80% to 90% of adults who haven't suffered trauma. The key to survival is early defibrillation and prompt CPR. First determine if the patient is unresponsive. Then call the EMS, who can provide early defibrillation. While waiting for EMS personnel, initiate CPR.

Nursing process step: Implementation
Client needs category: Physiological integrity
Client needs subcategory: Physiological adaptation
Taxonomic level: Comprehension

14. *Correct answer:* C

Endotracheal intubation should be performed by someone who is proficient at the procedure. Endotracheal intubation decreases the risk of aspiration. The patient should be ventilated with simple airway adjuncts before he's intubated. Defibrillation shouldn't be delayed to intubate a patient in cardiac arrest.

Nursing process step: Implementation
Client needs category: Physiological integrity
Client needs subcategory: Physiological adaptation
Taxonomic level: Application

15. *Correct answer:* B

A coronary artery bypass graft circumvents an occluded coronary artery with an autogenous graft (usually a segment of the saphenous vein from the leg or internal mammary artery), thereby restoring blood flow to the myocardium. Percutaneous transluminal coronary angioplasty uses a balloon-tipped catheter to dilate the coronary artery and compress the plaque against the vessel wall. Percutaneous transluminal valvuloplasty uses a balloon-tipped catheter to dilate calcified and stenotic valve leaflets. Valvular annuloplasty is the surgical repair or reconstruction of the valve leaflets and annulus.

Nursing process step: Planning
Client needs category: Physiological integrity
Client needs subcategory: Reduction of risk potential
Taxonomic level: Knowledge

16. *Correct answer:* **C**

Mr. Knowles shouldn't take aspirin for at least 7 days before surgery to reduce the risk of postoperative bleeding. Discontinuing furosemide may lead to pulmonary edema. Abrupt discontinuation of isosorbide may cause coronary vasospasm and increase the risk of myocardial infarction. Heparin is administered during cardiopulmonary bypass and shouldn't be stopped.

> *Nursing process step:* Planning
> *Client needs category:* Physiological integrity
> *Client needs subcategory:* Pharmacological and parenteral therapies
> *Taxonomic level:* Application

17. *Correct answer:* **D**

For the first few weeks after CABG surgery, patients commonly experience depression, fatigue, incisional chest discomfort, dyspnea, and anorexia. The depression typically resolves on its own without medical intervention. Confusion reflects neurologic dysfunction and should be further investigated. Syncope should be reported immediately, because it may result from decreased cardiac output, an abnormal condition after CABG surgery. Ankle edema rarely follows CABG surgery and may indicate right-sided heart failure, which should also be reported immediately.

> *Nursing process step:* Planning
> *Client needs category:* Psychosocial integrity
> *Client needs subcategory:* Psychosocial adaptation
> *Taxonomic level:* Application

18. *Correct answer:* **D**

Coronary artery disease develops when fatty deposits line the walls of the coronary arteries, impeding blood flow and therefore decreasing cardiac output. Thermoregulatory disturbances aren't usually associated with coronary artery disease unless accompanied by heart failure. Impaired gas exchange may occur if the blood's oxygen-carrying capacity was altered, as in anemia, chronic obstructive pulmonary disease, or carbon monoxide poisoning. There would be a risk of injury if the patient had sensory or motor deficits.

> *Nursing process step:* Analysis
> *Client needs category:* Physiological integrity
> *Client needs subcategory:* Reduction of risk potential
> *Taxonomic level:* Analysis

19. *Correct answer:* **C**

Hemodynamic stability is evident when blood pressure and pulse remain within normal limits, indicating efficient cardiac output. Confusion is evidence of altered cerebral perfusion; it may result from hemodynamic instability, but it wouldn't be the first symptom. BUN and creatinine levels are indicators of renal function. Skin breakdown would indicate poor peripheral perfusion.

> *Nursing process step:* Evaluation
> *Client needs category:* Physiological integrity
> *Client needs subcategory:* Reduction of risk potential
> *Taxonomic level:* Analysis

20. *Correct answer:* **D**

The recommended depth of chest compressions for an adult is 1½" to 2". The other options aren't within the recommended depth.

> *Nursing process step:* Implementation
> *Client needs category:* Physiological integrity
> *Client needs subcategory:* Physiological adaptation
> *Taxonomic level:* Knowledge

21. *Correct answer:* **B**

In ventricular fibrillation, the first shock should deliver 200 joules. If it fails to convert the rhythm, then a shock of 300 joules is given, followed by a shock of 360 joules, if necessary.

> *Nursing process step:* Implementation
> *Client needs category:* Physiological integrity
> *Client needs subcategory:* Physiological adaptation
> *Taxonomic level:* Knowledge

22. *Correct answer:* **C**

After the first three unsuccessful shocks, epinephrine is given I.V. or endotracheally and can be repeated every 3 to 5 minutes. No other single agent is more effective for treating persistent ventricular fibrillation. Sodium bicarbonate is given if the patient has known preexisting hyperkalemia, which wouldn't be possible in this case. Lidocaine would be tried after the next 3 shocks are given. Bretylium is tried next if lidocaine fails to convert the rhythm.

> *Nursing process step:* Implementation
> *Client needs category:* Physiological integrity
> *Client needs subcategory:* Pharmacological and parenteral therapies
> *Taxonomic level:* Comprehension

23. *Correct answer:* **C**

Blunt cardiac injury could occur leading to myocardial muscle contusion, cardiac chamber rupture, or valvular disruption. Other complications could include pneumothorax, fractured sternum or ribs, or pulmonary contusion. Spinal cord injury may result after he falls to the ground; spinal precautions should be used during treatment and transport. Abdominal or renal-pelvic injury probably wouldn't occur.

> *Nursing process step:* Assessment
> *Client needs category:* Physiological integrity
> *Client needs subcategory:* Physiological adaptation
> *Taxonomic level:* Analysis

24. *Correct answer:* **A**

They would benefit from a CPR course. Their son need not refrain from playing sports in the future, but the parents might consider having him wear a chest protector. Arrhythmias are most likely to develop during the first 24 hours following a cardiac contusion. Because lasting effects are rare, no cardiac medications are usually given after discharge, so drug interactions aren't a concern.

> *Nursing process step:* Planning
> *Client needs category:* Safe, effective care environment
> *Client needs subcategory:* Safety and infection control
> *Taxonomic level:* Application

25. *Correct answer:* **C**

Pericarditis is an inflammation of the fibroserous sac that envelops the heart. Unlike the pain of an MI, pericardial pain is often pleuritic and eases when the heart is pulled away from the diaphragmatic pleurae of the lungs. The hallmark indication of endocarditis is intermittent fever and malaise resulting from infection of the endocardium. Myocarditis has nonspecific symptoms that reflect the accompanying systemic infection.

> *Nursing process step:* Assessment
> *Client needs category:* Physiological integrity
> *Client needs subcategory:* Reduction of risk potential
> *Taxonomic level:* Application

26. *Correct answer:* **A**

A grating sound is heard with pericardial friction rub, which occurs as the heart moves; this is a classic sign of pericarditis. Murmurs are heard with valvular disorders. A loud first heart sound or opening snap is heard with mitral stenosis. A midsystolic click is heard with mitral valve prolapse.

> *Nursing process step:* Assessment
> *Client needs category:* Physiological integrity
> *Client needs subcategory:* Physiological adaptation
> *Taxonomic level:* Knowledge

27. *Correct answer:* **B**

Pericardial effusion (purulent serous or hemorrhagic exudate) is the major complication of pericarditis. Cardiac tamponade may occur if fluid accumulates rapidly, resulting in shock, cardiovascular collapse, and eventually death. Neoplasms aren't caused by pericarditis, but neoplasms can cause pericarditis. Pericarditis doesn't cause infiltrates or myalgia.

> *Nursing process step:* Assessment
> *Client needs category:* Physiological integrity
> *Client needs subcategory:* Reduction of risk potential
> *Taxonomic level:* Comprehension

28. *Correct answer:* **D**

Pericardiocentesis, the surgical aspiration of fluid from the pericardial cavity, is the treatment of choice for cardiac tamponade. Pericardiorrhaphy is the suturing of a pericardial wound. Pericardiolysis is done to free adhesions in the pericardium. Pericardectomy is the removal of the pericardium.

> *Nursing process step:* Planning
> *Client needs category:* Physiological integrity
> *Client needs subcategory:* Physiological adaptation
> *Taxonomic level:* Knowledge

29. *Correct answer:* **A**

Cardiogenic shock, sometimes called pump failure, is a condition of diminished cardiac output that severely impairs tissue perfusion. It occurs as a complication in nearly 15% of all patients hospitalized with acute MI. Thromboembolism could be a complication of MI, but the patient would probably complain of severe dyspnea and chest pain. Cardiomyopathy may lead to heart failure, but the onset is insidious and usually doesn't result from an acute MI. Cardiac tamponade may reveal some of the same symptoms, but most patients will have neck vein distention and paradoxical pulse and their lung fields will usually be clear when auscultated.

> *Nursing process step:* Assessment
> *Client needs category:* Physiological integrity
> *Client needs subcategory:* Reduction of risk potential
> *Taxonomic level:* Analysis

30. *Correct answer:* **B**

When the left ventricle contracts, blood leaves the heart and enters systemic circulation. Blood enters the heart in the right atrium. Coronary arteries receive blood, primarily during ventricular relaxation. The SA node is the heart's intrinsic pacemaker; electrical impulses originate there.

Nursing process step: Assessment
Client needs category : Physiological integrity
Client needs subcategory: Physiological adaptation
Taxonomic level: Knowledge

31. *Correct answer:* **C**

Cardiac output is the total amount of blood ejected by the heart per minute. It's determined by multiplying the patient's heart rate by his stroke volume. Stroke volume is the amount of blood ejected with each beat. Ejection fraction is the percent of left ventricular end-diastolic volume ejected during systole. Heart rate is the number of beats per minute.

Nursing process step: Assessment
Client needs category: Physiological integrity
Client needs subcategory: Physiological adaptation
Taxonomic level: Application

32. *Correct answer:* **B**

Dopamine increases stroke volume and cardiac output; it doesn't produce any of the other effects.

Nursing process step: Implementation
Client needs category: Physiological integrity
Client needs subcategory: Pharmacological and parenteral therapies
Taxonomic level: Comprehension

33. *Correct answer:* **A**

Thoracic aortic aneurysms commonly result from atherosclerosis, which weakens the aortic wall and gradually distends the vessel lumen. Hepatomegaly and dermatophytosis (a fungal skin infection) don't cause aortic aneurysms. Diabetes mellitus contributes to atherosclerosis but doesn't cause it.

Nursing process step: Assessment
Client needs category: Health promotion and maintenance
Client needs subcategory: Prevention and early detection of disease
Taxonomic level: Comprehension

34. *Correct answer:* **B**

An intimal tear in the ascending aorta initiates aortic dissection in about 60% of patients and requires prompt surgical intervention. Hypertension is a contributing factor in the development of an aneurysm. Coarctation (narrowing) of the aorta and polyphagia (excessive hunger) aren't complications of aneurysms.

Nursing process step: Assessment
Client needs category: Physiological integrity
Client needs subcategory: Reduction of risk potential
Taxonomic level: Application

35. *Correct Answer:* **D**

A heart valve prosthesis, such as a mitral valve replacement, is a major risk factor for infective endocarditis. Other risk factors include a history of heart disease (especially mitral valve prolapse), chronic debilitating disease, I.V. drug abuse, and immunosuppression. Although diabetes mellitus may predispose a person to cardiovascular disease, it isn't a major risk factor for infective endocarditis, nor is an appendectomy or pernicious anemia.

Nursing process step: Assessment
Client needs category: Health promotion and maintenance
Client needs subcategory: Prevention and early detection of disease
Taxonomic level: Comprehension

36. *Correct answer:* **B**

Prophylactic antibiotics should be given before, during, and after dental work to prevent endocarditis. Antianginals, antiemetics, or antidiuretics aren't routinely given, unless indicated by the patient's status.

Nursing process step: Planning
Client needs category: Physiological integrity
Client needs subcategory: Reduction of risk
Taxonomic level: Application

37. *Correct answer:* **C**

The nurse should ask the patient how long he's had the problem, how it affects his daily routine, when it began, and if anything relieves it. Leading questions should be avoided; whenever possible, familiar expressions should be used rather than medical terms. Educational background, medical insurance, and support systems all play a part in treatment, but aren't germane to patient assessment.

Nursing process step: Assessment
Client needs category: Health promotion and maintenance
Client needs subcategory: Prevention and early detection of disease
Taxonomic level: Comprehension

38. *Correct answer:* **A**

Right ventricular hypertrophy is a cardiac complication associated with COPD. Pulmonary hypertension associated with COPD increases the heart's workload. The right ventricle hypertrophies in an attempt to compensate. As right ventricular hypertrophy worsens, right-sided heart failure develops. The left ventricle isn't involved.

Nursing process step: Assessment
Client needs category: Physiological integrity
Client needs subcategory: Reduction of risk potential
Taxonomic level: Comprehension

39. *Correct answer:* **D**

Clinical signs of right-sided heart failure include jugular vein distention, dependent peripheral edema, hepatomegaly, splenomegaly, ascites, nausea, vomiting, weakness, dizziness and syncope. Respiratory acidosis, hypertension, and dyspnea are associated with left-sided heart failure.

Nursing process step: Assessment
Client needs category: Physiological integrity
Client needs subcategory: Physiological adaptation
Taxonomic level: Application

40. *Correct answer:* **C**

The patient with atrial fibrillation will have an ECG with erratic, irregular, and fibrillatory P waves. They aren't inverted. The QRS complexes are of uniform configuration and duration. The atrial and ventricular rhythms are grossly irregular.

Nursing process step: Assessment
Client needs category: Physiological integrity
Client needs subcategory: Physiological adaptation
Taxonomic level: Comprehension

41. *Correct answer:* **A**

The patient most likely has digitalis toxicity; withholding the digoxin and notifying the doctor is the first step in treatment. Continuing to administer digoxin may result in heart block. Obtaining a serum digoxin level doesn't treat the problem.

Nursing process step: Implementation
Client needs category: Physiological integrity
Client needs subcategory: Pharmacological and parenteral therapies
Taxonomic level: Application

42. *Correct answer:* **C**

Creatine and its isoenzyme are released into the bloodstream when myocardial tissue dies. The higher the level, the greater the damage to the myocardium. Pulmonary embolisms, ventricular arrhythmias, and cerebrovascular accidents don't affect CK-MB level.

Nursing process step: Planning
Client needs category: Physiological integrity
Client needs subcategory: Physiological adaptation
Taxonomic level: Application

43. *Correct answer:* **C**

Serum CK-MB levels can be detected 4 to 6 hours after the onset of chest pain. These levels peak within 12 to 18 hours and return to normal within 3 to 4 days.

Nursing process step: Assessment
Client needs category: Physiological integrity
Client needs subcategory: Physiological adaptation
Taxonomic level: Knowledge

44. *Correct answer:* **B**

When caring for the patient with a cardiac disorder, the rectal route should be avoided. Introducing a thermometer into the rectum may stimulate the vagus nerve, causing vasodilation and bradycardia. The oral, axillary, and tympanic routes are appropriate for measuring the temperature of cardiac patients.

Nursing process step: Implementation
Client needs category: Physiological integrity
Client needs subcategory: Physiological adaptation
Taxonomic level: Comprehension

45. *Correct answer:* **D**

Cardiac arrhythmias cause about 50% of deaths due to MI. Heart failure accounts for about 33% of post-MI deaths; cardiogenic shock, 9%. Pulmonary embolism, another potential complication of an MI, is less common.

Nursing process step: Assessment
Client needs category: Physiological adaptation
Client needs subcategory: Reduction of risk potential
Taxonomic level: Knowledge

46. *Correct answer:* **A**

Prinzmetal's or variant angina is triggered by coronary artery spasm. An unpredictable amount of activity may trigger unstable angina. Activities that increase myocardial oxygen demand may trigger predictable stable angina.

Nursing process step: Planning
Client needs category: Physiological integrity
Client needs subcategory: Reduction of risk potential
Taxonomic level: Comprehension

47. *Correct answer:* **B**

Calcium channel blockers reduce coronary artery spasm. Coronary artery blockers isn't a drug classification. Alpha-adrenergic blockers and ACE inhibitors don't produce this effect.

Nursing process step: Planning
Client needs category: Physiological integrity
Client needs subcategory: Pharmacological and parenteral therapies
Taxonomic level: Application

48. *Correct answer:* **C**

During PTCA, the patient receives heparin, an anticoagulant. Calcium channel blockers and nitrates may also be administered to reduce coronary artery spasm. An antibiotic isn't routinely given during PTCA. An anticonvulsant isn't indicated because PTCA doesn't increase the risk of seizures. An antihypertensive agent should be avoided during the procedure.

Nursing process step: Implementation
Client needs category: Physiological integrity
Client needs subcategory: Pharmacological and parenteral therapies
Taxonomic level: Application

49. *Correct answer:* **B**

Common signs and symptoms of cardiovascular dysfunction include shortness of breath, chest pain, palpitations, fainting, fatigue, and peripheral edema. Although irritability or confusion may occur if cardiovascular dysfunction leads to cerebral oxygen deprivation, this symptom more commonly reflects a respiratory or neurologic dysfunction. Insomnia rarely indicates a cardiovascular problem. Lower abdominal pain occurs with some GI disorders.

Nursing process step: Assessment
Client needs category: Physiological integrity
Client needs subcategory: Physiological adaptation
Taxonomic level: Application

50. *Correct answer:* **B**

Stage 1 is 140 to 159/90 to 99 mm Hg; stage 2 is 160 to 179/100 to 109 mm Hg; stage 3 is 180 to 209/110 to 119 mm Hg; and stage 4 is greater than or equal to 210/120 mm Hg.

Nursing process step: Assessment
Client needs category: Physiological integrity
Client needs subcategory: Physiological adaptation
Taxonomic level: Knowledge

51. *Correct answer:* **A**

Furosemide reduces circulating blood volume, which decreases the heart's work-load and lowers blood pressure. Furosemide doesn't block the sympathetic nervous system, cause peripheral vasodilation, or block renin angiotensin conversion.

> *Nursing process step:* Implementation
> *Client needs category:* Physiological integrity
> *Client needs subcategory:* Pharmacological and parenteral therapies
> *Taxonomic level:* Application

52. *Correct answer:* **D**

Untreated hypertension is the most common cause of malignant hypertension. Excessive catecholamine release (an effect of pheochromocytoma), pyelonephritis, and dissecting aortic aneurysm are less common causes.

> *Nursing process step:* Assessment
> *Client needs category:* Physiological integrity
> *Client needs subcategory:* Reduction of risk potential
> *Taxonomic level:* Knowledge

53. *Correct answer:* **A**

Arterial baroreceptors, which monitor arterial pressure, are found in the left ventricular wall, carotid sinus, and aorta. None exist in the right ventricular wall, dorsalis pedis artery, or common iliac artery.

> *Nursing process step:* Assessment
> *Client needs category:* Physiological integrity
> *Client needs subcategory:* Physiological adaptation
> *Taxonomic level:* Knowledge

54. *Correct answer:* **B**

The patient should be instructed to flex his calf muscles (to facilitate blood return to the heart), avoid alcohol, change positions slowly, eat a high-protein snack at night and grasp a stationary object when rising. Although the patient should rest between demanding activities and consume plenty of fluids and fiber to maintain a balanced diet, these measures don't directly relieve postural hypotension.

> *Nursing process step:* Planning
> *Client needs category:* Physiological integrity
> *Client needs subcategory:* Pharmacological and parenteral therapies
> *Taxonomic level:* Application

55. *Correct answer:* **C**

Severely elevated blood pressure damages the intima of small vessels, resulting in fibrin accumulation in the vessels, development of local edema, and possibly intravascular clotting. Therefore, cerebrovascular accident may occur when a clot suddenly impairs cerebral circulation in one or more blood vessels supplying the brain. Viral meningitis is inflammation of the meninges from a viral infection. A myoclonic seizure is caused by an electrical abnormality in the brain causing brief involuntary muscle jerks of the body or extremities. Status epilepticus is a continuous seizure state.

> *Nursing process step:* Planning
> *Client needs category:* Physiological integrity
> *Client needs subcategory:* Reduction of risk potential
> *Taxonomic level:* Comprehension

56. *Correct answer:* **A**

Serum lipid levels can be monitored and controlled by diet, exercise, and medication if necessary. Other risk factors that can be modified are cigarette smoking, sedentary lifestyle, stress, obesity, and an excessive intake of fats, carbohydrates, and salt. The other risk factors are non-modifiable, although coexisting disorders may be able to be controlled.

> *Nursing process step:* Planning
> *Client needs category:* Physiological integrity
> *Client needs subcategory:* Reduction of risk potential
> *Taxonomic level:* Application

57. *Correct answer:* **C**

The head of the patient's bed should be elevated to 15 to 30 degrees and his head should be turned facing the nurse. The nurse should place the pads of her index and middle fingers along the medial border of the sternocleidomastoid muscle and palpate his carotid pulse. The patient shouldn't have his neck hyperextended and shouldn't be placed in Trendelenburg's position.

> *Nursing process step:* Assessment
> *Client needs category:* Physiological integrity
> *Client needs subcategory:* Physiological adaptation
> *Taxonomic level:* Knowledge

58. *Correct answer:* **B**

Arterial occlusive disease, which narrows the carotid artery, is a common complication of atherosclerosis. Predisposing factors include smoking, hypertension, hyperlipidemia, and diabetes. The other conditions aren't directly related to arterial occlusive disease.

Nursing process step: Assessment
Client needs category: Physiological integrity
Client needs subcategory: Reduction of risk potential
Taxonomic level: Knowledge

59. *Correct answer:* **C**

Pain is the most common symptom of peripheral artery occlusion. It begins suddenly and occurs in the affected extremity. Other symptoms include pallor, pulselessness, paralysis, and paresthesia. The extremity would feel cool to the touch.

Nursing process step: Assessment
Client needs category: Physiological integrity
Client needs subcategory: Physiological adaptation
Taxonomic level: Knowledge

60. *Correct answer:* **D**

In carotid endarterectomy, the affected artery is incised and the plaque is dissected out. The artery is then patched with an autogenous saphenous vein or prosthetic material and closed. Embolectomy uses a balloon-tipped catheter to remove emboli. Following arthrectomy, stents are used as a mesh of wires that stretch and mold to the arterial wall to prevent re-occlusion. Patch grafting involves the use of an autogenous or Dacron graft to replace the thrombosed segment.

Nursing process step: Implementation
Client needs category: Physiological integrity
Client needs subcategory: Physiological adaptation
Taxonomic level: Knowledge

61. *Correct answer:* **A**

The priority assessment after surgery is assessing level of consciousness. Neurologic impairment indicates a blockage in cerebral blood flow. Skin temperature and color, intake and output, and dressing drainage need to be monitored, but they're not top priority for this patient.

Nursing process step: Assessment
Client needs category: Physiological integrity
Client needs subcategory: Reduction of risk potential
Taxonomic level: Application

62. *Correct answer:* **B**

In Raynaud's disease, episodic vasospasm occurs in the small peripheral arteries and arterioles, resulting in cyanosis and numbness in the extremities when the patient is exposed to cold or stress. In Buerger's disease, segmental lesions and thrombus produce intermittent claudication of the instep. Thrombophlebitis is inflammation and thrombus formation in a vein. Ménière's disease is an inner ear disorder.

> *Nursing process step:* Assessment
> *Client needs category:* Physiological integrity
> *Client needs subcategory:* Reduction of risk potential
> *Taxonomic level:* Knowledge

63. *Correct answer:* **B**

The patient should be taught to inspect her skin frequently and to seek immediate care for signs of skin breakdown or infection. Heart rate, blood pressure, and body temperature aren't affected by Raynaud's disease.

> *Nursing process step:* Planning
> *Client needs category:* Physiological integrity
> *Client needs subcategory:* Reduction of risk potential
> *Taxonomic level:* Knowledge

64. *Correct answer:* **B**

Hydralazine is a vasodilator. Sympatholytics reduce blood pressure by inhibiting or blocking motor and secretory action in the sympathetic nervous system. Examples include metoprolol (Aldomet) and clonidine (Catapres). Diuretics are used to increase urine volume and to maximize excretion of solutes and water. Examples include furosemide (Lasix), mannitol (Osmitrol), and bumetanide (Bumex). ACE inhibitors reduce blood pressure by interrupting the renin-angiotensin-aldosterone system. Examples include captopril (Capoten), enalapril (Vasotec), and quinapril (Accupril).

> *Nursing process step:* Planning
> *Client needs category:* Physiological integrity
> *Client needs subcategory:* Pharmacological and parenteral therapies
> *Taxonomic level:* Knowledge

65. *Correct answer:* **D**

Oral hydralazine should be taken with meals to promote absorption.

> *Nursing process step:* Implementation
> *Client needs category:* Physiological integrity
> *Client needs subcategory:* Pharmacological and parenteral therapies
> *Taxonomic level:* Knowledge

66. *Correct answer:* C

Hydralazine commonly produces such adverse reactions as headache, diarrhea, constipation, dizziness or light-headedness, orthostatic hypotension, and other effects. Dry eye syndrome, pharyngitis, and somnolence aren't adverse reactions associated with hydralazine.

Nursing process step: Implementation
Client needs category: Physiological integrity
Client needs subcategory: Pharmacological and parenteral therapies
Taxonomic level: Comprehension

NEUROSENSORY SYSTEM

QUESTIONS

1. An elderly patient may have sustained a basilar skull fracture after slipping and falling on an icy sidewalk. The nurse knows that basilar skull fractures:

    A. are the least significant type of skull fracture.
    B. may cause cerebrospinal fluid (CSF) leaks from the nose or ears.
    C. have no characteristic findings.
    D. are always surgically repaired.

2. Which of the following types of drugs might be given to control increased intracranial pressure (ICP)?

    A. Barbiturates
    B. Carbonic anhydrase inhibitors
    C. Anticholinergics
    D. Histamine receptor blockers

3. The nurse is teaching family members of a patient with a concussion about the early signs of increased intracranial pressure (ICP). Which of the following would she cite as an early sign of increased ICP?

    A. Decreased systolic blood pressure
    B. Headache and vomiting
    C. Inability to wake the patient with noxious stimuli
    D. Dilated pupils that don't react to light

4. Gary Adams is diagnosed with retinal detachment. Which intervention is the most important for this patient?

    A. Admitting him to the hospital on strict bed rest
    B. Patching both of his eyes
    C. Referring him to an ophthalmologist
    D. Preparing him for surgery

5. Dr. Harry Carson, a chemist, sustained a chemical burn to one eye. Which intervention takes priority for a patient with a chemical burn of the eye?

    A. Patch the affected eye and call the ophthalmologist.
    B. Administer a cycloplegic agent to reduce ciliary spasm.
    C. Immediately instill a topical anesthetic, then irrigate the eye with saline solution.
    D. Administer antibiotics to reduce the risk of infection.

6. The nurse is assessing a patient and notes a Brudzinski's sign and Kernig's sign. These are two classic signs of which of the following disorders?

A. Cerebrovascular accident (CVA)
B. Meningitis
C. Seizure disorder
D. Parkinson's disease

7. A patient is admitted to the hospital for a brain biopsy. The nurse knows that the most common type of primary brain tumor is:

   A. meningioma.
   B. angioma.
   C. hemangioblastoma.
   D. glioma.

8. The nurse should instruct the patient with Parkinson's disease to avoid which of the following?

   A. Walking in an indoor shopping mall
   B. Sitting on the deck on a cool summer evening
   C. Walking to the car on a cold winter day
   D. Sitting on the beach in the sun on a summer day

9. Jasmine Wilson suffered a cerebrovascular accident that left her unable to comprehend speech and unable to speak. This type of aphasia is known as:

   A. receptive aphasia.
   B. expressive aphasia.
   C. global aphasia.
   D. conduction aphasia.

10. Cynthia Knowlan complains that her headaches are occurring more frequently despite taking medications. Patients with a history of headaches should be taught to avoid:

   A. freshly prepared meats.
   B. citrus fruits.
   C. skim milk.
   D. chocolate.

11. Immediately following cerebral aneurysm rupture, the patient usually complains of:

   A. photophobia.
   B. explosive headache.
   C. seizures.
   D. hemiparesis.

12. Which of the following is a cause of embolic brain injury?

A. Persistent hypertension
B. Subarachnoid hemorrhage
C. Atrial fibrillation
D. Skull fracture

13. Although Ms. Gordon has a spinal cord injury, she can still have sexual intercourse. Discharge teaching should make her aware that:

A. she must remove her indwelling urinary catheter prior to intercourse.
B. she can no longer achieve orgasm.
C. positioning may be awkward.
D. she can still get pregnant.

14. Jennifer Durkin, age 25, suffered a cervical fracture requiring immobilization with halo traction. When caring for the patient in halo traction, the nurse must:

A. keep a wrench taped to the halo vest for quick removal if cardiopulmonary resuscitation is necessary.
B. remove the brace once a day to allow the patient to rest.
C. encourage the patient to use a pillow under the ring.
D. remove the brace so that the patient can shower.

15. The nurse asks a patient's husband if he understands why his wife is receiving nimodipine (Nimotop), since she suffered a cerebral aneurysm rupture. Which response by the husband indicates that he understands the drug's use?

A. "Nimodipine replaces calcium."
B. "Nimodipine promotes growth of blood vessels in the brain."
C. "Nimodipine reduces the brain's demand for oxygen."
D. "Nimodipine reduces vasospasm in the brain."

16. Many men who suffer spinal injuries continue to be sexually active. The teaching plan for a man with a spinal cord injury should include sexuality concerns. Which of the following injuries would most likely prevent erection and ejaculation?

A. C5
B. C7
C. T4
D. S4

17. Carol Finney, age 36, is a homemaker who frequently forgets to take her carbamazepine (Tegretol). As a result, she has been experiencing seizures. How can the nurse best help the patient remember to take her medication?

    A. Tell her to take her medication at bedtime.
    B. Instruct her to take her medication after one of her favorite television shows.
    C. Explain that she should take her medication with breakfast.
    D. Tell her to buy an alarm watch to remind her.

18. Miguel Rodriguez was diagnosed with pneumococcal meningitis. What response by the patient indicates that he understands the precautions necessary with this diagnosis?

    A. "I'm so depressed because I can't have any visitors for a week."
    B. "Thank goodness, I'll only be in isolation for 24 hours."
    C. "The nurse told me that my urine and stool are also sources of meningitis bacteria."
    D. "The doctor is a good friend of mine and won't keep me in isolation."

19. An early symptom associated with amyotrophic lateral sclerosis (ALS) includes:

    A. Fatigue while talking
    B. Change in mental status
    C. Numbness of the hands and feet
    D. Spontaneous fractures

SITUATION: *Ella Smith, age 34, is an unrestrained driver brought to the emergency department following a motor vehicle accident. She's unconscious and has a 6-cm laceration on her forehead.*

Questions 20 to 23 refer to this situation.

20. Ms. Smith is comatose, but when painful stimuli are applied she extends, adducts, and hyperpronates her upper extremities and has plantar flexion of the feet. This abnormal response is termed:

    A. decorticate response.
    B. decerebrate response.
    C. clonic-tonic activity.
    D. athetosis.

21. The Glasgow Coma Scale is used to assess Ms. Smith's level of consciousness. This tool evaluates:

    A. verbal, sensation, and motor responses.
    B. eye, motor, and verbal responses.
    C. verbal, pain, and reflex responses.
    D. eye, pain, and verbal responses.

22. If increased intracranial pressure (ICP) is suspected in this patient, which of the following diagnostic tests would be contraindicated?

    A. Intracranial computed tomography (CT) scan
    B. Skull radiography
    C. Lumbar puncture
    D. EEG

23. Ms. Smith is ordered a diagnostic test to measure electrical activity of the brain. This test is known as:

    A. an EEG.
    B. magnetic resonance imaging (MRI).
    C. a cerebral angiogram.
    D. a myelogram.

SITUATION: *Mrs. Jan Reed is transferred to the medical-surgical floor 3 days following a craniotomy for a cerebral aneurysm clipping.*

Questions 24 and 25 refer to this situation.

24. Which of the following should be included in Mrs. Reed's routine neurologic assessment?

    A. oculovestibular reflex
    B. orientation to time, place, and person
    C. hand strength only
    D. olfactory cranial nerve function

25. Mrs. Reed becomes confused and disoriented. An emergency computed tomography (CT) scan reveals cerebral vasospasm. Which of the following treatments would be most appropriate for this condition?

    A. Vasodilators
    B. Loop diuretics
    C. Intubation with hyperventilation
    D. Calcium channel blockers

SITUATION: *Mr. Thomas is transferred to the medical-surgical floor from the critical care unit where he's under observation for a closed head injury.*

Questions 26 to 28 refer to this situation.

26. When Mr. Thomas arrives on the medical-surgical floor, he's confused and disoriented. The nurse can encourage him to become oriented by:

    A. asking his family to stay away during visiting hours.

    B. keeping a clock, radio, TV, or newspaper in his room at all times.

    C. ignoring his behavior during nursing procedures.

    D. closing the window blinds during the day.

27. Mr. Thomas was started on phenytoin (Dilantin) to help prevent seizures, which can be a complication after head injury. Which of the following is a common adverse effect of the drug?

    A. Diarrhea

    B. Hyperalertness

    C. Loss of color vision

    D. Gingival hyperplasia

28. Because Mr. Thomas is at risk for developing further seizures, the nurse should:

    A. keep all side rails of the bed down.

    B. keep the height of the bed at the highest level possible.

    C. observe the patient frequently.

    D. keep a padded tongue blade at the bedside.

SITUATION: *Patrick Kelly, age 52, was an unrestrained driver who sustained a severe closed head injury. When rescue personnel arrived at the scene, his breathing was agonal and required intubation. They stabilized his neck in a cervical collar and placed him on a backboard.*

Questions 29 to 34 refer to this situation.

29. Mr. Kelly is placed on mechanical ventilation and hyperventilated. The nurse knows that this treatment is appropriate for the patient because it:

    A. increases the oxygen supply to the brain.

    B. increases cerebral blood volume.

    C. promotes vasoconstriction.

    D. dilates cerebral blood vessels.

30. Because Mr. Kelly sustained a head injury, the nurse knows she should do which of the following when suctioning him?

    A. Hyperoxygenate him before, during, and after suctioning.

    B. Suction his nasopharynx.

    C. Increase the delivered tidal volume prior to suctioning.

    D. Turn his head from side to side to facilitate suctioning.

31. Mr. Kelly has increased ICP. Which of the following interventions should the nurse use to try to reduce ICP?

    A. Keep the head of the bed flat.

    B. Maintain the hips in a flexed position.

    C. Avoid flexing the neck and hips.

    D. Keep the head of the bed elevated 60 degrees.

32. The doctor orders mannitol (Osmitrol) for Mr. Kelly. The reason for administering this drug is to:

    A. decrease blood pressure.

    B. decrease brain swelling.

    C. slow respirations and pulse.

    D. prevent further brain damage.

33. What nursing intervention takes top priority after administering Mr. Kelly's mannitol (Osmitrol) I.V.?

    A. Monitoring his intake and output

    B. Testing him for hyperglycemia

    C. Monitoring his activated partial thromboplastin time (APTT)

    D. Maintaining his airway

34. When the nurse is assessing Mr. Kelly, she notices a clear nasal drainage. The most appropriate nursing intervention would be to:

    A. notify the doctor immediately.

    B. test the drainage for glucose.

    C. examine the sinuses for inflammation.

    D. wipe his nose with facial tissues.

SITUATION: *James Young, age 46, arrives in the emergency department, complains of pain, and states that something is in his right eye. He has been working under his car. His right eye is tearing and red.*

Questions 35 and 36 refer to this situation.

35. Which of the following interventions takes top priority in the care of Mr. Young?

    A. Irrigating the eye with sterile saline solution

    B. Instilling ophthalmic antibiotic ointment

    C. Anesthetizing the cornea

    D. Manually removing the foreign body before irrigating

36. Mr. Young is given discharge instructions regarding his eye care. Which of the following statements shows that the patient understands the discharge instructions?

A. "I can save the topical anesthetic to use in the future."
B. "I'll need both eyes patched to prevent excessive eye movement."
C. "I'll need to see my doctor in a week."
D. "I'll be able to drive home as long as I'm careful."

SITUATION: *Jerome Peters is being treated for a severe brain injury that he sustained from an assault while walking his dog.*

Questions 37 to 39 refer to this situation.

37. Mr. Peters is comatose. His urine output is less than 30 ml/hour, his urine specific gravity is 1.029, and his serum sodium is 120 mEq/L. The nurse should expect to:

A. increase his fluid intake.
B. continue to monitor the patient.
C. administer hypertonic fluids.
D. irrigate his indwelling urinary catheter and increase the I.V. infusion rate.

38. Because Mr. Peters has syndrome of inappropriate diuretic hormone (SIADH) secretion, which of the following laboratory findings would the nurse expect to find?

A. Blood urea nitrogen (BUN) level of 45 mg/dl
B. Serum osmolality level of 250 mOsm/kg
C. Serum sodium level of 145 mEq/L
D. Urine specific gravity of 1.001

39. Mr. Peters' treatment plan should include which of the following to combat the fluid imbalances associated with syndrome of inappropriate antidiuretic hormone (SIADH) secretion?

A. Hypotonic saline solution
B. Fluid restriction
C. Colloids
D. 5% dextrose solution

SITUATION: *Kim Lee, age 32, has been experiencing localized seizures and personality and behavioral changes. She was admitted to the hospital for treatment of a suspected brain tumor.*

Questions 40 to 42 refer to this situation.

40. Because Ms. Lee has a history of localized seizures and personality and behavioral changes, her brain tumor is most likely located in the:

A. frontal lobe.
B. occipital lobe.
C. cerebellum.
D. brain stem.

41. Ms. Lee undergoes a craniotomy for removal of her brain tumor. The nurse notes that her dressing is saturated with blood. Which of the following interventions is most appropriate?

A. Replacing the dressing
B. Marking the area of drainage on the dressing
C. Reinforcing the dressing and notifying the doctor immediately
D. Doing nothing because this is a normal occurrence

42. When Ms. Lee returns from the operating room, she's placed in the semi-Fowler position with the head of the bed elevated 30 degrees. This is done to:

A. increase the circulating volume of blood to the brain.
B. facilitate venous return of blood from the brain.
C. maintain a patent airway.
D. prevent pulmonary congestion.

SITUATION: *Mr. Adams is a 75-year-old patient with a history of hypertension. He's admitted to the medical-surgical floor with a cerebrovascular accident.*

Questions 43 and 44 refer to this situation.

43. Mr. Adam's cerebrovascular accident has left him with homonymous hemianopsia on the left side. When caring for this patient, the nurse should be sure to:

A. speak clearly into his right ear.
B. approach him on the left side.
C. teach him to scan his visual field by turning his head back and forth.
D. teach him to chew slowly and thoroughly before swallowing.

44. Mr. Adams' recovery is uneventful. Discharge instructions include following a low-sodium diet. The nurse knows her teaching has been effective when Mr. Adams says:

A. "I know I should avoid eating oatmeal, frozen fruit, and fresh chicken."
B. "I'm so glad I can continue to eat fresh fish, pizza, and popcorn."
C. "I know I should avoid eating cold cereals, corn chips, and fresh fruit."
D. "I'm so glad I can still eat pasta, fresh chicken, and unsalted popcorn."

SITUATION: *Jordan Michaels is admitted to the medical-surgical floor after suffering a cerebrovascular accident. He has a history of hypertension and noncompliance with his therapeutic regimen.*

Questions 45 and 46 refer to this situation.

45. During the first 72 hours following a stroke, the nurse should position Mr. Michaels:

    A. in bed and lying on the side
    B. with the head of the bed elevated 30 degrees and his head in a midline neutral position
    C. with the head of the bed elevated 60 degrees and the knee gatch elevated
    D. flat in bed with his head elevated on a pillow.

46. Mr. Michaels's stroke has left him with diplopia. Which of the following nursing actions will help him visualize his environment?

    A. Teaching him to scan with his eyes from side to side
    B. Teaching him eye exercises to strengthen his eye muscles
    C. Placing all items within his visual field
    D. Patching the affected eye

SITUATION: *Mary Finster, age 76, was admitted to the medical-surgical floor with a cerebrovascular accident in the right hemisphere.*

Questions 47 to 50 refer to this situation.

47. Mrs. Finster's daughter states that before this episode her mother was experiencing periods of left-sided weakness that would resolve in less than a day. This type of neurologic problem is called:

    A. a completed cerebrovascular accident.
    B. a transient ischemic attack (TIA).
    C. a stroke-in-evolution.
    D. a progressive bleeding aneurysm.

48. Which of the following nursing diagnoses would be most appropriate for Mrs. Finster?

    A. Impaired verbal communication related to aphasia
    B. Impaired physical mobility related to right hemiparesis
    C. Risk for injury related to denial of deficits and impulsiveness
    D. Decreased cardiac output related to atrial arrhythmias

49. Mrs. Finster has dysphagia. Which nursing action might make swallowing most difficult for her?

    A. Feeding her clear liquids
    B. Positioning her upright
    C. Providing a diet of semisolid foods
    D. Adding a thickening agent to drinks

50. Mrs. Finster's cerebrovascular accident (CVA) resulted from the most common cause of ischemic brain injury, which is known as:

    A. thrombosis.
    B. cerebral hematoma.
    C. subarachnoid hemorrhage.
    D. cerebral hypertension.

SITUATION: *Peter James, a construction worker, fell 20' (6.1 m) and suffered a complete spinal cord injury at the level of his fourth thoracic vertebra. At admission, his vital signs were: blood pressure, 78/64 mm Hg; pulse, 48 beats/minute; respiratory rate, 32 breaths/minute.*

Questions 51 to 54 refer to this situation.

51. When assessing Mr. James, the nurse knows that a patient in spinal shock will present with which of the following signs and symptoms?

    A. Hypertension, headache, and flushing
    B. Hypotension, bradycardia, and sensation loss below the level of injury
    C. Hypotension, tachycardia, and sensation loss below the level of injury
    D. Diaphoresis, flushing, and tachycardia

52. In treating spinal shock, the nurse's first priority is to:

    A. place the patient in Trendelenburg's position.
    B. administer fluids via I.V. catheter.
    C. administer blood products.
    D. monitor the patient for further deterioration.

53. Mr. James complains of a headache. His blood pressure is 250/140 mm Hg, and he's diaphoretic. Which of the following nursing actions is most appropriate at this time?

    A. Placing the patient flat in bed
    B. Checking the indwelling urinary catheter for patency
    C. Increasing the I.V. fluid rate
    D. Administering oxygen

54. Mr. James requires medication given I.M. The nurse should administer this injection in which of the following muscles?

    A. Deltoid muscle
    B. Vastus lateralis muscle
    C. Ventral gluteal muscle
    D. Dorsal gluteal muscle

SITUATION: *Jane Capizzi was an unrestrained driver involved in a motor vehicle crash. She's complaining of neck pain and a cervical spine injury is suspected.*

Questions 55 and 56 refer to this situation.

55. Because Ms. Capizzi is suspected of having a cervical spine injury, initial intervention should include:

    A. transporting the patient in the position she was found without moving her extremities.
    B. transporting the patient with her arms flexed across her chest and her neck hyperextended to ensure airway patency.
    C. transporting the patient in a neutral position with a cervical collar applied.
    D. transporting the patient on her side with her head immobilized to prevent aspiration.

56. The minimum number of nurses required to logroll Ms. Capizzi is:

    A. two.
    B. three.
    C. four.
    D. five.

SITUATION: *Mr. Long, age 45, was a motorcycle driver involved in a crash with a car. At the scene he was placed on a backboard and a cervical collar was applied. He was transported to the local trauma center within 15 minutes of his injury.*

Questions 57 and 58 refer to this situation.

57. Mr. Long is being evaluated for a spinal cord injury and a complete spinal cord transection is suspected. Which of the following statements are true concerning a complete spinal cord transection?

    A. A complete spinal cord transection is also referred to as Brown-Sequard syndrome.
    B. There is a loss of all sensation on the opposite (contralateral) side of the lesion.
    C. Afferent impulses are unable to ascend from below the site of the lesion to the brain.
    D. Efferent impulses may descend on the same (ipsilateral) side of the lesion.

58. The drug of choice for treating spinal cord edema associated with Mr. Long's spinal cord injury is:

    A. mannitol (Osmitrol).
    B. methylprednisolone (Solu-Medrol).
    C. aspirin.
    D. meperidine (Demerol).

SITUATION: *Paul Leonne, age 83, was admitted to the medical-surgical floor with a cerebrovascular accident. He's comatose and receiving supportive care.*

Questions 59 and 60 refer to this situation.

59. When the nurse walks in to Mr. Leonne's room to assess him, he's having a tonic-clonic seizure. Which of the following drugs would the nurse expect to administer to Mr. Leonne?

    A. Phenytoin (Dilantin) I.V.
    B. Flumazenil (Romazicon) I.V.
    C. Carbamazepine (Tegretol) P.O.
    D. Lorazepam (Ativan) I.V.

60. Mr. Leonne's condition worsens and the nurse is assessing his corneal reflex. The best method for assessing corneal reflex is:

    A. touching the edge of the patient's cornea with a wisp of cotton.
    B. quickly moving a hand toward the patient's face.
    C. asking the patient to frown, smile, wrinkle his forehead, and puff out his cheeks.
    D. stroking a piece of cotton over the patient's face and asking him to respond when he feels it.

SITUATION: *Joanne Barrows, age 38, is admitted to the hospital for pain control. She has a history of migraine headaches that have progressively worsened. Her medical history includes ischemic heart disease.*

Questions 61 to 63 refer to this situation.

61. The nurse is completing Ms. Barrows's initial assessment. Which question would be most appropriate for identifying a precipitating factor?

    A. "Does the headache usually occur when you're in a dark room?"
    B. "Do you participate in frequent exercise programs?"
    C. "Is your diet high in saturated fat?"
    D. "Does the headache usually occur before you have your period?

62. Because of her history of ischemic heart disease, which of the following drugs should Ms. Barrows not be given for her migraine?

    A. Indomethacin (Indocin)
    B. Dihydroergotamine (D.H.E. 45)
    C. Prochlorperazine (Compazine)
    D. Sumatriptan succinate (Imitrex)

63. Ms. Barrows is prescribed propranolol (Inderal). After teaching her about the drug, the nurse sees a need for further teaching based on which of the following responses?

    A. "I'll take the last dose of the day at bedtime."
    B. "I'll slowly change my position from reclining to standing."
    C. "I'll take the drug with meals to help it absorb."
    D. "It's important for me to check my pulse for a fast heart rate."

SITUATION: *Elizabeth Moore is a 78-year-old patient diagnosed with Parkinson's disease. She was admitted to the hospital for medical management.*

Questions 64 and 65 refer to this situation.

64. Mrs. Moore is prescribed amantadine (Symadine) to treat her Parkinson's disease. Which of the following adverse reactions might she experience with long-term use of this drug?

    A. Livedo reticularis
    B. Liver cirrhosis
    C. Atrial arrhythmias
    D. Pleural effusions

65. Because a nursing diagnosis for a patient with Parkinson's disease is risk for altered nutrition less than body requirements, what foods would be most appropriate for Mrs. Moore?

    A. Frequent high-calorie hot liquids
    B. High-protein foods
    C. Foods high in L-tryptophan
    D. High-fiber foods

SITUATION: *Emma Bryant is a 65-year-old patient with a history of Alzheimer's disease admitted to the hospital for lower GI bleeding.*

Questions 66 and 67 refer to this situation.

66. What nursing intervention is most appropriate when encouraging Mrs. Bryant's independence and maintaining her safety?

    A. Keeping her bed in the lowest position with the lower side rails down

    B. Keeping her bed in the lowest position with all side rails up

    C. Making sure she knows where the nurse call bell is and how to use it

    D. Leaving a light on in the room so that she remembers where she's

67. Mrs. Bryant becomes very restless. The nurse is concerned that she may harm herself. Which of the following nursing interventions would best protect the patient?

    A. Applying a waist restraint under her gown

    B. Placing the patient in a special geriatric chair

    C. Distracting the patient with loud music

    D. Taking the patient for frequent walks

SITUATION: *Lori Gardener, age 37, was admitted to the medical-surgical floor with complaints of numbness and tingling in the legs that has recently progressed to the arms. Guillain-Barré syndrome is suspected.*

Questions 68 and 69 refer to this situation.

68. Which of the following questions is important to include when assessing Ms. Gardener?

    A. "Has anyone in your family ever had Guillain-Barré syndrome?"

    B. "Did you have an upper respiratory tract infection recently?"

    C. "Do you bruise easily?"

    D. "Have you been out of the country during the past 4 months?"

69. When assessing Ms. Gardener, what characteristic symptoms would the nurse expect to observe?

    A. Deteriorating level of consciousness

    B. Dilated pupils, facial numbness, and dysphagia

    C. Disorientation with inappropriate behavior and muscle weakness

    D. Ascending flaccid motor paralysis

ANSWER SHEET

	A B C D		A B C D		A B C D
1	○ ○ ○ ○	24	○ ○ ○ ○	47	○ ○ ○ ○
2	○ ○ ○ ○	25	○ ○ ○ ○	48	○ ○ ○ ○
3	○ ○ ○ ○	26	○ ○ ○ ○	49	○ ○ ○ ○
4	○ ○ ○ ○	27	○ ○ ○ ○	50	○ ○ ○ ○
5	○ ○ ○ ○	28	○ ○ ○ ○	51	○ ○ ○ ○
6	○ ○ ○ ○	29	○ ○ ○ ○	52	○ ○ ○ ○
7	○ ○ ○ ○	30	○ ○ ○ ○	53	○ ○ ○ ○
8	○ ○ ○ ○	31	○ ○ ○ ○	54	○ ○ ○ ○
9	○ ○ ○ ○	32	○ ○ ○ ○	55	○ ○ ○ ○
10	○ ○ ○ ○	33	○ ○ ○ ○	56	○ ○ ○ ○
11	○ ○ ○ ○	34	○ ○ ○ ○	57	○ ○ ○ ○
12	○ ○ ○ ○	35	○ ○ ○ ○	58	○ ○ ○ ○
13	○ ○ ○ ○	36	○ ○ ○ ○	59	○ ○ ○ ○
14	○ ○ ○ ○	37	○ ○ ○ ○	60	○ ○ ○ ○
15	○ ○ ○ ○	38	○ ○ ○ ○	61	○ ○ ○ ○
16	○ ○ ○ ○	39	○ ○ ○ ○	62	○ ○ ○ ○
17	○ ○ ○ ○	40	○ ○ ○ ○	63	○ ○ ○ ○
18	○ ○ ○ ○	41	○ ○ ○ ○	64	○ ○ ○ ○
19	○ ○ ○ ○	42	○ ○ ○ ○	65	○ ○ ○ ○
20	○ ○ ○ ○	43	○ ○ ○ ○	66	○ ○ ○ ○
21	○ ○ ○ ○	44	○ ○ ○ ○	67	○ ○ ○ ○
22	○ ○ ○ ○	45	○ ○ ○ ○	68	○ ○ ○ ○
23	○ ○ ○ ○	46	○ ○ ○ ○	69	○ ○ ○ ○

ANSWERS AND RATIONALES

1. *Correct answer:* **B**

A basilar skull fracture carries the risk of complications of dural tear, causing CSF leakage and damage to cranial nerves I, II, VII, and VIII. Classic findings in this type of fracture may include otorrhea, rhinorrhea, Battle's sign, and raccoon eyes. Surgical treatment isn't always required.

> *Nursing process step:* Assessment
> *Client needs category:* Physiological integrity
> *Client needs subcategory:* Physiological adaptation
> *Taxonomic level:* Knowledge

2. *Correct answer:* **A**

Barbiturates may be used to induce a coma in a patient with increased ICP. This decreases cortical activity and cerebral metabolism, reduces cerebral blood volume, decreases cerebral edema, and reduces the brain's need for glucose and oxygen. Carbonic anhydrase inhibitors are used to decrease ocular pressure or to decrease the serum pH in a patient with metabolic alkalosis. Anticholinergics have many uses including reducing GI spasms. Histamine receptor blockers are used to decrease stomach acidity.

> *Nursing process step:* Planning
> *Client needs category:* Physiological integrity
> *Client needs subcategory:* Pharmacological and parenteral therapies
> *Taxonomic level:* Application

3. *Correct answer:* **B**

Headache and projectile vomiting are early signs of increased ICP. Decreased systolic blood pressure, unconsciousness, and dilated pupils that don't react to light are considered late signs.

> *Nursing process step:* Implementation
> *Client needs category:* Physiological integrity
> *Client needs subcategory:* Reduction of risk potential
> *Taxonomic level:* Knowledge

4. *Correct answer:* **A**

Immediate bed rest is necessary to prevent further injury. Both eyes should be patched to avoid consensual eye movement and the patient should receive early referral to an ophthalmologist. If the macula is attached and central visual acuity is normal, an ophthalmologist should treat the condition immediately. Retinal reattachment can be accomplished by surgery only. If the macula is detached or threatened, surgery is urgent; prolonged detachment of the macula results in permanent loss of central vision.

Nursing process step: Implementation
Client needs category: Physiological integrity
Client needs subcategory: Reduction of risk potential
Taxonomic level: Knowledge

5. *Correct answer:* **C**

A chemical burn to the eye requires immediate instillation of a topical anesthetic followed by irrigation with copious amounts of saline solution. Irrigation should be done for 5 to 10 minutes, and then the pH of the eye should be checked. Irrigation should be continued until the pH of the eye is restored to neutral (pH 7.0). Double eversion of the eyelids should be performed to look for and remove material lodged in the cul-de-sac. A cycloplegic agent can then be used to reduce ciliary spasm, and an antibiotic ointment can be administered to reduce the risk of infection. Then the eye should be patched. Parenteral narcotic analgesia is often required for pain relief. An ophthalmologist should also be consulted.

Nursing process step: Implementation
Client needs category: Physiological integrity
Client needs subcategory: Reduction of risk potential
Taxonomic level: Knowledge

6. *Correct answer:* **B**

A positive response to one or both tests indicates meningeal irritation that is present with meningitis. Brudzinski's and Kernig's signs don't occur in CVA, seizure disorder, or Parkinson's disease.

Nursing process step: Assessment
Client needs category: Physiological integrity
Client needs subcategory: Reduction of risk potential
Taxonomic level: Application

7. *Correct answer:* **D**

Gliomas account for approximately 45% of all brain tumors. Meningiomas are the second most common, with 15%. Angiomas and hemangioblastomas are types of cerebral vascular tumors that account for 3% of brain tumors.

Nursing process step: Assessment
Client needs category: Health promotion and maintenance
Client needs subcategory: Prevention and early detection of disease
Taxonomic level: Comprehension

8. *Correct answer:* **D**

The patient with Parkinson's disease may be hypersensitive to heat, which increases the risk of hyperthermia, and he should be instructed to avoid sun exposure during hot weather.

> *Nursing process step:* Planning
> *Client needs category:* Health promotion and maintenance
> *Client needs subcategory:* Prevention and early detection of disease
> *Taxonomic level:* Application

9. *Correct answer:* **C**

Global aphasia occurs when all language functions are affected. Receptive aphasia, also known as Wernicke's aphasia, affects the ability to comprehend written or spoken words. Expressive aphasia, also known as Broca's aphasia, affects the patient's ability to form language and express thoughts. Conduction aphasia refers to abnormalities in speech repetition.

> *Nursing process step:* Assessment
> *Client needs category:* Physiological integrity
> *Client needs subcategory:* Basic care and comfort
> *Taxonomic level:* Knowledge

10. *Correct answer:* **D**

Patients with a history of headaches, especially migraines, should be taught to keep a food diary to identify potential food triggers. Typical headache triggers include alcohol, aged cheeses, processed meats, and chocolate- and caffeine-containing products.

> *Nursing process step:* Planning
> *Client needs category:* Health promotion and maintenance
> *Client needs subcategory:* Prevention and early detection of disease
> *Taxonomic level:* Application

11. *Correct answer:* **B**

An explosive headache or "the worst headache I've ever had" is typically the first presenting symptom of a bleeding cerebral aneurysm. Photophobia, seizures, and hemiparesis may occur later.

> *Nursing process step:* Assessment
> *Client needs category:* Physiological integrity
> *Client needs subcategory:* Physiological adaptation
> *Taxonomic level:* Knowledge

12. *Correct answer:* C

An embolic injury, caused by a traveling clot, may result from atrial fibrillation. Blood may pool in the fibrillating atrium and be released to travel up the cerebral artery to the brain. Persistent hypertension may place the patient at risk for a thrombotic injury to the brain. Subarachnoid hemorrhage and skull fractures aren't associated with emboli.

> *Nursing process step*: Assessment
> *Client needs category:* Health promotion and maintenance
> *Client needs subcategory:* Prevention and early detection of disease
> *Taxonomic level:* Knowledge

13. *Correct answer:* D

Women with spinal cord injuries who were sexually active may continue having sexual intercourse and must be reminded that they can still become pregnant. She may be fully capable of achieving orgasm. An indwelling urinary catheter may be left in place during sexual intercourse. Positioning will need to be adjusted to fit the patient's needs.

> *Nursing process step:* Planning
> *Client needs category:* Psychosocial integrity
> *Client needs subcategory:* Coping and adaptation
> *Taxonomic level:* Knowledge

14. *Correct answer:* A

The nurse must have a wrench taped on the vest at all times for quick halo removal in emergent situations. The brace isn't to be removed for any other reason until the cervical fracture is healed. Placing a pillow under the patient's head may alter the stability of the brace.

> *Nursing process step:* Implementation
> *Client needs category:* Physiological integrity
> *Client needs subcategory:* Reduction of risk potential
> *Taxonomic level:* Knowledge

15. *Correct answer:* D

Nimodipine is a calcium channel blocker that acts on cerebral blood vessels to reduce vasospasm. The drug doesn't increase the amount of calcium, affect cerebral vasculature growth, or reduce cerebral oxygen demand.

> *Nursing process step:* Evaluation
> *Client needs category:* Physiological integrity
> *Client needs subcategory:* Pharmacological and parenteral therapies
> *Taxonomic level:* Analysis

16. *Correct answer:* **D**

Men with spinal cord injury should be taught that the higher the level of the lesion, the better their sexual function will be. The sacral region is the lowest area on the spinal column and injury to this area will cause more erectile dysfunction.

> *Nursing process step:* Planning
> *Client needs category:* Psychosocial integrity
> *Client needs subcategory:* Coping and adaptation
> *Taxonomic level:* Knowledge

17. *Correct answer:* **C**

Tegretol should be taken with food to minimize GI distress. Taking it at meals will also establish a regular routine, which should help compliance.

> *Nursing process step:* Planning
> *Client needs category:* Physiological integrity
> *Client needs subcategory:* Pharmacological and parenteral therapies
> *Taxonomic level:* Knowledge

18. *Correct answer:* **B**

Patients with pneumococcal meningitis require respiratory isolation for the first 24 hours after treatment is initiated.

> *Nursing process step:* Evaluation
> *Client needs category:* Physiological integrity
> *Client needs subcategory:* Physiological adaptation
> *Taxonomic level:* Analysis

19. *Correct answer:* **A**

Early symptoms of ALS include fatigue while talking, dysphagia, and weakness of the hands and arms. ALS doesn't cause a change in mental status, paresthesia, or fractures.

> *Nursing process step:* Assessment
> *Client needs category:* Physiological adaptation
> *Client needs subcategory:* Physiological integrity
> *Taxonomic level:* Comprehension

20. *Correct answer:* **B**

In decerebrate response, or posturing, a painful stimulus causes teeth to be clenched; arms stiffly extended, adducted, and hyperpronated; and legs stiffly extended with plantar flexion of the feet. Decorticate posturing shows flexion of the arm, wrist, and fingers with adduction of the arm while the legs exhibit extension, internal rotation, and plantar flexion. Tonic-clonic activity is marked by rhythmic, rigid jerking and relaxation of the muscles during generalized seizure activity. Athetosis is irregular, slow, snakelike muscular movements.

Nursing process step: Assessment
Client needs category: Physiological integrity
Client needs subcategory: Physiological adaptation
Taxonomic level: Knowledge

21. *Correct answer:* B

The Glasgow Coma Scale evaluates the patient's best eye-opening, best verbal, and best motor responses.

Nursing process step: Assessment
Client needs category: Physiological integrity
Client needs subcategory: Physiological adaptation
Taxonomic level: Knowledge

22. *Correct answer:* C

Lumbar puncture is contraindicated with increased ICP. Removal of cerebral spinal fluid may decrease pressure in the spinal column sufficiently to cause the brain to herniate downward, resulting in death. Intracranial CT scans, skull radiography, and EEGs aren't invasive and so don't affect ICP.

Nursing process step: Planning
Client needs category: Physiological integrity
Client needs subcategory: Reduction of risk potential
Taxonomic level: Application

23. *Correct answer:* A

EEG measures the electrical activity of the brain. MRI produces cross-sectional images of the brain and spine in multiple planes. A cerebral angiogram allows visualization of blood vessels through injection of a radiopaque contrast medium. Myelography involves injection of a radiopaque contrast medium into the spinal subarachnoid space. CSF is removed for analysis at the time of myelography and is replaced by the heavier contrast medium, which gravitates toward the head or elsewhere within the spinal canal when the radiographic table is tilted.

Nursing process step: Implementation
Client needs category: Physiological integrity
Client needs subcategory: Reduction of risk potential
Taxonomic level: Knowledge

24. *Correct answer:* B

Noting orientation to time, place, and person should be part of every routine neurologic assessment. The doctor assesses for brain stem injury by checking the oculovestibular reflex. The patient's strength should be assessed in all extremities, not only the hands. Assessing the olfactory cranial nerve would be important in an initial or specialized assessment; it wouldn't be checked in a routine neurologic assessment.

Nursing process step: Assessment
Client needs category: Health promotion and maintenance
Client needs subcategory: Prevention and early detection of disease
Taxonomic level: Comprehension

25. *Correct answer:* **D**

Calcium channel blockers are the most appropriate treatment for the patient with cerebral vasospasm. They work by reducing the entry of calcium ions into cells, which is required for cerebral smooth-muscle contraction. The calcium channel blocker of choice for cerebral vasospasm is nimodipine (Nimotop). Other methods to decrease cerebral vasospasm include induced arterial hypertension with vasopressors and intravascular expansion with colloid solutions such as whole blood, plasma, or albumin. Intubation with hyperventilation is used to lower intracranial pressure.

Nursing process step: Implementation
Client needs category: Physiological integrity
Client needs subcategory: Pharmacological and parenteral therapies
Taxonomic level: Application

26. *Correct answer:* **B**

Patients may become more oriented if given cues such as a clock, radio, TV, or newspaper. The patient's family should be encouraged to visit. The nurse and family should talk with the patient, reorienting him to the current situation. Window blinds should be left open to keep the patient aware of day and night.

Nursing process step: Implementation
Client needs category: Psychosocial integrity
Client needs subcategory: Psychosocial adaptation
Taxonomic level: Knowledge

27. *Correct answer:* **D**

A common adverse effect of phenytoin is gingival hyperplasia. Other adverse effects may include constipation and drowsiness. Phenytoin doesn't affect color vision.

Nursing process step: Assessment
Client needs category: Physiological integrity
Client needs subcategory: Pharmacological and parenteral therapies
Taxonomic level: Knowledge

28. *Correct answer:* **C**

A patient at risk for seizures should be observed frequently for further seizure activity. Side rails should be kept up, with pads on the rails for additional protection. Bed height should always be set low to maintain safety. A padded tongue blade can cause injury if inserted into the patient's mouth during a seizure.

> *Nursing process step:* Implementation
> *Client needs category:* Physiological integrity
> *Client needs subcategory:* Reduction of risk potential
> *Taxonomic level:* Knowledge

29. *Correct answer:* **C**

The head-injured patient is placed on mechanical ventilation and hyperventilated to decrease the $Paco_2$ level, which promotes vasoconstriction and decreases intracranial pressure. Hyperventilation won't significantly increase the Pao_2 level.

> *Nursing process step:* Implementation
> *Client needs category:* Physiological integrity
> *Client needs subcategory:* Physiological adaptation
> *Taxonomic level:* Application

30. *Correct answer:* **A**

A head-injured patient should be hyperoxygenated before, during, and after suctioning to avoid hypoxia, which may increase intracranial pressure (ICP). Suctioning the nasopharynx is typically not necessary. Increasing the tidal volume on the ventilator increases the risk of lung trauma. Turning the head from side to side won't facilitate suctioning and may increase ICP.

> *Nursing process step:* Implementation
> *Client needs category:* Physiological integrity
> *Client needs subcategory:* Physiological adaptation
> *Taxonomic level:* Application

31. *Correct answer:* **C**

Neck and hip flexion should be avoided and the head of the bed should be maintained at 30 degrees to facilitate venous return and reduce ICP.

> *Nursing process step:* Implementation
> *Client needs category:* Physiological integrity
> *Client needs subcategory:* Physiological adaptation
> *Taxonomic level:* Application

32. *Correct answer:* **B**

Mannitol promotes osmotic diuresis, which decreases brain swelling and ICP. The drug may also lower blood pressure as it decreases fluid volume. Mannitol doesn't slow respirations and pulse.

> *Nursing process step:* Implementation
> *Client needs category:* Physiological integrity
> *Client needs subcategory:* Pharmacological and parenteral therapies
> *Taxonomic level:* Knowledge

33. *Correct answer:* **A**

Because mannitol promotes osmotic diuresis, the patient's intake and output should be monitored closely to evaluate the drug's effectiveness. Mannitol has no effect on the patient's serum glucose level, APTT, or airway.

> *Nursing process step:* Planning
> *Client needs category:* Physiological integrity
> *Client needs subcategory:* Pharmacological and parenteral therapies
> *Taxonomic level:* Application

34. *Correct answer:* **B**

Nasal drainage that occurs with a basilar skull fracture may indicate leaking cerebrospinal fluid. The nurse should check the drainage for glucose, or perform a halo test and then notify the doctor. It isn't necessary for the nurse to examine the sinuses for inflammation. If appropriate, the patient should be cautioned against blowing the nose and no type of nasal packing should be used.

> *Nursing process step:* Implementation
> *Client needs category:* Physiological integrity
> *Client needs subcategory:* Physiological adaptation
> *Taxonomic level:* Application

35. *Correct answer:* **C**

The first priority in caring for a patient with a foreign body in the eye is to relieve pain with an anesthetic solution. Anesthetizing the cornea allows for a more comfortable inspection and irrigation with saline solution. Ophthalmic antibiotic ointments are used after the foreign body is removed. If the foreign body isn't removed with irrigation, it should be removed manually.

> *Nursing process step:* Implementation
> *Client needs category:* Physiological integrity
> *Client needs subcategory:* Reduction of risk potential
> *Taxonomic level:* Knowledge

36. *Correct answer:* **B**

Consensual eye movement, which can result in increased injury, occurs if only the injured eye is patched. Therefore it's necessary for both eyes to be patched. Even though topical anesthetics effectively eliminate pain, they shouldn't be sent home with a patient because they can mask complications of the injury, risking additional eye damage. Because bilateral patching is usually performed, the patient can't drive home.

> *Nursing process step:* Evaluation
> *Client needs category:* Physiological integrity
> *Client needs subcategory:* Reduction of risk potential
> *Taxonomic level:* Application

37. *Correct answer:* **C**

The patient is exhibiting signs and symptoms of syndrome of inappropriate antidiuretic hormone (SIADH) due to his head injury. Hypertonic fluids should be administered to correct the associated hyponatremia. Classic signs of diabetes insipidus include: urine output greater than 300 ml/hour for 3 consecutive hours and a low specific gravity. Irrigation of the indwelling urinary catheter won't correct the low urine output because the symptoms are related to a hormonal problem not a catheter blockage. Fluid administration should be limited in the patient with SIADH.

> *Nursing process step:* Planning
> *Client needs category:* Physiological integrity
> *Client needs subcategory:* Reduction of risk potential
> *Taxonomic level:* Application

38. *Correct answer:* **B**

Serum osmolality level will be decreased in SIADH secretion due to fluid retention. Serum sodium level will also be decreased due to fluid retention and excretion of large volumes of sodium by the kidney. Urine specific gravity will be high due to decreased urine output. The BUN level isn't affected.

> *Nursing process step:* Assessment
> *Client needs category:* Physiological integrity
> *Client needs subcategory:* Physiological adaptation
> *Taxonomic level:* Knowledge

39. *Correct answer:* **B**

SIADH secretion is characterized by excessive amounts of antidiuretic hormone secreted from the posterior pituitary. Key features of antidiuretic hormone excess include water retention, hyponatremia, and low osmolality level. Treatment includes fluid restriction, administration of hypertonic saline solution, and demeclocycline (Declomycin).

Nursing process step: Planning
Client needs category: Physiological integrity
Client needs subcategory: Physiological adaptation
Taxonomic level: Application

40. *Correct answer:* **A**

Classic signs of a frontal lobe brain tumor include personality changes, inappropriate behavior, and seizures. Brain tumors located in the occipital lobe affect vision, cerebellar tumors affect gait, and brain stem tumors affect heart function and breathing.

Nursing process step: Assessment
Client needs category: Health promotion and maintenance
Client needs subcategory: Prevention and early detection of disease
Taxonomic level: Knowledge

41. *Correct answer:* **C**

If the dressing becomes saturated with blood, it should be reinforced and the doctor notified immediately. The patient may need to return to the operating room to stop the bleeding. The dressing shouldn't be removed because removing it might disturb clot formation. When there is a small amount of drainage on the dressing, the drainage area can be marked to easily identify an increase in drainage.

Nursing process step: Implementation
Client needs category: Physiological integrity
Client needs subcategory: Physiological adaptation
Taxonomic level: Application

42. *Correct answer:* **B**

The head of the patient's bed is elevated to facilitate venous return from the brain, which decreases intracranial pressure. Maintaining the patient in the semi-Fowler position with the head of her bed at 30 degrees doesn't increase circulating blood volume to the brain, maintain a patent airway, or prevent pulmonary congestion.

Nursing process step: Implementation
Client needs category: Physiological integrity
Client needs subcategory: Reduction of risk potential
Taxonomic level: Knowledge

43. *Correct answer:* **C**

Homonymous hemianopsia is loss of one-half of the visual field in both eyes (either the right half or left half). To compensate, the patient must be taught to scan his visual field by turning the head back and forth. Approaching the patient on the left side won't be effective because the vision loss is in both eyes. Homonymous hemianopsia doesn't affect hearing or swallowing.

Nursing process step: Implementation
Client needs category: Physiological integrity
Client needs subcategory: Basic care and comfort
Taxonomic level: Application

44. *Correct answer:* **D**

The nurse knows her teaching was effective when Mr. Adams states he can continue to eat pasta, fresh chicken, and unsalted popcorn. Pizza, cold cereals, and corn chips are all high in sodium. Oatmeal, frozen fruit, fresh chicken, pasta, fresh fish, and unsalted popcorn are all low in sodium.

Nursing process step: Evaluation
Client needs category: Physiological integrity
Client needs subcategory: Basic care and comfort
Taxonomic level: Analysis

45. *Correct answer:* **B**

The patient should be positioned in a midline neutral position with the head of his bed elevated to 30 degrees. This positioning will facilitate venous return from the brain. Positioning the patient flat in the bed or with neck or hip flexion may increase intracranial pressure because these positions don't promote venous return.

Nursing process step: Implementation
Client needs category: Physiological integrity
Client needs subcategory: Reduction of risk potential
Taxonomic level: Application

46. *Correct answer:* **D**

Diplopia, or double vision, is best corrected by having the patient wear an eye patch. Having the patient scan the visual field would be effective for homonymous hemianopsia rather than diplopia. Performing eye exercises and placing objects within the visual field won't correct the problem.

Nursing process step: Implementation
Client needs category: Physiological integrity
Client needs subcategory: Basic care and comfort
Taxonomic level: Application

47. *Correct answer:* **B**

A TIA elicits symptoms of a stroke, but they usually disappear within 24 hours. Deficits resulting from a completed stroke won't resolve in this short span of time (if ever). Symptoms of a stroke-in-evolution develop over a period of hours to days, and symptoms of a progressively bleeding aneurysm only increase in severity over time.

> *Nursing process step:* Assessment
> *Client needs category:* Physiological integrity
> *Client needs subcategory:* Physiological adaptation
> *Taxonomic level:* Knowledge

48. *Correct answer:* **C**

A patient with a right hemisphere CVA will exhibit poor judgment, lack of insight, impulsiveness, and denial of the affected side. A patient with a left hemisphere CVA may have aphasia and right hemiparesis. A CVA doesn't cause atrial arrhythmias.

> *Nursing process step:* Analysis
> *Client needs category:* Physiological integrity
> *Client needs subcategory:* Physiological adaptation
> *Taxonomic level:* Analysis

49. *Correct answer:* **A**

Patients with dysphagia (difficulty swallowing) shouldn't be given clear liquids. Thickened or semisolid foods are easier to swallow because they give the swallowing muscles more resistance to work against. Having the patient sit upright allows gravity to facilitate swallowing.

> *Nursing process step:* Implementation
> *Client needs category:* Physiological integrity
> *Client needs subcategory:* Basic care and comfort
> *Taxonomic level:* Application

50. *Correct answer:* **A**

Ischemic brain injury most commonly results from thrombosis caused by plaque buildup in the cerebral arteries. Cerebral hematoma and subarachnoid hemorrhage rarely cause CVA. Cerebral hypertension is a risk factor for a CVA, not a cause.

> *Nursing process step:* Assessment
> *Client needs category:* Physiological integrity
> *Client needs subcategory:* Physiological adaptation
> *Taxonomic level:* Knowledge

51. *Correct answer:* **B**

The patient in spinal shock (a form of distributive shock) will be hypotensive, bradycardic, and have sensation loss below the level of injury. Because of baroreceptor tone loss, the patient isn't tachycardic like patients who suffer from other types of shock. Hypertension, diaphoresis, and flushing aren't seen in shock states.

Nursing process step: Assessment
Client needs category: Physiological integrity
Client needs subcategory: Physiological adaptation
Taxonomic level: Knowledge

52. *Correct answer:* **B**

Treatment for spinal shock requires inserting an I.V. catheter to administer fluids into the abnormally dilated vascular system that results from spinal shock. Placing the patient in Trendelenburg's position won't affect his vital signs because there is a loss of vasomotor tone. Monitoring the patient won't affect the signs and symptoms of spinal shock.

Nursing process step: Implementation
Client needs category: Physiological integrity
Client needs subcategory: Pharmacological and parenteral therapies
Taxonomic level: Application

53. *Correct answer:* **B**

This patient is most likely experiencing autonomic dysreflexia, a complication that can occur after spinal cord injury. Treatment includes relieving the source of sympathetic stimulation — such as a distended bladder, constipation, pressure ulcers, wrinkles in the sheets, or ingrown toenails. Placing the patient flat in the bed and increasing the I.V. infusion rate will increase the patient's blood pressure. Oxygen administration may be beneficial but won't correct the problem.

Nursing process step: Implementation
Client needs category: Physiological integrity
Client needs subcategory: Physiological adaptation
Taxonomic level: Application

54. *Correct answer:* **A**

I.M. injections should be administered in the deltoid or abdominal muscles. Vastus lateralis or gluteal muscles will have decreased blood flow resulting from the spinal cord injury, so less medication will be absorbed from those sites.

Nursing process step: Planning
Client needs category: Physiological integrity
Client needs subcategory: Pharmacological and parenteral therapies
Taxonomic level: Knowledge

55. *Correct answer:* **C**

The patient should be transported on a backboard, in a neutral position with a hard cervical collar in place. Any other body position may cause further damage to the spinal cord.

> *Nursing process step:* Implementation
> *Client needs category:* Physiological integrity
> *Client needs subcategory:* Reduction of risk potential
> *Taxonomic level:* Knowledge

56. *Correct answer:* **B**

Three nurses are needed to safely logroll the patient: one to maintain proper head alignment during turning, and two others to maintain upper- and lower-body alignment.

> *Nursing process step:* Implementation
> *Client needs category:* Physiological integrity
> *Client needs subcategory:* Reduction of risk potential
> *Taxonomic level:* Comprehension

57. *Correct answer:* **C**

A complete spinal cord transection causes motor function and sensation loss on both sides of the body below the injury level. Brown-Sequard syndrome is a type of spinal cord injury resulting in ipsilateral paralysis or paresis and loss of touch, pressure, vibration, and proprioception, with contralateral loss of pain and temperature sensation.

> *Nursing process step:* Assessment
> *Client needs category:* Physiological integrity
> *Client needs subcategory:* Reduction of risk potential
> *Taxonomic level:* Knowledge

58. *Correct answer:* **B**

Methylprednisolone is the drug of choice for treating spinal cord edema associated with acute spinal injuries. To achieve maximum effectiveness, it should be administered I.V. as soon after the injury as possible. Mannitol is administered to treat cerebral edema. Aspirin and meperidine aren't indicated for treatment of central nervous tissue edema.

> *Nursing process step:* Planning
> *Client needs category:* Physiological integrity
> *Client needs subcategory:* Pharmacological and parenteral therapies
> *Taxonomic level:* Knowledge

59. *Correct answer:* **D**

Lorazepam is the drug of choice for treating tonic-clonic seizures. Lorazepam acts quickly and crosses the blood-brain barrier. It's preferred over diazepam because it has a longer duration of action. Phenytoin should be administered as a maintenance drug once the initial seizure activity is controlled by lorazepam. Carbamazepine is given to control seizures in the patient with a long-standing history of seizures. Flumazenil is used to reverse the effects of benzodiazepines.

> *Nursing process step:* Implementation
> *Client needs category:* Physiological integrity
> *Client needs subcategory:* Pharmacological and parenteral therapies
> *Taxonomic level:* Knowledge

60. *Correct answer:* **B**

Quickly moving a hand toward the patient's face will cause him to blink if his corneal reflex is intact. Touching the cornea with cotton may scratch the cornea and should be avoided. Assessing facial sensation and gestures doesn't elicit information about the corneal reflex.

> *Nursing process step:* Assessment
> *Client needs category:* Physiological integrity
> *Client needs subcategory:* Reduction of risk potential
> *Taxonomic level:* Application

61. *Correct answer:* **D**

Migraine headaches are generally triggered by certain events including changes in hormone levels during menses, pregnancy, stress, menopause, oral contraceptive use, ingestion of tyramine-containing foods (nuts, aged cheeses, alcohol, bananas), hunger, fatigue, too little or too much sleep, bright lights, and a stuffy room. Dark rooms, high-fat diets, or exercise don't typically trigger migraines.

> *Nursing process step:* Planning
> *Client needs category:* Physiological integrity
> *Client needs subcategory:* Reduction of risk potential
> *Taxonomic level:* Knowledge

62. *Correct answer:* **D**

Sumatriptan succinate is contraindicated in patients with coronary artery disease because it may increase the risk of coronary artery vasospasm. Indomethacin, dihydroergotamine, prochlorperazine, and sumatriptan succinate may be used to treat migraines in these patients.

> *Nursing process step:* Planning
> *Client needs category:* Physiological integrity
> *Client needs subcategory:* Pharmacological and parenteral therapies
> *Taxonomic level:* Application

63. *Correct answer:* **D**

Propranolol is a nonselective beta-adrenergic blocking agent that decreases heart rate. The patient should be taught to check her pulse and report a slow heart rate. The last dose of the day may be taken at bedtime. Changing positions slowly may reduce symptoms of postural hypotension. Propranolol should be taken with food to increase absorption.

> *Nursing process step:* Evaluation
> *Client needs category:* Physiological integrity
> *Client needs subcategory:* Pharmacological and parenteral therapies
> *Taxonomic level:* Analysis

64. *Correct answer:* **A**

Amantadine produces relatively few adverse reactions at usual dosages. However, long-term therapy may produce livedo reticularis (diffuse, mottled reddening of the skin usually confined to the lower extremities), which commonly is accompanied by mild ankle edema. Other relatively common adverse reactions include urine retention, orthostatic hypotension, anorexia, nausea, and constipation. Adverse central nervous system reactions may include inability to concentrate, confusion, light-headedness, anxiety, insomnia, irritability, dizziness, and hallucinations.

> *Nursing process step:* Assessment
> *Client needs category:* Physiological integrity
> *Client needs subcategory:* Pharmacological and parenteral therapies
> *Taxonomic level:* Knowledge

65. *Correct answer:* **D**

A high-fiber diet may combat constipation, which is a common complication associated with Parkinson's disease. Thin hot liquids may be difficult to swallow. A high-protein diet and one high in L-tryptophan may alter levodopa absorption and metabolism.

> *Nursing process step:* Planning
> *Client needs category:* Physiological integrity
> *Client needs subcategory:* Basic care and comfort
> *Taxonomic level:* Knowledge

66. *Correct answer:* **A**

To encourage independence and maintain safety the nurse should keep the patient's bed in the lowest position with the lower side rails down. Patients with Alzheimer's disease are unfamiliar with their surroundings and may get out of bed to locate a bathroom. Leaving all of the side rails up will increase the risk of injury because the patient may attempt to climb over the rails to get out of bed.

The patient won't remember to use the nurse call light before getting out of bed. Leaving a light on won't help the patient remember she's in the hospital.

Nursing process step: Planning
Client needs category: Physiological integrity
Client needs subcategory: Basic care and comfort
Taxonomic level: Knowledge

67. *Correct answer:* D

Taking the patient for frequent walks may reduce her restlessness and decrease her risk of harm. Distracting the patient with loud music may cause further agitation. Using restraints or a geriatric chair increases agitation and increases the risk of fall-related injuries.

Nursing process step: Implementation
Client needs category: Physiological integrity
Client needs subcategory: Reduction of risk potential
Taxonomic level: Knowledge

68. *Correct answer:* B

Of the patients diagnosed with Guillain-Barré syndrome, 60% to 70% have experienced an upper respiratory or GI viral infection 1 to 4 weeks before the onset of symptoms. Guillain-Barré syndrome isn't hereditary or related to exposure during foreign travel. It doesn't affect the clotting cascade.

Nursing process step: Assessment
Client needs category: Physiological integrity
Client needs subcategory: Reduction of risk potential
Taxonomic level: Knowledge

69. *Correct answer:* D

Guillain-Barré syndrome results from segmental loss of myelin along the peripheral nerve axon. Ascending flaccid motor paralysis is the most common presenting sign. This syndrome doesn't affect level of consciousness or pupil reactivity or cause disorientation with inappropriate behavior.

Nursing process step: Assessment
Client needs category: Physiological integrity
Client needs subcategory: Reduction of risk potential
Taxonomic level: Knowledge

CHAPTER 4

GASTROINTESTINAL SYSTEM

QUESTIONS

1. When caring for a patient with esophageal varices, the nurse knows that bleeding in this disorder usually stems from:

    A. esophageal perforation
    B. pulmonary hypertension
    C. portal hypertension
    D. peptic ulcers

2. Jean Ross is diagnosed with type A hepatitis. What special precautions should the nurse take when caring for this patient?

    A. Put on a mask and gown before entering the patient's room.
    B. Wear gloves and a gown when removing the patient's bedpan.
    C. Prevent the droplet spread of the organism.
    D. Use caution when bringing food to the patient.

3. Discharge instructions for a patient who has been operated on for colorectal cancer include irrigating the colostomy. The nurse knows her teaching is effective when the patient states he'll contact the doctor if:

    A. he experiences abdominal cramping while the irrigant is infusing
    B. he has difficulty inserting the irrigation tube into the stoma
    C. he expels flatus while the return is running out
    D. he's unable to complete the procedure in 1 hour

4. The nurse explains to the patient who has had an abdominal perineal resection that an indwelling urinary catheter must be kept in place for several days afterward because:

    A. it prevents urinary tract infection following surgery
    B. it prevents urine retention and resulting pressure on the perineal wound
    C. it minimizes the risk of wound contamination by the urine
    D. it determines whether the surgery caused bladder trauma

5. The first day after surgery the nurse finds no measurable fecal drainage from a patient's colostomy stoma. What is the most appropriate nursing intervention?

    A. Call the doctor immediately.
    B. Obtain an order to irrigate the stoma.
    C. Place the patient on bed rest and call the doctor.
    D. Continue the current plan of care.

6. If a patient's GI tract is functioning but he's unable to take foods by mouth, the preferred method of feeding is:

A. total parenteral nutrition
B. peripheral parenteral nutrition
C. enteral nutrition
D. oral liquid supplements

SITUATION: *Mary Chikovsky, age 82, is transferred to the hospital from a long-term care facility because of severe diarrhea. She's weak and dehydrated.*

Questions 7 to 10 refer to this situation.

7. While reading Mrs. Chikovsky's transfer sheet from the long-term care facility, the nurse suspects that one of Mrs. Chikovsky's medications may be causing the severe diarrhea. Which of the following could cause diarrhea?

    A. antacids with aluminum
    B. antibiotics
    C. anticholinergics
    D. narcotic analgesics

8. Which acid-base imbalance could Mrs. Chikovsky develop as a result of diarrhea?

    A. respiratory acidosis
    B. metabolic acidosis
    C. carbonic acid deficit
    D. metabolic alkalosis

9. Which of the following nursing diagnoses would be most appropriate for Mrs. Chikovsky at this time?

    A. knowledge deficit
    B. activity intolerance
    C. impaired skin integrity
    D. risk for infection

10. A barium enema and upper GI X-ray series are prescribed for Mrs. Chikovsky. The nurse administers enemas until the return is clear to prepare the patient for these diagnostic tests. Following the tests, Mrs. Chikovsky complains of weakness. Which of the following nursing diagnoses should receive priority?

    A. sensory/perceptual alterations (gustatory)
    B. colonic constipation
    C. fluid volume deficit
    D. altered nutrition less than body requirements

SITUATION: *Glenn Shapiro, age 45, is the president of a major corporation. He comes to the hospital complaining of abdominal pain. He's admitted with a suspected peptic ulcer.*

Questions 11 to 14 refer to this situation.

11. The nurse is completing Mr. Shapiro's initial assessment. Which physical examination technique would be used first when assessing the abdomen?

    A. percussion
    B. auscultation
    C. light palpation
    D. deep palpation

12. If Mr. Shapiro is diagnosed with a gastric ulcer, the nurse would expect his pain to occur:

    A. below the umbilicus
    B. at the umbilicus
    C. in the epigastric area
    D. after a high-fat meal

13. Mr. Shapiro is returned to his room after a fiber-optic esophagogastroduodenoscopy (EGD). He immediately requests some coffee. The most appropriate action by the nurse would be to:

    A. assess the patient's vital signs for orthostatic hypotension
    B. tell the patient he must wait for 1 hour, to allow his stomach to settle
    C. assess the patient's gag reflex
    D. tell the patient that the coffee will taste bitter from the local anesthesia he received

14. Mr. Shapiro's doctor prescribes sucralfate (Carafate). The nurse knows that sucralfate is given to:

    A. prevent additional bleeding
    B. inhibit the action of histamine
    C. inhibit the activity of the acid pump and block the formation of gastric acid
    D. protect the ulcer's surface by forming a barrier

SITUATION: *Dennis Bedard, a 45-year-old editor, has a bleeding gastric ulcer. Despite multiple blood transfusions, his hemoglobin is 7.6 g/dl and hematocrit is 28%. His doctor determines that surgical intervention is necessary.*

Questions 15 to 18 refer to this situation.

15. Mr. Bedard goes to the operating room for a partial gastrectomy. Postoperative nursing care would include:

    A. administering pain medications every 6 hours
    B. withholding fluids by mouth until the return of peristalsis
    C. positioning the patient in high Fowler's position
    D. flushing the nasogastric tube with sterile water

16. Mr. Bedard's doctor performed a partial gastrectomy with a vagotomy. What was the purpose of performing the vagotomy?

    A. to increase gastric emptying
    B. to regenerate the gastric mucosa
    C. to stop stress-related reactions
    D. to reduce acid production

17. Postoperatively, Mr. Bedard should be assessed for dumping syndrome, a complication of partial gastrectomy. Which of the following are early signs and symptoms of dumping syndrome?

    A. diaphoresis and tachycardia
    B. headache and constipation
    C. hunger and decreased bowel sounds
    D. hypoglycemia and blurred vision

18. How should the nurse instruct Mr. Bedard to decrease the effects of dumping syndrome?

    A. Tell the patient to drink plenty of water with each meal.
    B. Instruct the patient to eat three scheduled meals each day.
    C. Tell the patient to sit in a semirecumbent position during and immediately following meals.
    D. Teach the patient the importance of consuming a diet high in carbohydrates and low in protein.

SITUATION: *Henry Logan, age 47, is admitted with abdominal pain that increases with movement. He has a low-grade fever and his abdomen is rigid when palpated. The doctor suspects peritonitis.*

Questions 19 to 21 refer to this situation.

19. Mr. Logan has a nasogastric tube in place. He complains of thirst but can have nothing by mouth. The nurse should:

    A. increase his I.V. infusion rate
    B. use diversional activities to take his mind off his thirst
    C. provide frequent mouth care
    D. give him ice chips every 15 minutes

20. Which of the following laboratory test results would be present with peritonitis?

    A. serum potassium 4.2 mEq/L
    B. hematocrit 45%
    C. serum calcium 4.2 mEq/L
    D. white blood cell count 20,000/μl

21. Mr. Logan is at risk of developing which of the following complications associated with peritonitis?

    A. hypertension
    B. fluid overload
    C. septic shock
    D. diarrhea

SITUATION: *Jerry Spiegel is an 18-year-old patient admitted to the medical-surgical floor with acute onset of abdominal pain in the right lower quadrant.*

Questions 22 to 25 refer to this situation.

22. The doctor suspects that Mr. Spiegel has appendicitis. Which of the following is a classic sign of appendicitis that leads to his suspicion?

    A. urinary retention
    B. pain relieved by walking
    C. rebound abdominal tenderness
    D. increased lower bowel activity on auscultation

23. Mr. Spiegel requests a heating pad for his abdominal pain. Which would be the nurse's best verbal response?

    A. "I'll have to check with the doctor before giving you a heating pad."
    B. "Do you think you really need a heating pad, or can you wait?"
    C. "Were you applying heat to the area at home before coming here?"
    D. "Heat stimulates bowel activity, which can cause your appendix to rupture."

24. The most appropriate nursing diagnosis for Mr. Spiegel before surgery would be:

    A. constipation related to the inflammatory process
    B. knowledge deficit related to the disease process and anticipated surgery
    C. noncompliance with treatment regimen
    D. ineffective breathing pattern related to right lower quadrant pain

25. Mr. Spiegel has an appendectomy. Because the appendix had perforated, he had localized peritonitis. Postoperatively the nurse should position him in:

    A. high Fowler's position
    B. semi-Fowler's position
    C. Trendelenburg's position
    D. prone position

SITUATION: *Harriet Brown, age 82, was admitted to the medical-surgical floor from a long-term care facility with a possible bowel obstruction. Her blood pressure is 100/50 mm Hg, pulse 115 beats/minute, and respirations 22 breaths/minute.*

Questions 26 to 28 refer to this situation.

26. While at the long-term care facility, Mrs. Brown exhibited early signs of intestinal obstruction. Which of the following indicate this disorder?

    A. bowel sounds that are high-pitched, frequent, and rushing
    B. abdominal distention and rarely audible bowel sounds
    C. dull, aching pain throughout the entire abdomen
    D. sharp, epigastric pain that radiates to the back

27. A bowel obstruction can result from a mechanical or nonmechanical cause. Which of the following is a nonmechanical cause?

    A. hernia
    B. tumor
    C. adhesions
    D. paralytic ileus

28. Mrs. Brown has a bowel obstruction. Which of the following nursing interventions would be the most important when caring for her?

    A. weighing the patient daily
    B. measuring the patient's abdominal girth every shift
    C. administering narcotic analgesics as ordered
    D. forcing fluids

SITUATION: *Edward Hall, age 42, is admitted to the medical-surgical floor with a diagnosis of acute pancreatitis. His blood pressure is 136/76 mm Hg, pulse 96 beats/minute, respirations 21 breaths/minute, and temperature 101° F (38.3° C). His past medical history reveals hyperlipidemia and alcohol abuse.*

Questions 29 to 32 refer to this situation.

29. The doctor prescribes a nasogastric tube for Mr. Hall. Before inserting the tube, the nurse explains its purpose to the patient. Which of the following is the most accurate explanation?

A. "It empties the stomach of fluids and gas."
B. "It prevents spasms of the sphincter of Oddi."
C. "It prevents air from forming in the small and large intestines."
D. "It removes bile from the gall bladder."

30. Which of the following is the most accurate method of checking proper nasogastric tube placement?

A. assessing the patient's respirations and skin color
B. inserting the end of the tube in water and checking for bubbling
C. aspirating gastric contents with a syringe and checking the pH
D. injecting air into the tube with a syringe and listening for a rush of air

31. After the nasogastric tube is inserted, Mr. Hall vomits 200 ml. The nurse should immediately:

A. change the suction applied to the nasogastric tube from intermittent to continuous
B. advance the nasogastric tube 2″ (5 cm)
C. replace the nasogastric tube with a large one
D. irrigate the nasogastric tube with saline solution

32. Which of the following drugs can be used to treat Mr. Hall's severe abdominal pain?

A. meperidine (Demerol)
B. codeine
C. morphine
D. hydromorphone (Dilaudid)

SITUATION: *Paul Crumm, age 62, has a past medical history of diverticulosis. He has been complaining of left lower abdominal pain since eating sunflower seeds at a baseball game. He's admitted to the medical-surgical floor with a diagnosis of diverticulitis.*

Questions 33 to 37 refer to this situation.

33. The nurse understands that Mr. Crumm's diverticulitis occurred because:

A. fecal material or bacteria became trapped in the outpouchings of the mucosa
B. the outpouching in the mucosal lining perforated
C. the appendix ruptured and released bacteria and toxins into the peritoneum
D. a peritoneal lavage was preformed and the mucosal lining was irritated

34. The nurse would expect Mr. Crumm to exhibit which of the following signs and symptoms associated with diverticulitis?

    A. left lower abdominal pain and excessive rectal bleeding
    B. epigastric pain that radiates to the back, hypotension, and tachycardia
    C. nausea, vomiting, right lower quadrant rebound tenderness, and fever
    D. crampy, left lower quadrant pain and low-grade fever

35. The doctor has ordered a barium enema for Mr. Crumm. The nurse should include which of the following points when teaching the patient about this diagnostic test?

    A. "You may take nothing by mouth for 2 hours before the procedure."
    B. "You must take a stool softener the morning of the procedure."
    C. "You'll be in knee-chest position throughout the procedure."
    D. "You'll be given a bowel prep the night before the procedure"

36. The doctor orders psyllium (Metamucil) for Mr. Crumm. The nurse explains that psyllium is an example of which type of laxative?

    A. bulk-forming laxative
    B. lubricant laxative
    C. stool softener
    D. stimulant

37. The nurse teaches Mr. Crumm diet modification to avoid future episodes of diverticulitis. Which of the following statements confirms that teaching was effective?

    A. "I should eat at least one serving of meat every day."
    B. "I should avoid eating popcorn and nuts."
    C. "I can eat all the celery and fresh tomatoes I like."
    D. "I can still eat hot dogs and sausage as often as I like."

SITUATION: *Doris Dubin, age 21, has a history of ulcerative colitis. Although her condition had been stable for the past year, she now presents to the hospital with an acute exacerbation of the disease.*

    Questions 38 to 43 refer to this situation.

38. There are many differences between ulcerative colitis and Crohn's disease. Which of the following statements is true?

A. Crohn's disease involves the mucosal area only.

B. Crohn's disease can occur anywhere in the GI tract.

C. Ulcerative colitis affects the right ileum.

D. Ulcerative colitis may lead to fistulas.

39. When planning dietary teaching for Ms. Dubin, the nurse should recommend that she consume:

A. high-protein foods, such as eggs, meat, and cheese

B. whole milk and other dairy products

C. raw fruits and vegetables

D. products containing caffeine

40. Which of these nursing diagnoses should be given priority when caring for Ms. Dubin?

A. fluid volume deficit

B. activity intolerance

C. risk for impaired skin integrity

D. altered (GI) tissue perfusion

41. Because conservative treatment is no longer effective, Ms. Dubin is scheduled for a total colectomy with ileostomy. Which information is important for the nurse to include in her teaching plan?

A. The nurse should explain that the procedure isn't permanent.

B. The nurse should tell the patient that continence can be controlled.

C. The nurse should instruct the patient that she'll need to wear an appliance at all times.

D. The nurse should tell the patient that she'll have normal bowel movements.

42. Before surgery, enemas must be administered until the return is clear. Ms. Dubin complains of abdominal cramping during enema administration. The nurse should respond by:

A. giving the enema at a slower rate

B. continuing to administer the enema because the cramps will cease

C. stopping the enema until the cramps cease

D. stopping the enema

43. Postoperatively, the nurse teaches Ms. Dubin ileostomy care. Which of the following comments by the patient would indicate that she needs further instruction?

A. "The skin around the stoma should be cleaned with warm water and thoroughly dried."
B. "The appliance should be changed several times each day to control odors."
C. "The appliance should fit snugly to prevent leakage."
D. "When I change the appliance I should check the skin for irritation."

SITUATION: *John Roberts, a 62-year-old chemist with a family history of colorectal cancer, has a positive guaiac test. He's scheduled for a series of additional diagnostic tests.*

Questions 44 to 47 refer to this situation.

44. Mr. Roberts is scheduled for a colonoscopy. Which statement by the patient indicates the need for further teaching?

A. "A flexible tube will be inserted into my rectum."
B. "I'll be conscious but sedated during the procedure."
C. "I'm afraid to have general anesthesia for the procedure."
D. "I'll need to take a laxative and have enemas before the test."

45. Mr. Roberts receives midazolam (Versed) and fentanyl (Sublimaze) for conscious sedation during the colonoscopy. After the drug is given, the next nursing priority would be:

A. assessing for respiratory depression
B. managing abdominal discomfort
C. assessing for decreased bowel function
D. assessing for return of motor function

46. Mr. Roberts is diagnosed with bowel cancer requiring surgical intervention. Which of the following nursing actions would be most appropriate when preparing Mr. Roberts for surgery?

A. Reassure the patient that the results of the surgery will probably be positive.
B. Provide activities that distract the patient from worrying about surgery.
C. Encourage the patient and his family to express fears and concerns about surgery.
D. Tell the patient not to worry about being apprehensive because all patients experience such feelings.

47. Mr. Roberts required a colostomy to treat his cancer. When developing a colostomy care teaching plan, the nurse should recognize that teaching success can be greatly influenced by which of the following factors?

A. his wife's acceptance of his altered self-image
B. his acceptance of the colostomy
C. his acceptance of the impotence caused by the surgery
D. his ability to return to work and support his family

SITUATION: *Ruth Anne Moyer, age 66, required a colostomy for a ruptured diverticulum. She tolerated the surgery well and returned to the medical-surgical floor in stable condition.*

Questions 48 to 51 refer to this situation.

48. The nurse assesses Mrs. Moyer's colostomy stoma 2 days after surgery. Which of the following assessment findings would the nurse report to doctor?

    A. reddish-pink stoma
    B. brownish-black stoma
    C. blanched stoma
    D. edematous stoma

49. The nurse is teaching Mrs. Moyer colostomy care. To review, the nurse asks her when she should empty the colostomy bag. Teaching is effective if Mrs. Moyer replies:

    A. "Every time I see stool in the bag I should empty it."
    B. "I should empty the bag at least three times a day."
    C. "I should empty the bag when it's about one-third full."
    D. "I'll let my husband empty it. He doesn't mind."

50. The nurse is teaching Mrs. Moyer how to apply the colostomy appliance. How much skin should remain exposed between the stoma and the ring of the appliance?

    A. ⅛″ (3.17 mm)
    B. ¼″ (6.35 mm)
    C. ½″ (12.7 mm)
    D. 1″ (25.4 mm)

51. When evaluating the effectiveness of Mrs. Moyer's dietary teaching, which statement by the patient would indicate further teaching is needed?

    A. "Eggs, fish, beans, and cabbage may worsen colostomy odor."
    B. "If I eat something that is irritating, I should never eat that food again."
    C. "If I get diarrhea, I might need to cut down on fruits, coffee, or cola drinks."
    D. "If I get constipated, I should drink prune or apple juice."

SITUATION: *Andrea James, age 58, is admitted to the medical-surgical floor with complaints of gastroesophageal reflux, regurgitation, dysphagia, and belching. The doctor suspects a hiatal hernia.*

Questions 52 to 56 refer to this situation.

52. Mrs. James is scheduled for an esophagogastroduodenoscopy (EGD) procedure. The nurse explains that EGD:

    A. examines gastric fluid that is aspirated with a flexible tube

    B. directly visualizes the esophagus with a flexible fiber-optic endoscope

    C. is an esophageal X-ray that is taken while the patient swallows a barium solution

    D. visualizes the esophagus after a radioactive isotope is injected intravenously

53. After Mrs. James has had the esophagogastroduodenoscopy procedure, the most important nursing action would be to:

    A. assess her vital signs frequently

    B. assess her neck for cervical crepitus

    C. place her in a side-lying position to prevent aspiration

    D. give her an anesthetic lozenge for her sore throat

54. Mrs. James has a sliding esophageal hernia. The doctor prescribes an H_2-receptor antagonist. The nurse explains that H_2-receptor antagonists work by:

    A. decreasing the pressure in the lower esophageal sphincter (LES)

    B. coating the mucus membrane of the esophagus and stomach

    C. inhibiting secretion of gastric acid by the parietal cells

    D. neutralizing gastric acid

55. The nurse prepares to administer an H_2-receptor antagonist to Mrs. James. Which of the following drugs is an H_2-receptor antagonist?

    A. sucralfate (Carafate)

    B. omeprazole (Prilosec)

    C. metoclopramide (Reglan)

    D. cimetidine (Tagamet)

56. Discharge teaching for Mrs. James should include:

    A. telling her to recline for 1 hour after eating

    B. instructing her to increase fluid intake with meals

    C. explaining that she should elevate the head of her bed with 6″ to 8″ (15- to 20-cm) blocks

    D. telling her to eat three regular meals every day

SITUATION: *Leonard Mack is a 49-year-old truck driver admitted to the medical-surgical floor with rectal bleeding and severe rectal pain.*

Questions 57 and 58 refer to this situation.

57. Mr. Mack is diagnosed with hemorrhoids for which he'll be treated medically. This treatment will most likely include which of the following?

    A. a daily laxative regimen
    B. a well-balanced diet with cooked vegetables and fruits
    C. encouraging the patient to drink one glass of water with each meal
    D. a high-fiber diet

58. Mr. Mack's medical treatment wasn't effective, requiring a hemorrhoidectomy. Which statement by Mr. Mack indicates that postoperative teaching was effective?

    A. "I'm glad my surgery was successful because now I don't have to change my lifestyle."
    B. "I need to establish a bowel movement routine."
    C. "I'll need to give myself an enema every day."
    D. "I'll need to take a laxative every other day."

SITUATION: *Roger Balboa, age 28, is admitted to the medical-surgical floor with inguinal pain and bulging that occurred while he was lifting weights at the gym. He's diagnosed with an inguinal hernia.*

Questions 59 and 60 refer to this situation.

59. The nurse explains to Mr. Balboa that an inguinal hernia:

    A. is a protrusion of abdominal contents following a surgical procedure
    B. is caused by a defect or weakness in the rectus abdominis muscle
    C. is caused by a weakness in the opening where the vas deferens emerges
    D. is seen rarely in young healthy men

60. Mr. Balboa has undergone surgical repair of his hernia. Discharge teaching should include:

    A. telling the patient to avoid heavy lifting for 4 to 6 weeks
    B. instructing the patient to eat soft foods for 2 weeks
    C. telling the patient he has no activity limitations
    D. recommending that he drink eight glasses of water daily

SITUATION: *Dorothy Pearson, age 77, is admitted to the medical-surgical floor with abdominal pain and fullness. She states she hasn't had a bowel movement in 1 week. Her diet consisted of bread, pasta and sauce, and an occasional glass of water.*

Questions 61 to 63 refer to this situation.

61. An enema is prescribed for Mrs. Pearson. When administering the enema, the nurse should keep the solution container elevated:

    A. 6″ (15 cm) above the rectum
    B. 18″ (46 cm) above the rectum
    C. 24″ (61 cm) above the rectum
    D. level with the bed

62. After receiving the enema, Mrs. Pearson was relieved of the fullness and abdominal pain. The nurse suggests that she do which of the following to avoid recurrent constipation?

    A. drink 8 to 10 glasses of water every day
    B. take a laxative before bedtime every night
    C. get as much rest as possible
    D. suppress the first urge to defecate

63. Mrs. Pearson asks if she can use laxatives occasionally. The nurse knows that the safest laxative for long-term use is which of the following?

    A. mineral oil
    B. stimulant laxatives
    C. osmotic laxatives
    D. bulk-forming laxatives

SITUATION: *Patti Hayes, age 22, is admitted to the medical-surgical floor with a diagnosis of adult celiac disease.*

Questions 64 and 65 refer to this situation.

64. The nurse understands that a patient with adult celiac disease has poor absorption of fats and carbohydrates and an intolerance of:

    A. cereal gluten
    B. milk products
    C. fresh fruits
    D. vegetables

65. When assessing the patient with celiac disease, the nurse can expect to find which of the following?

     A. steatorrhea
     B. jaundiced sclerae
     C. clay-colored stools
     D. widened pulse pressure

ANSWER SHEET

	A B C D		A B C D		A B C D
1	○ ○ ○ ○	23	○ ○ ○ ○	45	○ ○ ○ ○
2	○ ○ ○ ○	24	○ ○ ○ ○	46	○ ○ ○ ○
3	○ ○ ○ ○	25	○ ○ ○ ○	47	○ ○ ○ ○
4	○ ○ ○ ○	26	○ ○ ○ ○	48	○ ○ ○ ○
5	○ ○ ○ ○	27	○ ○ ○ ○	49	○ ○ ○ ○
6	○ ○ ○ ○	28	○ ○ ○ ○	50	○ ○ ○ ○
7	○ ○ ○ ○	29	○ ○ ○ ○	51	○ ○ ○ ○
8	○ ○ ○ ○	30	○ ○ ○ ○	52	○ ○ ○ ○
9	○ ○ ○ ○	31	○ ○ ○ ○	53	○ ○ ○ ○
10	○ ○ ○ ○	32	○ ○ ○ ○	54	○ ○ ○ ○
11	○ ○ ○ ○	33	○ ○ ○ ○	55	○ ○ ○ ○
12	○ ○ ○ ○	34	○ ○ ○ ○	56	○ ○ ○ ○
13	○ ○ ○ ○	35	○ ○ ○ ○	57	○ ○ ○ ○
14	○ ○ ○ ○	36	○ ○ ○ ○	58	○ ○ ○ ○
15	○ ○ ○ ○	37	○ ○ ○ ○	59	○ ○ ○ ○
16	○ ○ ○ ○	38	○ ○ ○ ○	60	○ ○ ○ ○
17	○ ○ ○ ○	39	○ ○ ○ ○	61	○ ○ ○ ○
18	○ ○ ○ ○	40	○ ○ ○ ○	62	○ ○ ○ ○
19	○ ○ ○ ○	41	○ ○ ○ ○	63	○ ○ ○ ○
20	○ ○ ○ ○	42	○ ○ ○ ○	64	○ ○ ○ ○
21	○ ○ ○ ○	43	○ ○ ○ ○	65	○ ○ ○ ○
22	○ ○ ○ ○	44	○ ○ ○ ○		

ANSWERS AND RATIONALES

1. *Correct answer:* **C**

Increased pressure within the portal veins causes them to bulge, leading to rupture and bleeding into the lower esophagus. Bleeding associated with esophageal varices doesn't stem from esophageal perforation, pulmonary hypertension, or peptic ulcers.

> *Nursing process step:* Assessment
> *Client needs category:* Physiological integrity
> *Client needs subcategory:* Physiological adaptation
> *Taxonomic level:* Knowledge

2. *Correct answer:* **B**

The nurse should wear gloves and a gown when removing the patient's bedpan because the type A hepatitis virus occurs in stools. It may also occur in blood, nasotracheal secretions, and urine. Type A hepatitis isn't transmitted through the air by way of droplets. Special precautions aren't needed when feeding the patient, but disposable utensils should be used.

> *Nursing process step:* Planning
> *Client needs category:* Safe, effective care environment
> *Client needs subcategory:* Safety and infection control
> *Taxonomic level:* Comprehension

3. *Correct answer:* **B**

The patient should notify the doctor if he has difficulty inserting the irrigation tube into the stoma. Difficulty with insertion may indicate stenosis of the bowel. Abdominal cramping and expulsion of flatus may normally occur with irrigation. The procedure will often take an hour to complete.

> *Nursing process step:* Evaluation
> *Client needs category:* Physiological integrity
> *Client needs subcategory:* Reduction of risk potential
> *Taxonomic level:* Analysis

4. *Correct answer:* **B**

An indwelling urinary catheter is kept in place several days after this surgery to prevent urine retention that could place pressure on the perineal wound. An indwelling urinary catheter may be a source of postoperative urinary tract infection. Urine won't contaminate the wound. An indwelling urinary catheter won't necessarily show bladder trauma.

Nursing process step: Implementation
Client needs category: Physiological integrity
Client needs subcategory: Reduction of risk potential
Taxonomic level: Application

5. *Correct answer:* **D**

The colostomy may not function for 2 days or more (48 to 72 hours) after surgery. Therefore, the normal plan of care can be followed. Since no fecal drainage is expected for 48 to 72 hours after a colostomy (only mucous and serosanguineous), the doctor doesn't have to be notified and the stoma shouldn't be irrigated at this time.

Nursing process step: Implementation
Client needs category: Physiological integrity
Client needs subcategory: Reduction of risk potential
Taxonomic level: Application

6. *Correct answer:* **C**

If the patient's GI tract is functioning, enteral nutrition via a feeding tube is the preferred method. Peripheral and total parenteral nutrition places the patient at risk for infection. If the patient is unable to consume foods by mouth, oral liquid supplements are contraindicated.

Nursing process step: Planning
Client needs category: Physiological integrity
Client needs subcategory: Basic care and comfort
Taxonomic level: Comprehension

7. *Correct answer:* **B**

When a patient receives antibiotics the normal flora in the GI tract may be destroyed, allowing overgrowth of *Clostridium difficile,* which causes diarrhea. Antacids with aluminum, anticholinergics, and narcotic analgesics may all cause constipation.

Nursing process step: Assessment
Client needs category: Physiological integrity
Client needs subcategory: Pharmacological and parenteral therapies
Taxonomic level: Knowledge

8. *Correct answer:* **B**

Diarrhea causes the body to lose bicarbonate, which may cause metabolic acidosis. Respiratory acidosis is caused by alveolar hypoventilation. Carbonic acid excess occurs with respiratory alkalosis. Vomiting could lead to metabolic alkalosis.

Nursing process step: Assessment
Client needs category: Physiological integrity
Client needs subcategory: Reduction of risk potential
Taxonomic level: Analysis

9. *Correct answer:* **C**

Impaired skin integrity is the most appropriate nursing diagnosis for this patient because diarrhea is very irritating to the perianal skin. The other nursing diagnoses aren't appropriate at this time.

Nursing process step: Analysis
Client needs category: Physiological integrity
Client needs subcategory: Basic care and comfort
Taxonomic level: Application

10. *Correct answer:* **C**

The diagnostic test preparation can cause a deficit in the patient's fluid volume, causing her to feel weak. The patient doesn't have difficulty tasting food, so sensory/perceptual alterations (gustatory) would be inappropriate. The patient has diarrhea, not constipation. There is no indication of an altered nutritional status.

Nursing process step: Analysis
Client needs category: Physiological integrity
Client needs subcategory: Physiological adaptation
Taxonomic level: Analysis

11. *Correct answer:* **B**

Because percussion and palpation may alter bowel sounds, auscultation should be performed first to accurately evaluate preexisting bowel sounds.

Nursing process step: Assessment
Client needs category: Physiological integrity
Client needs subcategory: Reduction of risk potential
Taxonomic level: Comprehension

12. *Correct answer:* **C**

Pain in the epigastric area is associated with gastric ulcer disease. Pain below or at the umbilicus is associated with appendicitis. Abdominal pain that occurs after a high-fat meal is associated with cholecystitis.

Nursing process step: Assessment
Client needs category: Physiological integrity
Client needs subcategory: Basic care and comfort
Taxonomic level: Knowledge

13. *Correct answer:* **C**

The local anesthesia used during the procedure suppresses the gag reflex. The nurse must assess the patient to see that the gag reflex has returned before allowing the patient to have anything by mouth, such as coffee. It may take more than an hour for the gag reflex to return. EGD shouldn't cause orthostatic hypotension. Anesthesia may or may not affect the patient's ability to taste the coffee.

> *Nursing process step:* Assessment
> *Client needs category:* Physiological integrity
> *Client needs subcategory:* Reduction of risk potential
> *Taxonomic level:* Application

14. *Correct answer:* **D**

Sucralfate protects the ulcer's surface by forming a barrier so healing can take place. Bleeding isn't routinely present with peptic ulcer disease. Hista-mine blockers, such as cimetidine (Tagamet), famotidine (Pepcid), ranitidine (Zantac), and nizatidine (Axid), inhibit the action of histamine at the receptor sites of parietal cells, decreasing gastric acid secretion. Proton pump inhibitors, such as lansoprazole (Prevacid) and omeprazole (Prilosec), inhibit the activity of the acid (proton) pump to block the formation of gastric acid.

> *Nursing process step:* Implementation
> *Client needs category:* Physiological integrity
> *Client needs subcategory:* Pharmacological and parenteral therapies
> *Taxonomic level:* Knowledge

15. *Correct answer:* **B**

Postoperatively, the patient should have nothing by mouth until peristaltic activity returns, to decrease the risk of abdominal distention and obstruction. The patient will probably require pain medication more often then every 6 hours. The patient should be positioned for comfort (not necessarily high Fowler's position). The nasogastric tube isn't flushed, to avoid disturbing the suture line.

> *Nursing process step:* Planning
> *Client needs category:* Physiological integrity
> *Client needs subcategory:* Reduction of risk potential
> *Taxonomic level:* Application

16. *Correct answer:* **D**

A vagotomy reduces the production of stomach acids by decreasing cholinergic stimulation of parietal cells. The vagotomy also creates gastric stasis and reduces gastric emptying. Vagotomy won't regenerate gastric mucosa or stop stress-related reactions.

Nursing process step: Evaluation
Client needs category: Physiological integrity
Client needs subcategory: Reduction of risk potential
Taxonomic level: Comprehension

17. *Correct answer:* **A**

Signs and symptoms associated with dumping syndrome occur 5 to 30 minutes after eating and include diaphoresis, tachycardia, syncope, pallor, vertigo, diarrhea, nausea, abdominal cramping, and abdominal distention. Symptoms usually subside in 6 to 12 months. In dumping syndrome, large amounts of chyme rapidly enter the small intestine, causing fluid to move into the bowel lumen. This reduces plasma volume, causing the associated vasomotor symptoms of diaphoresis and tachycardia.

Nursing process step: Assessment
Client needs category: Physiological integrity
Client needs subcategory: Reduction of risk potential
Taxonomic level: Knowledge

18. *Correct answer:* **C**

The nurse should instruct the patient to sit in a semirecumbent position during and immediately following meals. This position helps delay stomach emptying. Drinking water with the meals increases abdominal distention. Six small meals high in protein and low in carbohydrates prevent large amount of food "dumping" into the duodenum.

Nursing process step: Planning
Client needs category: Physiological integrity
Client needs subcategory: Basic care and comfort
Taxonomic level: Application

19. *Correct answer:* **C**

Patients with nasogastric tubes frequently breathe through their mouth, causing dryness and a thirst sensation. Providing frequent mouth care can help combat this problem. The I.V. infusion rate shouldn't be changed without a doctor's order. The patient who is unable to have anything by mouth shouldn't have ice chips.

Nursing process step: Implementation
Client needs category: Physiological integrity
Client needs subcategory: Reduction of risk potential
Taxonomic level: Knowledge

20. *Correct answer:* **D**

The patient with peritonitis will typically have an elevated white blood cell count with a high neutrophil count. Hematocrit levels may be elevated from hemoconcentration. If vomiting is present, the patient may also have a low potassium level. Hypocalcemia may occur from syndromes that cause fat malabsorption.

> *Nursing process step:* Assessment
> *Client needs category:* Physiological integrity
> *Client needs subcategory:* Physiological adaptation
> *Taxonomic level:* Comprehension

21. *Correct answer:* **C**

The patient with peritonitis is at risk for developing septicemia, which, untreated, can lead to septic shock and death. The patient with septic shock is hypotensive, not hypertensive. The patient develops a fluid deficit from the fluid shift that occurs, which depletes circulating blood volume. Peritonitis inhibits peristalsis but doesn't cause diarrhea.

> *Nursing process step:* Assessment
> *Client needs category:* Physiological integrity
> *Client needs subcategory:* Reduction of risk potential
> *Taxonomic level:* Comprehension

22. *Correct answer:* **C**

Rebound tenderness in the right lower quadrant of the abdomen is a classic sign of appendicitis. Urinary retention may be present but isn't caused by appendicitis. Pain increases when the patient with appendicitis ambulates. Inflammation associated with appendicitis causes bowel activity to decrease.

> *Nursing process step:* Assessment
> *Client needs category:* Physiological integrity
> *Client needs subcategory:* Basic care and comfort
> *Taxonomic level:* Knowledge

23. *Correct answer:* **D**

Applying heat increases circulation to the abdominal area, which may cause the appendix to rupture.

> *Nursing process step:* Implementation
> *Client needs category:* Physiological integrity
> *Client needs subcategory:* Reduction of risk potential
> *Taxonomic level:* Application

24. *Correct answer:* **B**

The preoperative patient will have a knowledge deficit related to the disease process and anticipated surgery. Teaching the patient about both will relieve some of his anxiety. Since the patient sought treatment for his abdominal pain, he hasn't exhibited noncompliance. Lower quadrant abdominal pain doesn't affect the patient's breathing pattern.

Nursing process step: Analysis
Client needs category: Psychosocial integrity
Client needs subcategory: Coping and adaptation
Taxonomic level: Analysis

25. *Correct answer:* **B**

Placing the patient in semi-Fowler's position facilitates wound drainage and decreases the risk of subdiaphragmatic abscess. High Fowler's position may be too uncomfortable for the patient. The other positions won't facilitate drainage of the abdominal wound.

Nursing process step: Implementation
Client needs category: Physiological integrity
Client needs subcategory: Reduction of risk potential
Taxonomic level: Application

26. *Correct answer:* **A**

As the intestine attempts to propel its contents past the obstruction, peristaltic activity increases, producing bowel sounds that are high-pitched, frequent, and rushing. Abdominal distention and bowel sounds that occur rarely are manifestations of the late stages of intestinal obstruction. The pain associated with intestinal obstruction is crampy and spasmodic in nature. Sharp, epigastric pain that radiates to the back is characteristic of gallbladder pain or pancreatitis.

Nursing process step: Assessment
Client needs category: Physiological integrity
Client needs subcategory: Reduction of risk potential
Taxonomic level: Knowledge

27. *Correct answer:* **D**

Paralytic ileus, marked by loss of peristaltic activity, results from nonmechanical causes such as severe physiologic stress due to burns, peritonitis, or abdominal surgery. Hernia, tumor, and adhesions are examples of mechanical causes of intestinal obstruction.

Nursing process step: Assessment
Client needs category: Physiological integrity
Client needs subcategory: Physiological adaptation
Taxonomic level: Knowledge

28. *Correct answer:* **B**

Measuring and recording the patient's abdominal girth every shift assesses for increased abdominal distention associated with bowel obstruction. Weighing the patient daily doesn't help detect associated abdominal distention. Narcotic analgesics should be avoided because they decrease peristalsis, worsening the obstruction. Forcing fluids isn't appropriate for this patient because she'll be allowed nothing by mouth.

> *Nursing process step:* Implementation
> *Client needs category:* Physiological integrity
> *Client needs subcategory:* Reduction of risk potential
> *Taxonomic level:* Application

29. *Correct answer:* **A**

A nasogastric tube is inserted into the stomach to drain fluids and gas. A T tube collects bile drainage from the common bile duct. A nasogastric tube doesn't prevent spasms of the sphincter of Oddi or prevent air from forming in the small and large intestine.

> *Nursing process step:* Implementation
> *Client needs category:* Physiological integrity
> *Client needs subcategory:* Reduction of risk potential
> *Taxonomic level:* Comprehension

30. *Correct answer:* **C**

The most accurate method of checking proper nasogastric tube placement is aspirating gastric contents and checking the pH. If the pH is less than 3, the tube is in the stomach. Assessing the patient's respirations and skin color and inserting the end of the tube in water and checking for bubbling aren't accurate methods of confirming tube placement. The nurse can check nasogastric tube placement by injecting air into the tube with a syringe and listening for a rush of air, but this isn't the most accurate method.

> *Nursing process step:* Implementation
> *Client needs category:* Physiological integrity
> *Client needs subcategory:* Reduction of risk potential
> *Taxonomic level:* Knowledge

31. *Correct answer:* **D**

Vomiting after nasogastric tube insertion indicates that the tube isn't patent. The nurse should immediately irrigate the tube with saline solution to restore patency. If the tube is patent and the patient continues to vomit, the tube may need to be changed or repositioned or the suction may need to be increased.

Nursing process step: Implementation
Client needs category: Physiological integrity
Client needs subcategory: Reduction of risk potential
Taxonomic level: Application

32. *Correct answer:* A

Meperidine, a nonopioid analgesic, is the drug of choice for pain control in pancreatitis. Opioids can cause spasms of the sphincter of Oddi and exacerbate pain. The spasms block the normal flow of pancreatic enzymes and raise the levels of enzymes in the pancreas. Increased enzyme levels worsen autodigestion in the pancreas and increase pain.

Nursing process step: Implementation
Client needs category: Physiological integrity
Client needs subcategory: Pharmacological and parenteral therapies
Taxonomic level: Knowledge

33. *Correct answer:* A

Diverticulitis occurs when retained undigested food mixed with bacteria accumulates in the diverticulum (outpouching in the intestine), forming a hard mass of fecal matter. The mass cuts off blood supply to the diverticulum's thin walls, increasing its susceptibility to attack by colonic bacteria. Inflammation follows bacterial infection. If the diverticulum perforates, peritonitis develops. Peritonitis also develops as a result of appendix rupture. A peritoneal lavage could place the patient at risk for peritonitis, but it doesn't cause diverticulitis.

Nursing process step: Assessment
Client needs category: Physiological integrity
Client needs subcategory: Reduction of risk potential
Taxonomic level: Knowledge

34. *Correct answer:* D

Crampy, left lower quadrant pain and a low-grade fever are common symptoms of diverticulitis. The patient with diverticulitis may have some rectal bleeding with bouts of constipation, but bleeding isn't excessive. Epigastric pain that radiates to the back, hypotension, and tachycardia are associated with pancreatitis. Nausea, vomiting, right lower quadrant pain, and fever are associated with appendicitis.

Nursing process step: Assessment
Client needs category: Physiological integrity
Client needs subcategory: Reduction of risk potential
Taxonomic level: Knowledge

35. *Correct answer:* **D**

The patient will receive a bowel prep the night before the procedure to free the bowel of fecal material so it can be visualized on X-ray. The patient must also take nothing by mouth for 8 to 12 hours before the procedure. The patient will be asked to change positions during the procedure to facilitate passage of the barium.

> *Nursing process step:* Planning
> *Client needs category:* Physiological integrity
> *Client needs subcategory:* Reduction of risk potential
> *Taxonomic level:* Knowledge

36. *Correct answer:* **A**

Psyllium is a bulk-forming laxative that absorbs water and expands to increase bulk and moisture content of stool, thus encouraging peristalsis and bowel movement. Mineral oil (Fleet mineral oil) is an example of a lubricant laxative. It works by increasing water retention in the stool by creating a barrier between the colon wall and feces that prevents colonic reabsorption of fecal water. Docusate sodium (Colace) is an example of a stool softener. It works by reducing surface tension of interfacing liquid contents of the bowel. This detergent activity promotes incorporation of additional liquid into the stool, thus forming a softer mass. Castor oil (Emulsoil) is a stimulant laxative that increases peristalsis probably by direct affect on the smooth muscle of the intestine.

> *Nursing process step:* Implementation
> *Client needs category:* Physiological integrity
> *Client needs subcategory:* Pharmacological and parenteral therapies
> *Taxonomic level:* Knowledge

37. *Correct answer:* **B**

The patient with diverticular disease should be encouraged to eat foods high in fiber to add bulk to the stool and speed its passage through the bowel. These foods include fresh fruits with skin, such as apples, pears, grapes, and plums. The patient should be taught to avoid foods high in roughage, such as popcorn, raw celery, and nuts, which can accumulate in the diverticular sacs and mix with bacteria, causing inflammation. Eating hot dogs and sausage doesn't worsen diverticular disease, but they are high in saturated fats and should be consumed with moderation.

> *Nursing process step:* Evaluation
> *Client needs category:* Physiological integrity
> *Client needs subcategory:* Reduction of risk potential
> *Taxonomic level:* Application

38. *Correct answer:* **B**

Crohn's disease can occur anywhere in the GI tract, but it usually occurs in the distal ileum. Crohn's disease affects the full thickness of the bowel wall. Ulcerative colitis affects the rectum and colon, ending at the ileocecal junction. Fistulas are a complication of Crohn's disease.

> *Nursing process step:* Assessment
> *Client needs category:* Physiological integrity
> *Client needs subcategory:* Reduction of risk potential
> *Taxonomic level:* Comprehension

39. *Correct answer:* **A**

Patients with ulcerative colitis should be encouraged to consume foods high in protein and calories to promote healing. Fat intake should be limited, especially if steatorrhea is present. Patients should also be encouraged to avoid raw fruits and vegetables, dried fruit and beans, whole grains, bran, seeds, and nuts to reduce bowel movements. Caffeinated and carbonated beverages should be avoided because they stimulate intestinal peristalsis.

> *Nursing process step:* Planning
> *Client needs category:* Physiological integrity
> *Client needs subcategory:* Basic care and comfort
> *Taxonomic level:* Comprehension

40. *Correct answer:* **A**

Fluid volume deficit would be the priority nursing diagnosis for the patient with ulcerative colitis because excessive fluids are lost due to frequent diarrhea. The diarrhea may cause *impaired skin integrity* and *activity intolerance,* but the priority is managing fluid volume.

> *Nursing process step:* Analysis
> *Client needs category:* Physiological integrity
> *Client needs subcategory:* Reduction of risk potential
> *Taxonomic level:* Analysis

41. *Correct answer:* **C**

The nurse should instruct the patient that she'll need to wear an ostomy appliance at all times, because liquid will drain continuously from the ileostomy. A total colectomy with ileostomy is a permanent procedure; once performed it can't be reversed. The patient won't have normal bowel movements, and continence can't be controlled.

> *Nursing process step:* Planning
> *Client needs category:* Psychosocial integrity
> *Client needs subcategory:* Coping and adaptation
> *Taxonomic level:* Knowledge

42. *Correct answer:* **A**

Giving the enema slowly will reduce the cramps and allow the patient to tolerate and retain greater volume. Continuing at the same rate will cause more cramping. It shouldn't be necessary to stop the procedure.

> *Nursing process step:* Implementation
> *Client needs category:* Physiological integrity
> *Client needs subcategory:* Reduction of risk potential
> *Taxonomic level:* Knowledge

43. *Correct answer:* **B**

Changing the appliance several times a day can cause impaired skin integrity. The patient should clean the skin around the stoma with warm water, dry it thoroughly, and check for irritation. She should make sure that the appliance fits snugly to prevent leakage.

> *Nursing process step:* Evaluation
> *Client needs category:* Physiological integrity
> *Client needs subcategory:* Basic care and comfort
> *Taxonomic level:* Analysis

44. *Correct answer:* **C**

A colonoscopy is the visual examination of the lining of the large intestine with a flexible fiber-optic endoscope. The patient is given sedation during the procedure but isn't anesthetized. The large intestine must be thoroughly cleansed to be clearly visible. The patient is given a laxative the evening before the procedure; if fecal results still aren't clear, a suppository or tap water enema may be given.

> *Nursing process step:* Evaluation
> *Client needs category:* Physiological integrity
> *Client needs subcategory:* Reduction of risk potential
> *Taxonomic level:* Analysis

45. *Correct answer:* **A**

The greatest concern when monitoring the patient who has received conscious sedation is the risk of respiratory depression. Conscious sedation should also relieve any associated abdominal discomfort. There is no reduction in peristalsis or motor function.

> *Nursing process step:* Assessment
> *Client needs category:* Physiological integrity
> *Client needs subcategory:* Reduction of risk potential
> *Taxonomic level:* Application

46. *Correct answer:* **C**

The nurse should encourage the patient and his family to verbalize their feelings and concerns. Telling the patient that the outcome will be positive gives him false reassuran e because there are no guarantees that the results will be positive. Providing distraction doesn't give the patient the opportunity to deal with his feelings. Telling the patient not to worry minimizes his concerns.

> *Nursing process step:* Implementation
> *Client needs category:* Psychosocial integrity
> *Client needs subcategory:* Coping and adaptation
> *Taxonomic level:* Application

47. *Correct answer:* **B**

Teaching can be futile if the patient hasn't accepted the colostomy. Nonacceptance from his wife, impotence, and the inability to continue working can interfere with the teaching process but not as much as his own nonacceptance of the procedure.

> *Nursing process step:* Assessment
> *Client needs category:* Psychosocial integrity
> *Client needs subcategory:* Coping and adaptation
> *Taxonomic level:* Application

48. *Correct answer:* **B**

A stoma that appears brownish-black in color indicates that there is a lack of blood supply to the stoma and necrosis is likely. Two days postoperatively, the stoma will be edematous and reddish-pink. A blanched or pale stoma indicates possible decreased blood flow, and it should be assessed regularly.

> *Nursing process step:* Assessment
> *Client needs category:* Physiological integrity
> *Client needs subcategory:* Reduction of risk potential
> *Taxonomic level:* Application

49. *Correct answer:* **C**

The patient should empty the colostomy bag whenever it's about one-third full. If the bag is allowed to get too full, it may cause the appliance to separate from the skin and cause leakage. The bag may need to be emptied more than three times a day. The patient should be encouraged to manage her colostomy herself if she's physically able.

> *Nursing process step:* Evaluation
> *Client needs category:* Physiological integrity
> *Client needs subcategory:* Basic care and comfort
> *Taxonomic level:* Analysis

50. *Correct answer:* **A**

Approximately ⅛″ of skin should be exposed to prevent skin breakdown. If the ring of the appliance is placed too closely to the stoma, it may compromise circulation to the stoma. If too much skin is exposed to the colostomy drainage, skin breakdown can occur.

> *Nursing process step:* Implementation
> *Client needs category:* Physiological integrity
> *Client needs subcategory:* Reduction of risk potential
> *Taxonomic level:* Knowledge

51. *Correct answer:* **B**

If a food is irritating, the patient shouldn't eliminate it totally from her diet but should try it again at a later time in a smaller quantity. The other options are all correct.

> *Nursing process step:* Evaluation
> *Client needs category:* Physiological integrity
> *Client needs subcategory:* Basic care and comfort
> *Taxonomic level:* Knowledge

52. *Correct answer:* **B**

An EGD uses a fiber-optic endoscope to directly visualize the esophagus. Gastric pH analysis is done by aspirating fluid from a flexible nasogastric tube. A barium swallow is an esophageal X-ray that is taken as the patient swallows a barium solution. A computed tomography scan of the esophagus visualizes the esophagus after a radioactive isotope is injected intravenously.

> *Nursing process step:* Implementation
> *Client needs category:* Physiological integrity
> *Client needs subcategory:* Reduction of risk potential
> *Taxonomic level:* Comprehension

53. *Correct answer:* **A**

The nurse should assess the patient's vital signs frequently; changes in vital signs signal possible esophageal perforation. Cervical crepitus is seen if air from the mediastinum moves into the soft tissues of the neck. Positioning the patient and administering lozenges don't take priority over assessing vital signs.

> *Nursing process step:* Implementation
> *Client needs category:* Physiological integrity
> *Client needs subcategory:* Reduction of risk potential
> *Taxonomic level:* Application

54. *Correct answer:* **C**

H_2-receptor antagonists inhibit the histamine action at the H_2-receptor sites in the gastric parietal cells. Anticholinergic drugs decrease LES pressure. Sucralfate (Carafate) is a mucosal protectant. Antacids neutralize gastric acid.

> *Nursing process step:* Implementation
> *Client needs category:* Physiological integrity
> *Client needs subcategory:* Pharmacological and parenteral therapies
> *Taxonomic level:* Knowledge

55. *Correct answer:* **D**

Cimetidine is an H_2-receptor antagonist; sucralfate is a mucosal protectant; omeprazole is a proton pump inhibitor; and metoclopramide stimulates upper GI tract motility.

> *Nursing process step:* Planning
> *Client needs category:* Physiological integrity
> *Client needs subcategory:* Pharmacological and parenteral therapies
> *Taxonomic level:* Knowledge

56. *Correct answer:* **C**

The nurse should instruct the patient to elevate the head of her bed on 6″ to 8″ blocks. The elevation will prevent the esophageal hernia from sliding upward and causing discomfort, regurgitation, and belching. Reclining after meals may cause the hernia to slide up and cause symptoms. Eating smaller meals and not increasing fluid intake at meals prevents the stomach from filling, which can add to the discomfort.

> *Nursing process step:* Planning
> *Client needs category:* Physiological integrity
> *Client needs subcategory:* Basic care and comfort
> *Taxonomic level:* Application

57. *Correct answer:* **D**

The patient should be encouraged to consume a high-fiber diet, which facilitates peristalsis and decreases the need to strain when defecating. Straining at stool worsens hemorrhoids. Daily laxatives can lead to laxative dependence. Fresh fruits and vegetables contain more fiber and should be chosen over cooked vegetables. The patient should drink 8 to 10 glasses of water each day.

> *Nursing process step:* Planning
> *Client needs category:* Physiological integrity
> *Client needs subcategory:* Basic care and comfort
> *Taxonomic level:* Comprehension

58. *Correct answer:* **B**

The patient should establish a daily bowel movement routine (such as going to the bathroom each morning after breakfast) to prevent constipation and reduce the risk of hemorrhoids. Surgery doesn't prevent possible recurrence, so lifestyle changes are necessary. With a proper diet, enemas and laxatives aren't necessary.

> *Nursing process step:* Evaluation
> *Client needs category:* Physiological integrity
> *Client needs subcategory:* Reduction of risk potential
> *Taxonomic level:* Analysis

59. *Correct answer:* **C**

An inguinal hernia is located in the groin area and is caused by a weakness in the opening in the abdominal wall where the vas deferens passed through the abdominal wall. A hernia that occurs at the site of a previous surgical procedure is a ventral hernia. A weakness or defect in the rectus abdominis is an umbilical hernia. Inguinal hernias occur three times more commonly in men than women.

> *Nursing process step:* Implementation
> *Client needs category:* Physiological integrity
> *Client needs subcategory:* Reduction of risk potential
> *Taxonomic level:* Comprehension

60. *Correct answer:* **A**

The patient should avoid heavy lifting for 4 to 6 weeks after surgery to prevent stress on the inguinal area. No special diet is necessary for this patient. Recommending eight glasses of water per day is good advice for most patients, but it isn't a priority for the patient with a hernia repair.

> *Nursing process step:* Planning
> *Client needs category:* Physiological integrity
> *Client needs subcategory:* Reduction of risk potential
> *Taxonomic level:* Application

61. *Correct answer:* **B**

The enema solution container should be no higher than 18″ above the rectum. Placing the container higher than 18″ will cause the solution to infuse at a fast rate and cause abdominal cramping. If the solution container is level with the bed, the solution won't infuse into the rectum. Placing the container 6″ above the rectum may not provide enough pressure for the fluid to enter the rectum.

> *Nursing process step:* Planning
> *Client needs category:* Physiological integrity
> *Client needs subcategory:* Reduction of risk potential
> *Taxonomic level:* Knowledge

62. *Correct answer:* **A**

The patient should be encouraged to drink 8 to 10 glasses of water every day to avoid constipation. Water helps maintain bowel motility and soften stools. The patient shouldn't be encouraged to take a laxative every night. Laxative overuse contributes to constipation. The patient should get plenty of exercise to increase bowel motility. Encouraging the patient to respond to the first urge to defecate promotes regular bowel habits.

Nursing process step: Planning
Client needs category: Physiological integrity
Client needs subcategory: Basic care and comfort
Taxonomic level: Comprehension

63. *Correct answer:* **D**

Bulk-forming laxatives provide bulk that draws water into the intestine and softens stool, making it safest for long-term use. Mineral oil can reduce fat-soluble vitamin absorption. Stimulant and osmotic laxatives may suppress the normal bowel reflexes if used for long periods.

Nursing process step: Planning
Client needs category: Physiological integrity
Client needs subcategory: Pharmacological and parenteral therapies
Taxonomic level: Comprehension

64. *Correct answer:* **A**

Celiac disease is a hereditary disorder in which the person is sensitive to gluten and therefore cannot tolerate foods that contain wheat, rye, barley, or oats. Milk products, fresh fruits, and vegetables can be eaten by a patient with celiac disease.

Nursing process step: Planning
Client needs category: Physiological integrity
Client needs subcategory: Basic care and comfort
Taxonomic level: Knowledge

65. *Correct answer:* **A**

Because celiac disease destroys the absorbing surface of the intestine, fat isn't absorbed but is passed in the stool. Steatorrhea is bulky, fatty stools that have a foul odor. Jaundiced sclerae result from elevated bilirubin levels. Clay-colored stools are seen with biliary disease when bile flow is blocked. Celiac disease doesn't cause a widened pulse pressure.

Nursing process step: Assessment
Client needs category: Physiological integrity
Client needs subcategory: Physiological adaptation
Taxonomic level: Application

CHAPTER 5

RENAL
SYSTEM

QUESTIONS

1. Which type of solution causes water to shift from the cells into the plasma?

    A. hypertonic
    B. hypotonic
    C. isotonic
    D. alkaline

2. Particles move from an area of greater osmolarity to one of lesser osmolarity through:

    A. active transport
    B. osmosis
    C. diffusion
    D. filtration

3. Which assessment finding indicates dehydration?

    A. tenting of chest skin when pinched
    B. rapid filling of hand veins
    C. a pulse that isn't easily obliterated
    D. neck vein distention

4. Which nursing intervention would most likely lead to a hypo-osmolar state?

    A. performing nasogastric tube irrigation with normal saline solution
    B. weighing the patient daily
    C. administering tap water enema until the return is clear
    D. encouraging the patient with excessive perspiration to drink broth

5. Which assessment finding would indicate an extracellular fluid volume deficit?

    A. bradycardia
    B. a central venous pressure of 6 mm Hg
    C. pitting edema
    D. an orthostatic blood pressure change

6. A patient with metabolic acidosis has a preexisting problem with the kidneys. Which other organ helps regulate blood pH?

    A. liver
    B. pancreas
    C. lungs
    D. heart

7. The nurse considers the patient anuric if the patient:

    A. voids during the nighttime hours
    B. has a urine output of less than 100 ml in 24 hours
    C. has a urine output of at least 100 ml in 2 hours
    D. has pain and burning on urination

8. Which nursing action is appropriate to prevent infection when obtaining a sterile urine specimen from an indwelling urinary catheter?

    A. aspirate urine from the tubing port using a sterile syringe and needle
    B. disconnect the catheter from the tubing and obtain urine
    C. open the drainage bag and pour out some urine
    D. wear sterile gloves when obtaining urine

9. After undergoing a transurethral resection of the prostate to treat benign prostatic hypertrophy, a patient is returned to the room with continuous bladder irrigation in place. One day later, the patient reports bladder pain. What should the nurse do first?

    A. increase the I.V. flow rate
    B. notify the doctor immediately
    C. assess the irrigation catheter for patency and drainage
    D. administer meperidine (Demerol) as prescribed

10. A patient comes to the hospital complaining of sudden onset of sharp, severe pain originating in the lumbar region and radiating around the side and toward the bladder. The patient also reports nausea and vomiting and appears pale, diaphoretic, and anxious. The doctor tentatively diagnoses renal calculi and orders flat-plate abdominal X-rays. Renal calculi can form anywhere in the urinary tract. What is their most common formation site?

    A. kidney
    B. ureter
    C. bladder
    D. urethra

11. A patient comes to the hospital complaining of severe pain in the right flank, nausea, and vomiting. The doctor tentatively diagnoses right ureterolithiasis (renal calculi). When planning this patient's care, the nurse should assign highest priority to which nursing diagnosis?

    A. pain
    B. risk for infection
    C. altered urinary elimination
    D. altered nutrition: less than body requirements

12. The nurse is reviewing the report of a patient's routine urinalysis. Which of the following values should the nurse consider abnormal?

    A. specific gravity of 1.002
    B. urine pH of 3
    C. absence of protein
    D. absence of glucose

13. A patient with suspected renal insufficiency is scheduled for a comprehensive diagnostic work-up. After the nurse explains the diagnostic tests, the patient asks which part of the kidney "does the work." Which answer is correct?

    A. the glomerulus
    B. Bowman's capsule
    C. the nephron
    D. the tubular system

14. During a shock state, the renin-angiotensin-aldosterone system exerts which of the following effects on renal function?

    A. decreased urine output, increased reabsorption of sodium and water
    B. decreased urine output, decreased reabsorption of sodium and water
    C. increased urine output, increased reabsorption of sodium and water
    D. increased urine output, decreased reabsorption of sodium and water

15. While assessing a patient who complained of lower abdominal pressure, the nurse notes a firm mass extending above the symphysis pubis. The nurse suspects:

    A. a urinary tract infection
    B. renal calculi
    C. an enlarged kidney
    D. a distended bladder

SITUATION: *Two weeks after being diagnosed with a streptococcal infection, Harriet Franz is admitted to the medical-surgical floor with acute glomerulonephritis.*

Questions 16 and 17 refer to this situation.

16. On initial assessment of Mrs. Franz, the nurse detects one of the classic signs of acute glomerulonephritis of sudden onset. Such signs include:

     A. generalized edema, especially of the face and periorbital area
     B. green-tinged urine
     C. moderate to severe hypotension
     D. polyuria

17. Which immediate action should the nurse take when caring for Mrs. Franz?

     A. Place her on bed rest, which must be maintained for 10 to 12 days.
     B. Provide a high-protein, fluid-restricted diet.
     C. Prepare to assist with insertion of a Tenckhoff catheter for hemodialysis.
     D. Place the patient on a sheepskin and monitor for increasing edema.

SITUATION: *George Garland has had a history of renal insufficiency. His renal function has worsened and he's admitted to the hospital for treatment of chronic renal failure.*

Questions 18 to 23 refer to this situation.

18. In chronic renal failure, symptoms may not become apparent until later stages of the disease because:

     A. liver hormones mask the symptoms
     B. the kidneys have great functional reserve
     C. other body systems take over some of the kidney's functions
     D. the adrenal glands compensate for the kidney's decreased function

19. The nurse knows that chronic renal failure increases Mr. Garland's risk for:

     A. water and sodium retention secondary to a severe decrease in the glomerular filtration rate
     B. a decreased serum phosphate level secondary to kidney failure
     C. an increased serum calcium level secondary to kidney failure
     D. metabolic alkalosis secondary to retention of hydrogen ions

20. Mr. Garland's serum calcium level is low. Low serum calcium levels in renal failure may be caused by:

     A. decreased amounts of parathyroid hormone
     B. decreased activation of vitamin D
     C. demineralization of bone
     D. decreased levels of phosphorus

21. The doctor creates an arteriovenous fistula in Mr. Garland's left arm for dialysis. Which nursing measure is necessary to maintain the fistula?

    A. instructing the patient not to exercise his arm
    B. avoiding blood pressure measurements in the left arm
    C. observing for cannula separation at the connection site
    D. applying a dry, sterile dressing daily

22. Which observation involving Mr. Garland's fistula would require the nurse to notify the doctor?

    A. blood flow detected while palpating the fistula site
    B. blood flow observed through the cannula
    C. absence of an audible bruit while auscultating the graft
    D. straw-colored blood flow observed through the cannula

23. Mr. Garland is ready for discharge. The nurse should reinforce which dietary instruction?

    A. "Be sure to eat meat at every meal."
    B. "Monitor your fruit intake and eat plenty of bananas."
    C. "Restrict your salt intake."
    D. "Drink plenty of fluids."

SITUATION: *Alex Robinson, a 62-year-old police officer, is admitted to the hospital with benign prostatic hyperplasia (BPH).*

Questions 24 to 29 refer to this situation.

24. Nursing assessment of the patient with BPH would most likely reveal:

    A. dysuria, urinary hesitancy, and dribbling
    B. flank pain and decreased caliber of urine stream
    C. urinary frequency, nocturia, and decreased force of urine stream
    D. hematuria, urinary hesitancy, and pyuria

25. The doctor inserts an indwelling urinary catheter to relieve Mr. Robinson's urine retention. Which nursing action would help maintain the drainage system's patency?

    A. restricting fluids to 500 ml per day
    B. taping the catheter to the inner aspect of the thigh
    C. positioning the tubing with dependent loops
    D. keeping the drainage bag below bladder level

26. Mr. Robinson requires prostate gland removal. Before providing preoperative and postoperative instructions to the patient, the nurse asks the surgeon which prostatectomy procedure will be done. What is the most widely used procedure for prostate gland removal?

A. transurethral resection of the prostate (TURP)
B. suprapubic prostatectomy
C. retropubic prostatectomy
D. transurethral laser incision of the prostate

27. The doctor schedules Mr. Robinson for a transurethral resection of the prostate (TURP)under spinal anesthesia. Before surgery, the nurse should tell the patient that:

A. he may receive continuous bladder irrigation after the procedure
B. the procedure may cause impotence
C. sterility is a common complication of this procedure
D. the doctor will remove the entire prostate during the procedure

28. Because of the position Mr. Robinson must assume during transurethral resection of the prostate (TURP), the nurse should assess him postoperatively for:

A. incision site infection
B. thrombophlebitis
C. atelectasis
D. water intoxication

29. The fourth day after the procedure, the doctor removes Mr. Robinson's indwelling urinary catheter. Later that day, he complains of "wetting" himself. Which nursing intervention is most appropriate?

A. advising the patient to contract his perineal muscles periodically
B. restricting his fluid intake
C. applying a condom catheter
D. suggesting that the patient void as soon as the urge comes

SITUATION: *Carol Manning, a 35-year-old homemaker, is admitted with signs and symptoms of urinary tract infection.*

Questions 30 to 32 refer to this situation.

30. Mrs. Manning's doctor diagnoses acute pyelonephritis. Which clinical manifestations should the nurse expect?

A. lower abdominal pain, dysuria, and urinary frequency
B. pyuria, hematuria, and groin pain
C. flank pain, urinary frequency, and an elevated white blood cell (WBC) count
D. urinary frequency and casts in the urine

31. What anatomic fact should the nurse keep in mind when palpating Mrs. Manning's kidneys?

    A. The left kidney usually is slightly higher than the right one.
    B. The kidneys are situated just above the adrenal glands.
    C. The average kidney is approximately 2″ (5 cm) long and ¾″ to 1″ (2 to 3 cm) wide.
    D. The kidneys lie between the 10th and 12th thoracic vertebrae.

32. The doctor orders co-trimoxazole (Bactrim) and phenazopyridine hydrochloride (Pyridium) for Mrs. Manning. Which therapeutic effects should this combination of drugs have?

    A. pain relief and decreased WBC count
    B. equal fluid intake and output
    C. polyuria with a reddish stain
    D. increased complaints of bladder spasm after 20 minutes

SITUATION: *Samuel Adams, age 64, has a history of chronic renal failure. He's admitted to the hospital with these findings: blood pressure 190/110 mm Hg, pulse 122 beats/minute, respirations 32 breaths/minute, neck vein distention, and crackles are auscultated in lung bases.*

Questions 33 to 36 refer to this situation.

33. Which of these laboratory tests is the most accurate indicator of Mr. Adams's renal function?

    A. blood urea nitrogen
    B. creatinine clearance
    C. serum creatinine
    D. urinalysis

34. Which nursing diagnosis should receive highest priority when caring for Mr. Adams?

    A. fear
    B. urinary retention
    C. fluid volume excess
    D. toileting self-care deficit

35. Mr. Adams develops hyperkalemia. Which finding indicates hyperkalemia?

    A. crackles in the bases of the lungs
    B. fever
    C. Chvostek's sign
    D. muscle weakness and paresthesia

36. Mr. Adams receives hemodialysis and his condition stabilizes. The doctor orders aluminum hydroxide (Amphojel) with each meal. This drug is given to:

    A. remove protein wastes of metabolism
    B. bind phosphorus in the GI tract
    C. exchange sodium for potassium in the colon
    D. inhibit development of a stress ulcer

SITUATION: *Debbie Jones returns from the operating room after a small-bowel resection. Her vital signs are stable and her urine output averages 30 ml/hour.*

Questions 37 to 43 refer to this situation.

37. Which nursing intervention would best prevent Ms. Jones from developing acute renal failure in the postoperative period?

    A. having the patient deep breathe and cough every hour to prevent lung congestion
    B. taking vital signs every 2 hours to identify impending hemorrhage and shock
    C. turning the patient every 2 hours to prevent skin breakdown
    D. monitoring I.V. fluids every 4 hours to prevent fluid overload

38. The nurse is reviewing Ms. Jones's fluid intake and output record. What is the normal relationship between fluid intake and urine output?

    A. fluid intake should be double the urine output
    B. fluid intake should approximately equal the urine output
    C. fluid intake should be half the urine output
    D. fluid intake should be inversely proportional to the urine output

39. The nurse documents that Ms. Jones is oliguric. Oliguria is defined as:

    A. a urine output of greater than 1,500 ml in 24 hours
    B. no urine output in 24 hours
    C. a urine output of less than 75 ml in 24 hours
    D. a urine output of less than 500 ml in 24 hours

40. Ms. Jones is in the oliguric phase of acute renal failure. Which of the following actions should the nurse take when caring for this patient?

    A. encourage a low-carbohydrate diet
    B. observe for signs and symptoms of osteodystrophy
    C. help the patient maintain a fluid restriction
    D. encourage the patient to ambulate

41. When assessing Ms. Jones, the nurse would expect her skin to be:

    A. dry and cracked
    B. bruised and discolored
    C. pale and bruised
    D. pale and pruritic

42. Ms. Jones begins peritoneal dialysis. Which outcome should the nurse expect from this procedure?

    A. decreased blood urea nitrogen (BUN)
    B. stimulated urine formation from external kidney pressure
    C. increased serum glucose concentration
    D. removal of excess serum parathyroid hormone

43. Ms. Jones experiences shortness of breath while undergoing peritoneal dialysis. What action should the nurse take first?

    A. elevate the head of the bed and observe the patient
    B. slow the instillation of the dialyzing solution
    C. check the patient's vital signs and weight and document the findings
    D. drain the fluid from the peritoneal cavity and notify the doctor

SITUATION: *Marion Wells, age 50, is admitted to the hospital with a diagnosis of chronic glomerulonephritis.*

Questions 44 to 46 refer to this situation.

44. When caring for Mrs. Wells, which of the following would the nurse recognize as a characteristic finding of chronic glomerulonephritis?

    A. a blood pressure over 130/85 mm Hg
    B. blood urea nitrogen (BUN) level over 60 mg/dl
    C. slightly swollen joints
    D. apprehension

45. Mrs. Wells mentions that she likes salty foods. The nurse should warn her to avoid foods containing sodium because:

    A. reducing sodium promotes urea nitrogen excretion
    B. reducing sodium improves her glomerular filtration rate
    C. reducing sodium increases potassium absorption
    D. reducing sodium decreases edema

46. Mrs. Wells's discharge teaching should include which of the following concerns?

A. the need for a nephrectomy
B. the need for a high-protein diet
C. the need to protect against infection
D. the need for foot care

SITUATION: *Lester Johnson, age 66, is a retired factory worker. He's admitted to the hospital for cystoscopic examination to assess for bladder cancer. Cystoscopy confirms the diagnosis. After inserting an indwelling urinary catheter, Mr. Johnson's doctor prescribes chemotherapy and schedules him for a cystectomy with ileal conduit urinary diversion.*

Questions 47 to 49 refer to this situation.

47. Which of the following findings prompted Mr. Johnson to seek treatment initially?

A. painless hematuria
B. a change in voiding pattern
C. abrupt weight gain
D. weakness

48. The purpose of Mr. Johnson's chemotherapy is to:

A. eliminate the need for surgery
B. augment the treatment regimen
C. reduce pain and anxiety before surgery
D. sterilize the bowel before surgery

49. The nurse should include which of the following points in Mr. Johnson's preoperative teaching?

A. the need to perform stoma self-care immediately after surgery
B. the need to remain on bed rest for 3 days following surgery
C. the procedure creates a stoma and he must wear a pouch afterward
D. the patient will be able to control urine passage through the stoma

SITUATION: *Kirby Fisher, age 42, complains of fatigue, weakness, and palpitations. After several diagnostic tests, the doctor determines that these symptoms are caused by hypophosphatemia.*

Questions 50 to 52 refer to this situation.

50. The most common cause of hypophosphatemia is:

    A. acute renal failure
    B. chronic alcoholism
    C. alkalosis
    D. chronic renal failure

51. Assessment of Mr. Fisher would most likely reveal:

    A. numbness around the mouth
    B. clinical manifestations of hypercalcemia
    C. carpopedal spasm
    D. muscle twitching and cramping

52. Mr. Fisher's initial treatment should include the administration of:

    A. potassium phosphate (Neutra-Phos-K)
    B. acetazolamide (Diamox)
    C. aluminum hydroxide (Amphojel)
    D. vitamins

SITUATION: *Because of difficulties with hemodialysis, Lamar Brighton is admitted to the hospital for insertion of a Tenckhoff catheter and continuous ambulatory peritoneal dialysis.*

Question 53 to 57 refer to this situation.

53. Which nursing diagnosis is most important for Mr. Brighton while he undergoes continuous ambulatory peritoneal dialysis?

    A. altered urinary elimination
    B. activity intolerance
    C. toileting self-care deficit
    D. risk for infection

54. Mr. Brighton has developed faulty red blood cell (RBC) production. The nurse should monitor him for:

    A. nausea and vomiting
    B. dyspnea and tachypnea
    C. fatigue and weakness
    D. thrush and fever

55. The doctor prescribes recombinant epoetin alfa (Epogen) for Mr. Brighton. Which of the following should the nurse teach him about this drug?

A. This drug will help with the bleeding problems associated with kidney damage.

B. Epoetin alfa should reduce fatigue and improve energy levels.

C. Taking this drug may reduce the need for dialysis.

D. Once a good blood level is established, the injectable form will be changed to an oral form.

56. Mr. Brighton is at risk for developing which of the following adverse reactions caused by epoetin alfa?

    A. blurred vision

    B. hypertension

    C. constipation

    D. urine retention

57. As part of Mr. Brighton's discharge teaching, which of the following symptoms indicate peritonitis and should be reported at once to the doctor?

    A. blood-tinged dialysate outflow with abdominal pain

    B. brown dialysate outflow with an urge to move the bowels

    C. amber dialysate outflow with urinary incontinence

    D. cloudy dialysate outflow with abdominal pain

SITUATION: *Jermaine Lawrence, age 35, is admitted to the hospital for a kidney transplant. He has a history of hypertension and chronic renal failure.*

Questions 58 to refer 62 to this situation.

58. The nurse assesses Mr. Lawrence shortly after kidney transplant surgery. Which postoperative finding should the nurse report to the doctor immediately?

    A. serum potassium level of 4.9 mEq/L

    B. serum sodium level of 135 mEq/L

    C. temperature of 99.2° F (37.3° C)

    D. urine output of 20 ml/hour

59. When changing Mr. Lawrence's sterile surgical dressing, what should the nurse do first?

    A. wash her hands

    B. apply sterile gloves

    C. remove the old dressing with clean gloves

    D. open sterile packages and moisten dressings with sterile saline

60. Following his kidney transplant, Mr. Lawrence must take cyclosporine (Sandimmune) daily along with several other immunosuppressants. How may cyclosporine produce its therapeutic effects?

A. by eliminating antigen-reactive T cells in peripheral blood
B. by inhibiting ribonucleic acid synthesis
C. by inhibiting helper T cells and suppressor T cells
D. by antagonizing metabolism of the amino acid purine

61. The nurse should warn Mr. Lawrence that cyclosporine may interact with which of the following commonly prescribed antibiotics?

A. tetracycline
B. ampicillin
C. penicillin
D. erythromycin

62. The nurse should teach Mr. Lawrence about adverse reactions to cyclosporine. What is the most severe adverse reaction that may occur?

A. bone marrow suppression
B. pulmonary edema
C. drug fever
D. nephrotoxicity

ANSWER SHEET

	A B C D		A B C D		A B C D
1	○ ○ ○ ○	22	○ ○ ○ ○	43	○ ○ ○ ○
2	○ ○ ○ ○	23	○ ○ ○ ○	44	○ ○ ○ ○
3	○ ○ ○ ○	24	○ ○ ○ ○	45	○ ○ ○ ○
4	○ ○ ○ ○	25	○ ○ ○ ○	46	○ ○ ○ ○
5	○ ○ ○ ○	26	○ ○ ○ ○	47	○ ○ ○ ○
6	○ ○ ○ ○	27	○ ○ ○ ○	48	○ ○ ○ ○
7	○ ○ ○ ○	28	○ ○ ○ ○	49	○ ○ ○ ○
8	○ ○ ○ ○	29	○ ○ ○ ○	50	○ ○ ○ ○
9	○ ○ ○ ○	30	○ ○ ○ ○	51	○ ○ ○ ○
10	○ ○ ○ ○	31	○ ○ ○ ○	52	○ ○ ○ ○
11	○ ○ ○ ○	32	○ ○ ○ ○	53	○ ○ ○ ○
12	○ ○ ○ ○	33	○ ○ ○ ○	54	○ ○ ○ ○
13	○ ○ ○ ○	34	○ ○ ○ ○	55	○ ○ ○ ○
14	○ ○ ○ ○	35	○ ○ ○ ○	56	○ ○ ○ ○
15	○ ○ ○ ○	36	○ ○ ○ ○	57	○ ○ ○ ○
16	○ ○ ○ ○	37	○ ○ ○ ○	58	○ ○ ○ ○
17	○ ○ ○ ○	38	○ ○ ○ ○	59	○ ○ ○ ○
18	○ ○ ○ ○	39	○ ○ ○ ○	60	○ ○ ○ ○
19	○ ○ ○ ○	40	○ ○ ○ ○	61	○ ○ ○ ○
20	○ ○ ○ ○	41	○ ○ ○ ○	62	○ ○ ○ ○
21	○ ○ ○ ○	42	○ ○ ○ ○		

ANSWERS AND RATIONALES

1. *Correct answer:* **A**

A hypertonic solution causes water to shift from the cells into the plasma because the hypertonic solution has a greater osmotic pressure than the cells. A hypotonic solution has a lower osmotic pressure than that of the cells. It causes fluid to shift into the cells, possibly resulting in rupture. An isotonic solution, which has the same osmotic pressure as the cells, wouldn't cause any shift. A solution's alkalinity is related to the hydrogen ion concentration, not its osmotic effect.

> *Nursing process step:* Implementation
> *Client needs category:* Physiological integrity
> *Client needs subcategory:* Pharmacological and parenteral therapies
> *Taxonomic level:* Comprehension

2. *Correct answer:* **C**

Particles move from an area of greater osmolarity to one of lesser osmolarity through diffusion. Active transport is the movement of particles through energy expenditure from other sources such as enzymes. Osmosis is the movement of a pure solvent through a semipermeable membrane from an area of greater osmolarity to one of lesser osmolarity until equalization occurs. The membrane is impermeable to the solute but permeable to the solvent. Filtration is the process by which fluid is forced through a membrane by a difference in pressure; small molecules pass through, but large ones don't.

> *Nursing process step:* Not applicable
> *Client needs category:* Not applicable
> *Client needs subcategory:* Not applicable
> *Taxonomic level:* Comprehension

3. *Correct answer:* **A**

Tenting of chest skin when pinched indicates decreased skin elasticity due to dehydration. Hand veins fill slowly with dehydration, not rapidly. A pulse that isn't easily obliterated and neck vein distention indicate fluid overload, not dehydration.

> *Nursing process step:* Assessment
> *Client needs category:* Health promotion and maintenance
> *Client needs subcategory:* Prevention and early detection of disease
> *Taxonomic level:* Application

4. *Correct answer:* **C**

Administering a tap water enema until return is clear would most likely contribute to a hypo-osmolar state. Because tap water is hypotonic, it would be absorbed by the body, diluting the body fluid concentration and lowering osmolality. Weighing the patient is the easiest, most accurate method to determine fluid changes. Therefore, it helps identify rather than contribute to fluid imbalance. Nasogastric tube irrigation with normal saline solution wouldn't cause a shift in fluid balance. Drinking broth wouldn't contribute to a hypo-osmolar state because it doesn't replace sodium and water lost through excessive perspiration.

> *Nursing process step:* Evaluation
> *Client needs category:* Physiological integrity
> *Client needs subcategory:* Reduction of risk potential
> *Taxonomic level:* Knowledge

5. *Correct answer:* D

An orthostatic blood pressure indicates an extracellular fluid volume deficit. (The extracellular compartment consists of both the intravascular compartment and interstitial space.) A fluid volume deficit within the intravascular compartment would cause tachycardia, not bradycardia or orthostatic blood pressure change. A central venous pressure of 6 mm Hg is in the high normal range, indicating adequate hydration. Pitting edema indicates fluid volume overload.

> *Nursing process step:* Assessment
> *Client needs category:* Physiological integrity
> *Client needs subcategory:* Reduction of risk potential
> *Taxonomic level:* Knowledge

6. *Correct answer:* **C**

The respiratory and renal systems act as compensatory mechanisms to counteract acid-base imbalances. The lungs alter the carbon dioxide levels in the blood by increasing or decreasing the rate and depth of respirations, thereby increasing or decreasing carbon dioxide elimination. The liver, pancreas, and heart play no part in compensating for acid-base imbalances.

> *Nursing process step:* Evaluation
> *Client needs category:* Health promotion and maintenance
> *Client needs subcategory:* Prevention and early detection of disease
> *Taxonomic level:* Comprehension

7. *Correct answer:* **B**

Anuria refers to a urine output of less than 100 ml in 24 hours. The baseline for urine output and renal function is 30 ml of urine per hour. A urine output of at least 100 ml in 2 hours is within normal limits. Voiding at night is called nocturia. Pain and burning on urination is called dysuria.

Nursing process step: Assessment
Client needs category: Physiological integrity
Client needs subcategory: Reduction of risk potential
Taxonomic level: Comprehension

8. *Correct answer:* **A**

To obtain urine properly, the nurse should aspirate it from a port, using a sterile syringe after cleaning the port. Opening a closed urine drainage system increases the risk of urinary tract infection. Standard precautions specify the use of gloves during contact with body fluids; however, sterile gloves aren't necessary.

Nursing process step: Implementation
Client needs category: Safe, effective care environment
Client needs subcategory: Safety and infection control
Taxonomic level: Comprehension

9. *Correct answer:* **C**

Although postoperative pain is expected, the nurse should ensure that other factors, such as an obstructed irrigation catheter, aren't the cause of the pain. After assessing catheter patency, the nurse should administer an analgesic such as meperidine as prescribed. Increasing the I.V. flow rate may worsen the pain. Notifying the doctor isn't necessary unless the pain is severe or unrelieved by the prescribed medication.

Nursing process step: Implementation
Client needs category: Physiological integrity
Client needs subcategory: Reduction of risk potential
Taxonomic level: Analysis

10. *Correct answer:* **A**

Renal calculi most commonly form in the kidney. They may remain there or become lodged anywhere along the urinary tract. The ureter, bladder, and urethra are less common sites of renal calculi formation.

Nursing process step: Assessment
Client needs category: Physiological integrity
Client needs subcategory: Reduction of risk potential
Taxonomic level: Comprehension

11. *Correct answer:* **A**

Ureterolithiasis typically causes such acute, severe pain that the patient can't rest and becomes increasingly anxious. Therefore, the nursing diagnosis of *pain* takes highest priority. *Risk for infection* and *altered urinary elimination* are appropriate once the patient's pain is controlled. *Altered nutrition: less than body requirements* isn't appropriate at this time.

> *Nursing process step:* Planning
> *Client needs category:* Physiological integrity
> *Client needs subcategory:* Reduction of risk potential
> *Taxonomic level:* Analysis

12. *Correct answer:* **B**

Normal urine pH is 4.5 to 8; therefore, a urine pH of 3 is abnormal and may indicate such conditions as renal tuberculosis, pyrexia, phenylketonuria, alkaptonuria, and acidosis. Urine specific gravity normally ranges from 1.002 to 1.035, making the patient's value normal. Normally, urine contains no protein, glucose, ketones, bilirubin, bacteria, casts, or crystals.

> *Nursing process step:* Assessment
> *Client needs category:* Physiological integrity
> *Client needs subcategory:* Reduction of risk potential
> *Taxonomic level:* Comprehension

13. *Correct answer:* **C**

The nephron is the kidney's functioning unit. The glomerulus, Bowman's capsule, and tubular system are components of the nephron.

> *Nursing process step:* Assessment
> *Client needs category:* Physiological integrity
> *Client needs subcategory:* Reduction of risk potential
> *Taxonomic level:* Knowledge

14. *Correct answer:* **A**

As a response to shock, the renin-angiotensin-aldosterone system alters renal function by decreasing urine output and increasing reabsorption of sodium and water. Reduced renal perfusion stimulates the renin-angiotensin-aldosterone system in an effort to conserve circulating volume.

> *Nursing process step:* Evaluation
> *Client needs category:* Physiological integrity
> *Client needs subcategory:* Physiological adaptation
> *Taxonomic level:* Analysis

15. *Correct answer:* **D**

The bladder isn't usually palpable unless it's distended. The feeling of pressure is usually relieved with urination. Reduced bladder tone due to general anesthesia is a common postoperative complication that causes difficulty in voiding. A urinary tract infection and renal calculi aren't palpable. The kidneys aren't palpable above the symphysis pubis.

Nursing process step: Analysis
Client needs category: Health promotion and maintenance
Client needs subcategory: Prevention and early detection of disease
Taxonomic level: Analysis

16. *Correct answer:* **A**

Generalized edema, especially of the face and periorbital area, is a classic sign of acute glomerulonephritis of sudden onset. Other classic signs and symptoms include hematuria, proteinuria, fever, chills, weakness, pallor, anorexia, nausea, and vomiting. Green-tinged urine is not present with acute glomerulonephritis. The patient also may have moderate to severe hypertension, oliguria or anuria, headache, reduced visual acuity, and abdominal or flank pain.

Nursing process step: Assessment
Client needs category: Physiological integrity
Client needs subcategory: Reduction of risk potential
Taxonomic level: Knowledge

17. *Correct answer:* **A**

The nurse must enforce immediate bed rest for a patient with glomerulonephritis to ensure a complete recovery and help prevent complications. Depending on disease severity, the patient may require fluid, sodium, potassium, and protein restrictions. Because of the risk of altered urinary elimination related to oliguria, this patient may require hemodialysis or plasmapheresis for several weeks until renal function improves; however, a Tenckhoff catheter is used in peritoneal dialysis, not hemodialysis. Although comfort measures such as placing the patient on a sheepskin are important, they don't take precedence.

Nursing process step: Implementation
Client needs category: Physiological integrity
Client needs subcategory: Reduction of risk potential
Taxonomic level: Knowledge

18. *Correct answer:* **B**

Because of the great functional reserve of the kidneys, chronic renal failure develops more slowly than acute renal failure and signs and symptoms don't appear until later stages of the disease. Liver hormones don't mask symptoms of renal failure, and other body systems don't compensate for the kidney's decreased function.

Nursing process step: Assessment
Client needs category: Physiological integrity
Client needs subcategory: Reduction of risk potential
Taxonomic level: Comprehension

19. *Correct answer:* **A**

A patient with chronic renal failure is at risk for fluid imbalance—dehydration if the kidneys fail to concentrate urine, or fluid retention if the kidneys fail to produce urine. Electrolyte imbalances associated with chronic renal failure result from the kidney's inability to excrete phosphorus; such imbalances may lead to hyperphosphatemia with reciprocal hypocalcemia. Chronic renal failure may cause metabolic acidosis, not metabolic alkalosis, secondary to the kidney's inability to excrete hydrogen ions.

> *Nursing process step:* Evaluation
> *Client needs category:* Physiological integrity
> *Client needs subcategory:* Reduction of risk potential
> *Taxonomic level:* Knowledge

20. *Correct answer:* **B**

Decreased activation of vitamin D in renal failure reduces GI absorption of calcium. Although demineralization of bone can occur with renal failure, the condition is due to repeated episodes of hypocalcemia. Patients with renal failure have elevated phosphate levels with correspondingly low calcium levels.

> *Nursing process step:* Evaluation
> *Client needs category:* Physiological integrity
> *Client needs subcategory:* Reduction of risk potential
> *Taxonomic level:* Knowledge

21. *Correct answer:* **B**

The nurse shouldn't take blood pressure measurements in the left arm because this may compromise circulation to the fistula; clot formation may occur, reducing the fistula's patency or rendering it useless. The patient should exercise the arm to promote circulation through the fistula. Because the fistula is internal, the nurse wouldn't be able to observe any separation of the cannula at the connection site. Applying a dry, sterile dressing is unnecessary once the incision is healed.

> *Nursing process step:* Implementation
> *Client needs category:* Physiological integrity
> *Client needs subcategory:* Reduction of risk potential
> *Taxonomic level:* Application

22. *Correct answer:* **C**

The nurse should hear turbulent blood flow through the vessels using the bell of the stethoscope; absent bruit indicates a nonpatent fistula, requiring the nurse to notify the doctor. Blood flow detected while palpating the fistula site indicates that the fistula is patent; notifying the doctor wouldn't be necessary. Because an arteriovenous fistula doesn't require an external cannula, blood flow — regardless of color — wouldn't be visible.

Nursing process step: Planning
Client needs category: Physiological integrity
Client needs subcategory: Reduction of risk potential
Taxonomic level: Comprehension

23. *Correct answer:* **C**

In a patient with chronic renal failure, unrestricted intake of sodium, protein, potassium, and fluid may lead to a dangerous accumulation of electrolytes and protein metabolic products, such as amino acids and ammonia. Therefore, the patient must limit his intake of sodium, meat (high in protein), bananas (high in potassium), and fluid (because the kidneys can't secrete adequate urine).

Nursing process step: Implementation
Client needs category: Physiological integrity
Client needs subcategory: Basic care and comfort
Taxonomic level: Application

24. *Correct answer:* **C**

Urinary frequency, nocturia, and decreased force and caliber of the urine stream are common clinical manifestations of BPH; they result from urethral obstruction. Dysuria, urinary hesitancy, dribbling, and pyuria are associated with irritation possibly from infection. Flank pain is common with kidney inflammation, not BPH. Hematuria indicates cancer of the prostate, not BPH.

Nursing process step: Assessment
Client needs category: Physiological integrity
Client needs subcategory: Reduction of risk potential
Taxonomic level: Comprehension

25. *Correct answer:* **D**

Keeping the drainage bag below bladder level allows steady drainage from gravity. Forcing (not restricting) fluids maintains urine volume, causing steady movement of urine through the drainage system and preventing clogs. Taping the indwelling urinary catheter to the inner aspect of the thigh prevents tension on the urinary meatus; it wouldn't help maintain system patency. Dependent loops should be avoided to help prevent drainage stagnation and possible clogging.

Nursing process step: Implementation
Client needs category: Physiological integrity
Client needs subcategory: Reduction of risk potential
Taxonomic level: Knowledge

26. *Correct answer:* **A**

TURP is the most widely used procedure for prostate gland removal. Because it requires no incision, TURP is especially suitable for men with relatively minor prostate enlargements and for those who are poor surgical risks. Suprapubic prostatectomy, retropubic prostatectomy, and transurethral laser incision of the prostate are less common procedures, and all require incisions.

> *Nursing process step:* Implementation
> *Client needs category:* Physiological integrity
> *Client needs subcategory:* Reduction of risk potential
> *Taxonomic level:* Knowledge

27. *Correct answer:* **A**

Continuous bladder irrigation is common after TURP; it promotes the removal of clots from the bladder. Impotence is a potential complication with perineal prostatic resection, not TURP. Because the testes aren't removed during the procedure, sterility is uncommon. The doctor doesn't remove the entire prostate during TURP.

> *Nursing process step:* Planning
> *Client needs category:* Physiological integrity
> *Client needs subcategory:* Reduction of risk potential
> *Taxonomic level:* Knowledge

28. *Correct answer:* **B**

Thrombophlebitis is a potential complication after TURP because the patient must assume the lithotomy position for a prolonged period; this causes pressure at the popliteal area, which may lead to venous stasis and resulting thrombophlebitis. Incision site infection isn't a potential complication of the procedure because there is no open incision site. Atelectasis isn't a common complication of TURP; it's more likely after a perineal prostatectomy or a procedure requiring inhaled general anesthetics. Water intoxication may result from continuous bladder irrigation during the procedure, but this isn't related to the patient's position.

> *Nursing process step:* Assessment
> *Client needs category:* Physiological integrity
> *Client needs subcategory:* Reduction of risk potential
> *Taxonomic level:* Application

29. *Correct answer:* **A**

Perineal muscle contraction helps reestablish bladder sphincter tone and control voiding. Unless contraindicated, fluids should be forced, not restricted, after transurethral resection of the prostate to maintain renal function. Applying a condom catheter will prevent soiling, but it won't reestablish sphincter control.

Stopping and starting the urine stream would be more effective in reestablishing sphincter control than voiding when the urge occurs.

Nursing process step: Implementation
Client needs category: Physiological integrity
Client needs subcategory: Reduction of risk potential
Taxonomic level: Application

30. *Correct answer:* **C**

Flank pain, urinary frequency, and elevated WBCs are common clinical manifestations of pyelonephritis. Lower abdominal pain, dysuria, urinary frequency, and groin pain are associated with cystitis. Pyuria, hematuria, and casts in the urine are common with glomerulonephritis.

Nursing process step: Assessment
Client needs category: Physiological integrity
Client needs subcategory: Reduction of risk potential
Taxonomic level: Comprehension

31. *Correct answer:* **A**

The left kidney usually is slightly higher than the right one. An adrenal gland lies atop each kidney, not the other way round. The average kidney measures approximately 4″ (11 cm) long, 2″ (5 cm) wide, and 1″ (2.5 cm) thick. The kidneys are located retroperitoneally, in the posterior aspect of the abdomen, on either side of the vertebral column. They lie between the 12th thoracic and 3rd lumbar vertebrae.

Nursing process step: Assessment
Client needs category: Physiological integrity
Client needs subcategory: Reduction of risk potential
Taxonomic level: Knowledge

32. *Correct answer:* **A**

This combination's therapeutic effect includes pain relief and a decreased WBC count; phenazopyridine is an analgesic, and co-trimoxazole is an antibiotic. The drugs don't affect fluid intake or output; however, because co-trimoxazole is a sulfa preparation, the patient's fluid intake should be increased to prevent crystallization in the urine. Phenazopyridine causes a reddish stain in the urine, but this effect has no therapeutic value. The patient's complaints of bladder spasm should decrease, not increase, after administration of phenazopyridine.

Nursing process step: Evaluation
Client needs category: Physiological integrity
Client needs subcategory: Pharmacological and parenteral therapies
Taxonomic level: Comprehension

33. *Correct answer:* **B**

Creatinine clearance closely correlates with the kidneys' glomerular filtration rate and tubular excretion ability. Results from blood urea nitrogen, serum creatinine, and urinalysis may be influenced by various conditions and aren't specific to renal disease.

> *Nursing process step:* Assessment
> *Client needs category:* Physiological integrity
> *Client needs subcategory:* Reduction of risk potential
> *Taxonomic level:* Knowledge

34. *Correct answer:* **C**

A patient with renal failure is unable to eliminate sufficient fluid, which increases the risk of fluid overload and the resulting respiratory and electrolyte problems. The patient is exhibiting signs of *fluid volume excess. Fear* and *toileting self-care deficit* may be problems but aren't as high a priority because they aren't life-threatening. *Urinary retention* may be a cause of renal failure but isn't as urgent a concern as fluid volume excess.

> *Nursing process step:* Analysis
> *Client needs category:* Physiological integrity
> *Client needs subcategory:* Reduction of risk potential
> *Taxonomic level:* Analysis

35. *Correct answer:* **D**

Potassium, an intracellular cation, is necessary for neuromuscular function; muscle weakness and paresthesia are symptoms of hyperkalemia, a common complication of chronic renal failure. Fever isn't related to hyperkalemia. A positive Chvostek's sign indicates hypocalcemia, not hyperkalemia.

> *Nursing process step:* Assessment
> *Client needs category:* Physiological integrity
> *Client needs subcategory:* Reduction of risk potential
> *Taxonomic level:* Application

36. *Correct answer:* **B**

Aluminum hydroxide (Amphojel) is given to control serum phosphorus. This drug neutralizes gastric acidity and binds with phosphates in the GI tract to increase phosphorus excretion. With chronic renal failure, unfiltered waste products of metabolism such as protein accumulate in the blood; however, aluminum hydroxide has no effect on the excretion of protein or other waste products. This drug doesn't exchange sodium for potassium; sodium polystyrene sulfonate (Kayexalate) has this effect. Chronic renal failure doesn't necessarily lead to stress ulcers. Antacids don't inhibit ulcers but reduce gastric acidity, which increases with a peptic ulcer.

Nursing process step: Implementation
Client needs category: Physiological integrity
Client needs subcategory: Pharmacological and parenteral therapies
Taxonomic level: Knowledge

37. *Correct answer:* **B**

Unresolved shock from hemorrhage leads to decreased vascular volume. This causes inadequate hydrostatic pressure for glomerular filtration, resulting in acute renal failure. Lung congestion isn't a complication of postoperative renal failure. Turning the patient every 2 hours prevents skin breakdown, not renal failure. Fluid overload results from renal failure; it doesn't cause it.

Nursing process step: Implementation
Client needs category: Physiological integrity
Client needs subcategory: Reduction of risk potential
Taxonomic level: Application

38. *Correct answer:* **B**

Normally, fluid intake should be approximately equal to urine output. Any other relationship signals an abnormality. For example, fluid intake that is double the urine output indicates fluid retention. Fluid intake that is half the urine output indicates dehydration. Normally, fluid intake isn't inversely proportional to urine output.

Nursing process step: Assessment
Client needs category: Physiological integrity
Client needs subcategory: Reduction of risk potential
Taxonomic level: Application

39. *Correct answer:* **D**

Oliguria is defined as a urine output of less than 500 ml in 24 hours. A urine output of greater than 1,500 ml in 24 hours is well within normal limits. A urine output of less than 75 ml in 24 hours or no urine output at all is termed anuria.

Nursing process step: Implementation
Client needs category: Physiological integrity
Client needs subcategory: Physiological adaptation
Taxonomic level: Comprehension

40. *Correct answer:* **C**

The nurse should help the patient maintain a fluid restriction. The degree of restriction varies depending on kidney output; the patient should consume only enough fluid to replace what is lost. Carbohydrates are an essential nutrient and shouldn't be restricted. If the carbohydrate intake is inadequate, the body metabolizes protein for energy. Osteodystrophy is a complication of chronic renal failure, not acute renal failure. Bed rest is recommended to conserve energy, reduce the metabolic rate, and decrease edema. Ambulation should be restricted during the early oliguric phase.

> *Nursing process step:* Implementation
> *Client needs category:* Physiological integrity
> *Client needs subcategory:* Reduction of risk potential
> *Taxonomic level:* Application

41. *Correct answer:* D

Decreased renal function may cause pale skin due to a low hemoglobin level, and pruritus from the presence of calcium deposits in the skin. The patient wouldn't have dry and cracked, or bruised or discolored skin as a result of renal failure.

> *Nursing process step:* Assessment
> *Client needs category:* Physiological integrity
> *Client needs subcategory:* Reduction of risk potential
> *Taxonomic level:* Comprehension

42. *Correct answer:* A

The nurse should expect decreased BUN after peritoneal dialysis. This procedure removes waste products from the body when the kidneys aren't functioning properly. Although the instillation of fluid into the peritoneal cavity increases intra-abdominal pressure, peritoneal dialysis doesn't stimulate urine formation; nor does it affect the level of serum glucose or parathyroid hormone.

> *Nursing process step:* Evaluation
> *Client needs category:* Physiological integrity
> *Client needs subcategory:* Physiological adaptation
> *Taxonomic level:* Comprehension

43. *Correct answer:* A

The nurse should elevate the head of the bed and observe the patient for improved breathing. Elevation reduces the pressure on the diaphragm caused by fluid accumulation in the abdomen, which can cause shortness of breath. Because slowing the instillation wouldn't greatly reduce pressure on the thorax, this action wouldn't help the patient's breathing. Checking vital signs and weight and documenting these findings provides data, but this situation requires immediate nursing intervention. Draining the fluid and notifying the doctor wouldn't be necessary initially if elevating the patient's head improves breathing. If circulatory overload is suspected, the nurse should notify the doctor.

Nursing process step: Implementation
Client needs category: Physiological integrity
Client needs subcategory: Reduction of risk potential
Taxonomic level: Application

44. *Correct answer:* **B**

The normal BUN level is 6 to 20 mg/dl; an elevated level indicates renal failure, a result of glomerular inflammation in chronic glomerulonephritis. A blood pressure of 130/85 mm Hg is considered normal in a 50-year-old woman. Swollen joints aren't characteristic of chronic glomerulonephritis. Apprehension is normal for a newly admitted patient, but it isn't specifically related to this disease.

Nursing process step: Assessment
Client needs category: Physiological integrity
Client needs subcategory: Reduction of risk potential
Taxonomic level: Analysis

45. *Correct answer:* **D**

Reducing sodium intake reduces fluid retention. Fluid retention increases blood volume, which changes blood vessel permeability and allows plasma to move into interstitial tissue, causing edema. Urea nitrogen excretion can be increased only by improved renal function. Sodium intake doesn't affect the glomerular filtration rate. Potassium absorption is improved only by increasing the glomerular filtration rate; it isn't affected by sodium intake.

Nursing process step: Implementation
Client needs category: Physiological integrity
Client needs subcategory: Basic care and comfort
Taxonomic level: Application

46. *Correct answer:* **C**

To prevent further exacerbations of chronic glomerulonephritis, the patient must protect herself against infections, which increase the metabolic rate and result in more waste products; their excretion is decreased because of impaired kidney function. Recurrent infections also predispose the kidneys to greater damage. Even if the patient has renal failure, a nephrectomy wouldn't necessarily be indicated. A high-protein diet is contraindicated because of impaired removal of protein wastes. Foot problems aren't associated with chronic glomerulonephritis.

Nursing process step: Planning
Client needs category: Physiological integrity
Client needs subcategory: Reduction of risk potential
Taxonomic level: Application

47. *Correct answer:* **A**

Painless hematuria is the first clinical manifestation in most patients with bladder tumors. A change in voiding pattern commonly results from renal failure or
prostate enlargement. Abrupt weight gain is caused by fluid retention, a symptom of renal failure or heart failure. Weakness is a nonspecific symptom of many
disorders; it isn't commonly seen with bladder tumors.

> *Nursing process step:* Assessment
> *Client needs category:* Physiological integrity
> *Client needs subcategory:* Reduction of risk potential
> *Taxonomic level:* Comprehension

48. *Correct answer:* **B**

Chemotherapy augments the patient's treatment regimen; it destroys tumor cells
before surgical removal of the tumor, reducing the risk that cancer may spread or
recur. Chemotherapy in bladder cancer typically isn't curative and doesn't eliminate the need for surgery. Chemotherapeutic agents have no analgesic or sedative
actions; they don't reduce pain or anxiety. Bowel sterilization isn't necessary before a cystectomy.

> *Nursing process step:* Implementation
> *Client needs category:* Physiological integrity
> *Client needs subcategory:* Pharmacological and parenteral therapies
> *Taxonomic level:* Comprehension

49. *Correct answer:* **C**

The nurse should ensure that the patient understands that a stoma will be
formed and that he'll need to wear a pouch. The nurse will care for the stoma
immediately after surgery; self-care will begin when the patient is physically able.
The patient will be encouraged to get out of bed the first day after surgery to prevent complications of immobility. Urine flow can't be controlled through a
stoma.

> *Nursing process step:* Planning
> *Client needs category:* Physiological integrity
> *Client needs subcategory:* Basic care and comfort
> *Taxonomic level:* Knowledge

50. *Correct answer:* **B**

Hypophosphatemia is most commonly caused by chronic alcoholism. The alcoholic patient's nutrition is typically poor, causing an inadequate phosphate intake. Other causes include malabsorption problems, starvation, and total parenteral nutrition. Acute and chronic renal failure causes hyperphosphatemia because the failing kidneys can't excrete phosphates. Alkalosis accelerates phosphate
passage from the serum into cells, but this rarely occurs.

Nursing process step: Assessment
Client needs category: Physiological integrity
Client needs subcategory: Reduction of risk potential
Taxonomic level: Knowledge

51. *Correct answer:* **B**

Because phosphate and calcium have an inverse relationship, the calcium level is high when the phosphate is low. Therefore, the clinical manifestations of hypercalcemia and hypophosphatemia are the same (mental confusion, muscle weakness, anorexia, nausea, and impaired reflexes). Numbness around the mouth, carpopedal spasm, and muscle twitching and cramping are signs of the opposite situation — hyperphosphatemia and hypocalcemia.

Nursing process step: Assessment
Client needs category: Physiological integrity
Client needs subcategory: Reduction of risk potential
Taxonomic level: Comprehension

52. *Correct answer:* **A**

Treatment for hypophosphatemia should include administering potassium phosphate until phosphate levels return to normal. The doctor may order sodium phosphate or potassium phosphate I.V. if hypophosphatemia is severe. Acetazolamide and aluminum hydroxide aren't given because they would further decrease the phosphate level. Vitamin replacement wouldn't be part of the patient's initial therapy because it wouldn't eliminate low phosphate levels — phosphate is a mineral, not a vitamin.

Nursing process step: Implementation
Client needs category: Physiological integrity
Client needs subcategory: Pharmacological and parenteral therapies
Taxonomic level: Application

53. *Correct answer:* **D**

Because the peritoneal dialysis catheter and regular exchanges of the dialysis bag give bacteria a direct portal of entry into the body, the patient is at risk for infection. The remaining options may be pertinent but don't take precedence over this nursing diagnosis. If the patient develops peritoneal infections, continuous ambulatory peritoneal dialysis may no longer be effective in clearing the body's waste products.

Nursing process step: Analysis
Client needs category: Physiological integrity
Client needs subcategory: Reduction of risk potential
Taxonomic level: Application

54. *Correct answer:* **C**

RBCs carry oxygen throughout the body. Decreased production of them diminishes cellular oxygen, thereby causing fatigue and weakness. Nausea and vomiting may occur in chronic renal failure but aren't caused by faulty RBC production. Dyspnea and tachypnea are associated with fluid excess. Thrush and fever signal infection and aren't signs of faulty RBC production.

> *Nursing process step:* Assessment
> *Client needs category:* Physiological integrity
> *Client needs subcategory:* Reduction of risk potential
> *Taxonomic level:* Application

55. *Correct answer:* **B**

Epoetin alfa stimulates the bone marrow to increase red blood cell production, thus helping to resolve anemia and improving activity tolerance. The drug has no effect on bleeding or the need for dialysis. It's administered by subcutaneous injection; no oral form is available.

> *Nursing process step:* Implementation
> *Client needs category:* Physiological integrity
> *Client needs subcategory:* Pharmacological and parenteral therapies
> *Taxonomic level:* Application

56. *Correct answer:* **B**

Hypertension is the most common adverse reaction to epoetin alfa. It may occur even in previously hypotensive patients. Other adverse reactions reported in more than 5% of patients during clinical trials include headache, arthralgia, nausea, edema, fatigue, diarrhea, vomiting, chest pain, skin reactions at the injection site, asthenia, and dizziness. Blurred vision, constipation, and urine retention aren't adverse reactions associated with epoetin alfa.

> *Nursing process step:* Assessment
> *Client needs category:* Physiological integrity
> *Client needs subcategory:* Pharmacological and parenteral therapies
> *Taxonomic level:* Comprehension

57. *Correct answer:* **D**

Cloudy dialysate outflow with abdominal pain indicates peritonitis. Blood-tinged outflow may indicate abdominal bleeding or uremic coagulopathy. Brown outflow is associated with bowel perforation and usually occurs in the first exchange of the dialysate fluid. Amber outflow is a sign of bladder perforation and occurs during the first exchange of dialysate.

Nursing process step: Planning
Client needs category: Physiological integrity
Client needs subcategory: Reduction of risk potential
Taxonomic level: Comprehension

58. *Correct answer:* **D**

Because kidney transplantation increases the risk of transplant rejection, infection, and other serious complications, the nurse should monitor the patient's urinary function closely. A decrease from the normal urine output of 30 ml/hour is significant and warrants notifying the doctor immediately. The remaining options reflect normal assessment findings.

Nursing process step: Assessment
Client needs category: Physiological integrity
Client needs subcategory: Physiological adaptation
Taxonomic level: Application

59. *Correct answer:* **A**

To prevent the spread of microorganisms, the nurse always should wash her hands before providing patient care. The remaining options reflect correct technique but should be performed after hand washing.

Nursing process step: Implementation
Client needs category: Safe, effective care environment
Client needs subcategory: Safety and infection control
Taxonomic level: Knowledge

60. *Correct answer:* **C**

Experimental data suggest that cyclosporine inhibits helper T cells and suppressor T cells.

Nursing process step: Assessment
Client needs category: Physiological integrity
Client needs subcategory: Pharmacological and parenteral therapies
Taxonomic level: Knowledge

61. *Correct answer:* **D**

An interaction between cyclosporine and erythromycin may increase the serum cyclosporine level. There are no known interactions between cyclosporine and tetracycline, ampicillin, or penicillin.

Nursing process step: Assessment
Client needs category: Physiological integrity
Client needs subcategory: Pharmacological and parenteral therapies
Taxonomic level: Comprehension

62. *Correct answer:* **D**

The most severe adverse reaction to cyclosporine is nephrotoxicity, usually characterized by increased blood urea nitrogen and serum creatinine levels. Bone marrow suppression is an adverse reaction to the immunosuppressant azathioprine. Drug fever and pulmonary edema are adverse reactions that may occur with the immunosuppressant lymphocyte immune globulin.

Nursing process step: Assessment
Client needs category: Physiological integrity
Client needs subcategory: Pharmacological and parenteral therapies
Taxonomic level: Comprehension

CHAPTER 6

MUSCULOSKELETAL AND INTEGUMENTARY SYSTEMS

QUESTIONS

1. Which of the following deformities is described as a lateral curvature of the thoracic spine?

 A. kyphosis
 B. scoliosis
 C. lordosis
 D. genu valgum

SITUATION: *Cynthia Firestone, age 33, was involved in a house fire in which she suffered a burn injury to her left hand and arm. She was admitted to the hospital for wound care and fluid resuscitation.*

Questions 2 and 3 refer to this situation.

2. Ms. Firestone's burn is described as white and leathery with no blisters. Which degree of severity is this burn?

 A. first-degree burn
 B. second-degree burn
 C. third-degree burn
 D. fourth-degree burn

3. What is the most important, immediate goal of therapy for Ms. Firestone?

 A. maintaining fluid, electrolyte, and acid-base balance
 B. planning for rehabilitation and discharge
 C. providing emotional support to the patient and family
 D. preserving full range of motion to all affected joints

SITUATION: *A 28-year-old female nurse is seen in the employee health department for mild itching and rash of both hands.*

Questions 4 to 6 refer to this situation.

4. During the assessment interview, questions should focus on:

 A. possible medication allergies
 B. current life stressors she may be experiencing
 C. chemicals she may be using and use of latex gloves
 D. any recent changes made in laundry detergent or bath soap

5. Contact dermatitis is initially suspected. The diagnosis is confirmed if the rash appears:

    A. erythematous with raised papules
    B. dry and scaly with flaking skin
    C. inflamed with weeping and crusting lesions
    D. excoriated with multiple fissures

6. The rash's appearance confirms the diagnosis of contact dermatitis. This nurse will most likely be instructed to avoid using latex gloves and to treat the existing rash with:

    A. oral corticosteroids
    B. phototherapy
    C. topical corticosteroids
    D. lanolin-based hand cream

SITUATION: *Sydney Randolph, a 45-year-old automotive mechanic, comes to his doctor's office with a 20-year history of psoriasis vulgaris. He comes because the exacerbation of psoriasis on his hands is making it difficult for him to work.*

Questions 7 to 9 refer to this situation.

7. What type of skin lesion would the nurse see when inspecting Mr. Randolph's hands?

    A. multiple vesicles of which some may appear pustular
    B. depigmented white patches of skin that appear atrophied, with superficial ulcers
    C. scaly, erythematous patches that vary in size
    D. bright-red macules and papules with clearly demarcated margins

8. In the past, Mr. Randolph has used coal tar preparations to treat his skin lesions. He no longer finds this treatment effective. The nurse should question him to see if he is:

    A. removing loose scales before applying the coal tar cream
    B. applying the coal tar cream to surrounding tissue to prevent enlargement of lesions
    C. concurrently taking oral corticosteroids to enhance the coal tar's effectiveness
    D. applying the coal tar cream before work for all-day protection

9. Mr. Randolph tells the nurse that his finger joints are stiff and sore in the morning. The nurse should respond by:

A. inquiring further about this problem because psoriatic arthritis can accompany psoriasis vulgaris
B. suggesting he take aspirin for relief because it's probably early rheumatoid arthritis
C. validating his complaint but assuming it's a side effect of his vocation
D. asking him if he has been diagnosed or treated for carpal tunnel syndrome

SITUATION: *Jane Simon, a school cafeteria worker, comes to the doctor's office complaining of severe scalp itching. Upon inspection the nurse finds nail marks on the scalp and small, light-colored, round specks attached to the hair shafts close to the scalp.*

Questions 10 and 11 refer to this situation.

10. These findings suggest that Mrs. Simon suffers from:

A. scabies
B. head lice
C. tinea capitis
D. impetigo

11. To treat head lice, Mrs. Simon should be instructed to:

A. saturate her hair with vinegar for 30 minutes, massage vigorously, and then wash with hot water and shampoo
B. wash her hair with a pediculicide and then comb thoroughly with a fine-toothed comb
C. apply an antibacterial cream to scalp lesions
D. shave her head because that is the only way the problem can be completely eradicated

SITUATION: *Elva Martinez, age 75, is admitted to the hospital with a compression fracture of two vertebrae. After viewing spinal X-rays, the doctor diagnoses osteoporosis.*

Questions 12 and 13 refer to this situation.

12. Which of the following could have helped prevent osteoporosis in Mrs. Martinez?

A. postmenopausal hormone replacement therapy
B. increasing her daily calcium intake to 500 mg
C. a low-cholesterol diet
D. participating in sports, such as swimming, cycling, and golfing

13. Which of the following diagnostic tests would best evaluate the severity of Mrs. Martinez's osteoporosis?

    A. magnetic resonance imaging
    B. computed tomography scan
    C. dual-energy X-ray absorptiometry
    D. bone scan

SITUATION: *Mary Johnson, who has a history of severe osteoarthritis, has been admitted to the hospital for a right hip replacement.*

Questions 14 to 16 refer to this situation.

14. Ms. Johnson asks the nurse, "What's the difference between osteoarthritis and rheumatoid arthritis?" The nurse's response is correct when she states:

    A. "Osteoarthritis is a noninflammatory joint disease. Rheumatoid arthritis is an inflammatory joint disease."
    B. "Osteoarthritis and rheumatoid arthritis are very similar, but osteoarthritis affects the smaller joints and rheumatoid arthritis affects the larger, weight-bearing joints."
    C. "Osteoarthritis affects joints on both sides of the body, and rheumatoid arthritis is usually unilateral."
    D. "Osteoarthritis is more common in women, and rheumatoid arthritis is more common in men."

15. As the nurse develops a postoperative nursing care plan for Ms. Johnson, she knows that Ms. Johnson is at risk for developing complications associated with immobility. Which of the following is the most common postoperative complication of total hip replacement surgery?

    A. pneumonia
    B. thromboembolism
    C. hemorrhage
    D. wound infection

16. Postoperative care should include measures to prevent dislocation of Ms. Johnson's new hip prosthesis. Which of the following interventions would achieve this objective?

    A. keeping the affected leg in a position of adduction
    B. using pressure relief measures, other than turning, to prevent pressure ulcers
    C. placing the leg in abduction
    D. keeping the hip flexed by placing pillows under the patient's knee

SITUATION: *Arthur Brown, who is paraplegic due to a T6 spinal cord injury, is admitted the medical-surgical floor with a stage 4 pressure ulcer on his right hip. The doctor also suspects osteomyelitis.*

Questions 17 and 18 refer to this situation.

17. What are the characteristics of a stage 4 pressure ulcer?

   A. It is an area of nonblanching erythema.
   B. It is an area of skin loss involving the dermis with a shallow crater-like appearance.
   C. It is an area of full-thickness skin loss with a deep lesion that extends down through the subcutaneous tissue.
   D. It is an area of full-thickness skin loss with exposure of muscle tissue, the hip bone, and surrounding support structures.

18. Which of the following statements made by Mr. Brown in response to teaching indicates he understands how this episode of osteomyelitis will be treated?

   A. "I will probably need to have part of the bone — if not the entire hip joint — removed."
   B. "I will need I.V. antibiotic therapy for 4 to 6 weeks."
   C. "After a week on I.V. antibiotics, I will probably go home on oral antibiotics."
   D. "You will need to irrigate my wound with antibiotic solution, but I won't be on oral or intravenous antibiotics."

SITUATION: *Nick Smith, age 18, is admitted to the hospital with a possible fractured tibia. The doctor orders X-rays to determine the type and location of the fracture.*

Questions 19 and 20 refer to this situation.

19. The X-ray shows that the bone is in alignment but a fracture line extends around the ankle. This type of fracture is called a:

   A. comminuted fracture
   B. Colles' fracture
   C. transverse fracture
   D. greenstick fracture

20. Nick has a short leg cast applied. His mother is instructed how to perform cast care and neurovascular checks at home. She calls the emergency department 6 hours later and states her son's pain has increased, especially when his leg is elevated, and his pain is unrelieved by prescription analgesics. The nurse should:

A. instruct her to tell her son to keep his leg elevated and apply ice continuously

B. instruct her to call the doctor immediately

C. tell her this is normal and the pain should lessen in 24 to 48 hours

D. tell her to give ibuprofen (Motrin) with his pain medication to enhance its effectiveness

SITUATION: *Matti Cation is a 40-year-old patient recovering from a motor vehicle accident. She has fractures involving both legs and her pelvis. Skeletal traction was applied to her right femur.*

Questions 21 and 22 refer to this situation.

21. Ms. Cation asks the nurse why her leg is in skeletal traction instead of being placed in a cast. Which of the following would be the nurse's best response?

A. "A cast cannot be placed on your leg because of the location of the fracture."

B. "Your leg will be in traction until it heals so it remains in perfect alignment."

C. "Skeletal traction will align the bones so they can be surgically repaired using special nails and plates."

D. "All femoral fractures are treated with skeletal traction."

22. Ms. Cation becomes restless and confused 5 days after admission. She complains of dyspnea and her temperature is 103° F (39.4° C). These symptoms indicate she has probably developed:

A. an infection

B. atelectasis

C. pneumonia

D. fat embolism syndrome

SITUATION: *Jason Wilson, age 20, is having a synthetic fiberglass cast placed on his arm for a fractured radius.*

Questions 23 to 25 refer to this situation.

23. Ten minutes after the cast is placed on his arm, Jason complains of a heat sensation under the cast. The nurse should:

A. perform a neurovascular assessment of his fingers to make sure the cast is not too tight
B. suspect an allergic reaction to the cast material and alert the doctor immediately
C. explain that this is a normal thermal reaction that occurs while a synthetic cast is drying
D. apply ice immediately because the water used to moisten the cast material was too hot

24. To decrease the risk of compartment syndrome, Jason should be instructed to:

    A. elevate his arm
    B. wriggle his fingers frequently
    C. take a mild analgesic
    D. take frequent deep breaths

25. Jason returns 6 weeks later to have his cast removed. He should be instructed to call the doctor if:

    A. full range of motion and strength don't return within 2 to 4 weeks
    B. his wrist feels stiff and weak
    C. his hand is swollen in the morning
    D. his skin is very red, dry, and mottled

SITUATION: *Jim Smith, age 18, is evaluated for a knee injury. He states his knee swells after exercise and sometimes "catches" when attempting flexion.*

Questions 26 to 28 refer to this situation.

26. When the nurse flexes Jim's knee, she feels a grating sensation. This is called:

    A. kinesthesia
    B. claudication
    C. fasciculations
    D. crepitus

27. Which diagnostic test will most likely be ordered to evaluate the internal structures of the knee?

    A. myelogram
    B. magnetic resonance imaging (MRI)
    C. computed tomography (CT) scan
    D. gallium scan

28. A loose piece of cartilage is found in Jim's knee and arthroscopic removal is recommended. Jim agrees to have the surgical procedure and asks how long his recovery period will be. Which of the following patient-teaching responses is most accurate?

    A. "Bed rest will be necessary for 48 hours after surgery."
    B. "Non-weight-bearing walking with crutches will be necessary for 1 week."
    C. "A limited amount of walking will be allowed the first few days after surgery."
    D. "Normal activities may be resumed immediately."

SITUATION: *Pam Renfrue complains of numbness in her fingers and bilateral wrist pain that is at its worst when she awakes.*

Questions 29 and 30 refer to this situation.

29. The nurse asks her to perform Phalen's test—placing the backs of her hands together and flexing her wrists for 30 seconds. Which result would indicate the test was positive?

    A. pain in the wrists
    B. numbness in the thumb, index, and middle fingers
    C. muscle twitching of the inner wrists
    D. inability to maintain this position for the specified 30 seconds

30. Phalen's test is done to help diagnose carpal tunnel syndrome. Which of the following occupations would put Ms. Renfrue at risk for developing carpal tunnel syndrome?

    A. registered nurse
    B. day care provider
    C. waitress
    D. secretary

SITUATION: *Helen Sweeney is brought to the emergency department by ambulance after falling at home. X-rays confirm the diagnosis of displaced fracture of the neck of the left femur.*

Questions 31 to 34 refer to this situation.

31. As a result of this injury, Ms. Sweeney complains of severe pain in the hip region; concurrently, her left leg would be:

    A. internally rotated and shortened
    B. internally rotated and lengthened
    C. externally rotated and shortened
    D. externally rotated and lengthened

32. Which of the following interventions should be done first to mobilize Ms. Sweeney quickly and avoid medical complications?

    A. placing a sandbag or a trochanter roll on the outside of the leg
    B. scheduling early surgical intervention
    C. applying Buck's traction to her leg
    D. teaching her how to walk with crutches

33. Aseptic necrosis is a common complication after surgical repair of fractures of the neck of the femur because:

    A. the vascular supply may be damaged with the fracture
    B. the patient cannot bear any weight on the leg
    C. the patient is usually elderly
    D. surgical repair takes a long time

34. During her postoperative period, which of the following should Mrs. Sweeney be encouraged to do?

    A. decrease fluid intake to avoid the need to urinate
    B. perform foot flexion exercises to prevent clot formation
    C. stay in bed as much as possible to conserve energy
    D. avoid using assistive devices for walking

SITUATION: *Senior nursing students have been asked to present information about osteoporosis to a women's club. After researching the topic, they decide on the information they want to present.*

Questions 35 to 37 refer to this situation.

35. Risk factors associated with the development of osteoporosis include:

    A. being an overweight black American female
    B. being an underweight Caucasian female
    C. taking estrogen replacement therapy
    D. participating in an aerobic exercise program

36. A patient may have osteoporosis unknowingly because:

    A. most women die before it becomes a problem
    B. fractures resulting from osteoporosis are rare
    C. there is no way to determine the mineral content of bone
    D. there are no clear warning signs and symptoms

37. To prevent or treat osteoporosis, adequate calcium intake:

A. is essential throughout the life span
B. is only necessary after menopause
C. can only be obtained by supplements
D. is important only until bone density peaks

SITUATION: *John Sampson has had a below-the-knee amputation of the left leg. He was diagnosed with diabetes mellitus 20 years ago and has been treated for peripheral vascular disease for the last 5 years.*

Questions 38 to 40 refer to this situation.

38. Preparing Mr. Sampson, physically and psychologically, to cope with his life as an amputee should begin:

    A. when he arrives at a rehabilitation facility
    B. when the decision to amputate is made
    C. when he stops grieving over the loss of his leg
    D. when his need for pain medication decreases

39. Immediately after surgery, Mr. Sampson should be assessed for which of the following complications?

    A. a pressure ulcer on the stump
    B. excessive bleeding
    C. flexion contracture
    D. neuroma

40. Postoperative teaching for Mr. Sampson should include:

    A. telling him to avoid touching the stump
    B. instructing him to keep the stump elevated on a pillow
    C. stressing the importance of wrapping the stump with elastic bandages
    D. explaining that phantom limb pain will persist for the rest of his life

SITUATION: *William Leahy was diagnosed with osteoarthritis of his left hip 15 years ago. Since that time, he has been treated conservatively. Now his pain is almost constant and he is unable to do most of the activities that give quality to his life. He has been referred to an orthopedic surgeon for total hip replacement.*

Questions 41 to 44 refer to this situation.

41. Before surgery, Mr. Leahy donates 1 unit of blood that may be administered to him in the perioperative or postoperative period. This type of blood transfusion is called:

    A. homologous
    B. allogeneic
    C. leukocyte-poor
    D. autologous

42. For how long before surgery should the nurse tell Mr. Leahy to discontinue any drugs containing aspirin and nonsteroidal anti-inflammatory drugs?

    A. 7 to 10 days before surgery
    B. 2 days before surgery
    C. 3 to 5 days before surgery
    D. 30 days before surgery

43. Because of the high risk of deep vein thrombosis and pulmonary embolism after orthopedic surgery, Mr. Leahy is given the anticoagulant warfarin (Coumadin). The dosage of warfarin:

    A. varies, based on the partial thromboplastin time (PTT)
    B. varies, based on the prothrombin time (PT)
    C. is given I.V.
    D. is the same throughout the postoperative period

44. Mr. Leahy is taught hip dislocation precautions postoperatively. This includes cautioning him to:

    A. keep his knees lower than his hips when sitting
    B. bathe by sitting in the tub
    C. keep the knee of his operated leg rolled inward
    D. bend from the waist to put on socks and shoes

SITUATION: *Melvina Higgins, a 49-year-old merchandise buyer, fell at work and landed with full force on her outstretched right hand. She was brought to the hospital with a swollen, painful, and deformed right wrist. X-ray of the wrist revealed a displaced Colles' fracture. An unsuccessful attempt was made to reduce the displacement in the emergency department, so Mrs. Higgins was admitted for surgical repair.*

Questions 45 and 46 refer to this situation.

45. An external fixator was placed during surgery. The surgeon explains that this method of repair:

    A. has a very low complication rate
    B. maintains reduction and overall hand function
    C. is less bothersome than a cast
    D. is best for older people

46. Mrs. Higgins is discharged the day after surgery. Her discharge instructions should include:

    A. telling her not to use her right hand to avoid dislodging the external fixator pins

    B. explaining the need to keep her right hand elevated above her head at all times to reduce swelling

    C. telling her to report any increase in drainage from the pin sites

    D. explaining that she should expect swelling, redness, and pain around the pin sites

SITUATION: *During a touch football game, Andrew Peters is tackled and injures his left knee. His knee X-ray shows no bone damage. He is discharged with crutches. Because pain and swelling have persisted, he is scheduled for an anterior cruciate ligament repair.*

Questions 47 to 50 refer to this situation.

47. Immediately following soft tissue injury, the doctor prescribes treatment that follows the acronym "RICE," which stands for:

    A. Rest, Immobilization, Compression, Exercise

    B. Relax, Ice, Conserve energy, Elevation

    C. Rest, Ice, Compression, Elevation

    D. Rigid fixator, Immobilization, Compression, Exercise

48. Mr. Peters undergoes arthroscopy. Which of the following statements is true about arthroscopy?

    A. It involves injecting dye into a joint and taking X-rays.

    B. It is useful for diagnosing joint problems only.

    C. It is useful for diagnosing and treating joint conditions.

    D. It usually involves a lengthy hospitalization.

49. Mr. Peters suffered a tear of the anterior cruciate ligament. Ligaments function by connecting:

    A. bone to bone

    B. muscle to bone

    C. muscle to muscle

    D. tendons to bone

50. Following arthroscopy, discharge teaching for Mr. Peters should include monitoring and reporting:

A. decreased sensation below the knee
B. problems related to anesthesia
C. insomnia
D. weight gain

SITUATION: *Ida Bonsall, a 72-year-old patient, sustains a fracture of her right hip in a fall at a nursing home. Her surgery is delayed until she can be medically stabilized.*

Questions 51 and 52 refer to this situation.

51. Buck's traction is applied to Mrs. Bonsall's right leg. Which of the following is true about Buck's traction?

    A. The head of the bed should be elevated.
    B. Her heel should be resting on the bed.
    C. The use of an overhead trapeze should be discouraged.
    D. The leg in traction must not be elevated on a pillow.

52. The nurse should be aware of which of following when assessing Mrs. Bonsall?

    A. risk of skin breakdown
    B. risks associated with immobility
    C. risk of respiratory complications
    D. risk of venous thrombus formation

SITUATION: *Harry Ross has been undergoing conservative treatment for a herniated nucleus pulposus at L5 - S1, which was diagnosed by magnetic resonance imaging. Because of worsening symptoms, he required a lumbar laminectomy.*

Questions 53 to 55 refer to this situation.

53. While managing Mr. Ross postoperatively the nurse should:

    A. discourage him from doing any range-of-motion exercises
    B. have him sit up in a chair as much as possible
    C. logroll him from side to side
    D. elevate the head of his bed to a 90-degree angle

54. Because of the risk for nerve root injury during laminectomy surgery, Mr. Ross's neurovascular assessment:

    A. should be performed by the nurse every 2 hours for the first 24 hours
    B. should be performed only by the doctor
    C. is not reliable in identifying complications
    D. can be discontinued after 24 hours

55. Discharge teaching for Mr. Ross should emphasize that:

    A. strenuous exercise will strengthen the paraspinal muscles
    B. driving an automobile shouldn't cause problems
    C. rest periods are not necessary because resting causes loss of strength
    D. excessive activity could result in pain caused by spasm of the paraspinal muscles

SITUATION: *Anna Myers, age 76, is brought to the hospital by her daughter. Mrs. Myers spent a sleepless night after experiencing sudden, acute pain in her thoracic spine when she turned over in bed. X-rays reveal a compression fracture at the T6 level.*

    Questions 56 to 58 refer to this situation.

56. Before the doctor decides whether Mrs. Myers's fracture should be treated surgically or conservatively, he should perform an assessment to determine if the fracture is:

    A. stable or unstable
    B. caused by osteoporosis
    C. limited to one vertebrae
    D. interfering with her breathing

57. Mrs. Myers will be treated conservatively at home. Discharge instructions include remaining on bed rest for how long?

    A. 2 weeks
    B. until she can be admitted to a long-term care facility
    C. until she no longer needs analgesics
    D. until the acute pain subsides

58. Mrs. Myers and her daughter should be informed that the combination of bed rest and analgesics puts her at risk for developing:

    A. insomnia
    B. constipation
    C. indigestion
    D. pressure ulcers

ANSWER SHEET

	A B C D		A B C D		A B C D
1	○ ○ ○ ○	21	○ ○ ○ ○	41	○ ○ ○ ○
2	○ ○ ○ ○	22	○ ○ ○ ○	42	○ ○ ○ ○
3	○ ○ ○ ○	23	○ ○ ○ ○	43	○ ○ ○ ○
4	○ ○ ○ ○	24	○ ○ ○ ○	44	○ ○ ○ ○
5	○ ○ ○ ○	25	○ ○ ○ ○	45	○ ○ ○ ○
6	○ ○ ○ ○	26	○ ○ ○ ○	46	○ ○ ○ ○
7	○ ○ ○ ○	27	○ ○ ○ ○	47	○ ○ ○ ○
8	○ ○ ○ ○	28	○ ○ ○ ○	48	○ ○ ○ ○
9	○ ○ ○ ○	29	○ ○ ○ ○	49	○ ○ ○ ○
10	○ ○ ○ ○	30	○ ○ ○ ○	50	○ ○ ○ ○
11	○ ○ ○ ○	31	○ ○ ○ ○	51	○ ○ ○ ○
12	○ ○ ○ ○	32	○ ○ ○ ○	52	○ ○ ○ ○
13	○ ○ ○ ○	33	○ ○ ○ ○	53	○ ○ ○ ○
14	○ ○ ○ ○	34	○ ○ ○ ○	54	○ ○ ○ ○
15	○ ○ ○ ○	35	○ ○ ○ ○	55	○ ○ ○ ○
16	○ ○ ○ ○	36	○ ○ ○ ○	56	○ ○ ○ ○
17	○ ○ ○ ○	37	○ ○ ○ ○	57	○ ○ ○ ○
18	○ ○ ○ ○	38	○ ○ ○ ○	58	○ ○ ○ ○
19	○ ○ ○ ○	39	○ ○ ○ ○		
20	○ ○ ○ ○	40	○ ○ ○ ○		

ANSWERS AND RATIONALES

1. *Correct answer:* **B**

Scoliosis is a lateral deformity of the thoracic spine. This deformity becomes apparent during adolescence. Kyphosis is a vertical curvature of the spine, or "humpback." Lordosis is an increase in curvature of the lumbar spine. Genu valgum is internal angling of the knees, or "knock-knees."

> *Nursing process step:* Assessment
> *Client needs category:* Health promotion and maintenance
> *Client needs subcategory:* Prevention and early detection of disease
> *Taxonomic level:* Knowledge

2. *Correct answer:* **C**

First-degree burns are superficial and involve the epidermis only. There is local pain and redness but no blistering. Second-degree burns appear red and moist with blister formation and are painful. Third-degree burns may appear white, red, or black and are dry and leathery with no blisters. There may be little pain because nerve endings have been destroyed. Fourth-degree burns involve underlying muscle and bone tissue.

> *Nursing process step:* Assessment
> *Client needs category:* Physiological integrity
> *Client needs subcategory:* Physiological adaptation
> *Taxonomic level:* Knowledge

3. *Correct answer:* **A**

Although all of the goals are important, the most immediate and life-sustaining goal is to maintain fluid, electrolyte, and acid-base balance. This helps prevent potentially life-threatening complications, including shock, disseminated intravascular coagulation, respiratory failure, heart failure, and acute tubular necrosis.

> *Nursing process step:* Planning
> *Client needs category:* Physiological integrity
> *Client needs subcategory:* Reduction of risk potential
> *Taxonomic level:* Application

4. *Correct answer:* **C**

Because the itching and rash are localized, an environmental cause in the workplace should be suspected. With the advent of universal precautions, many nurses are experiencing allergies to latex gloves. Allergies to medications, laundry detergents, or bath soaps or a dermatologic reaction to stress usually elicit a more generalized or widespread rash.

Nursing process step: Assessment
Client needs category: Safe, effective care environment
Client needs subcategory: Safety and infection control
Taxonomic level: Comprehension

5. *Correct answer:* **A**

Contact dermatitis is caused by exposure to a physical or chemical allergen such as cleaning products, skin care products, and latex gloves. Initial symptoms of itching, erythema, and raised papules occur at the site of exposure and can begin within an hour of exposure. Allergic reactions tend to be red and not scaly or flaky. Weeping, crusting lesions are also uncommon unless the reaction is quite severe or has been present for a long time. Excoriation is more common in skin disorders associated with a moist environment.

Nursing process step: Assessment
Client needs category: Safe, effective care environment
Client needs subcategory: Safety and infection control
Taxonomic level: Application

6. *Correct answer:* **C**

Since the rash is still mild and limited to the hands and wrists, topical corticosteroids would be the treatment of choice. Oral corticosteroids are used for severe disorders that become systemic. Phototherapy is ineffective for contact dermatitis, and hand creams that decrease air exchange can prolong or worsen the rash.

Nursing process step: Planning
Client needs category: Physiological integrity
Client needs subcategory: Pharmacological and parenteral therapies
Taxonomic level: Application

7. *Correct answer:* **C**

Psoriasis vulgaris, a chronic condition, presents with scaly and erythematous patches of skin and is usually seen on the scalp, elbows, knees, and sacrum. The skin becomes thicker in these areas and may develop an overgrowth of skin at the site of previous injuries (Koebner's phenomenon). This may explain why Mr. Randolph's psoriasis is worse on his hands because the lesions are repeatedly abraded. Since this disease produces flakes or scales, vesicles would not be expected. Psoriatic lesions are irregular and poorly demarcated.

Nursing process step: Assessment
Client needs category: Physiological integrity
Client needs subcategory: Reduction of risk potential
Taxonomic level: Knowledge

8. *Correct answer:* **A**

Coal tar treatments are more effective if dead, scaly skin is first removed. Application should be restricted to the lesions because it can cause staining of surrounding skin. While psoriasis may be treated by topical or locally injected corticosteroids, systemic corticosteroids provide little or no benefit. Coal tar cream is best applied at bedtime to allow it to work overnight.

> *Nursing process step:* Evaluation
> *Client needs category:* Physiological integrity
> *Client needs subcategory:* Pharmacological and parenteral therapies
> *Taxonomic level:* Analysis

9. *Correct answer:* **A**

Anyone with psoriasis vulgaris who reports joint pain should be evaluated for psoriatic arthritis. Approximately 15% to 20% of individuals with psoriasis will also develop psoriatic arthritis, which can be painful and cause deformity. Carpal tunnel syndrome causes sensory and motor changes in the fingers rather than localized pain in the joints.

> *Nursing process step:* Assessment
> *Client needs category:* Physiological integrity
> *Client needs subcategory:* Reduction of risk potential
> *Taxonomic level:* Application

10. *Correct answer:* **B**

The light-colored spots attached to the hair shafts are nits, which are the eggs of head lice. They cannot be brushed off the hair shaft like dandruff. Scabies is a contagious dermatitis caused by the itch mite, *Sarcoptes scabiei,* which lives just beneath the skin. Tinea capitis, or ringworm, causes patchy hair loss and circular lesions with healing centers. Impetigo is an infection caused by *Staphylococcus* or *Streptococcus,* manifested by vesicles or pustules that form a thick, honey-colored crust.

> *Nursing process step:* Assessment
> *Client needs category:* Physiological integrity
> *Client needs subcategory:* Reduction of risk potential
> *Taxonomic level:* Knowledge

11. *Correct answer:* **B**

Mrs. Simon should be instructed to wash her hair with a pediculicide, an agent designed to kill lice. After shampooing she should comb her hair with a fine-toothed comb to remove the nits or eggs from the hair shafts. Shaving her head removes the lice and nits but is not a cosmetically pleasing way to eradicate the problem. Washing the hair with vinegar would be ineffective and could be irritating to scalp lesions. Antibacterials are also ineffective against lice infestation.

Nursing process step: Implementation
Client needs category: Physiological integrity
Client needs subcategory: Pharmacological and parenteral therapies
Taxonomic level: Application

12. *Correct answer:* A

Hormone replacement therapy using estrogen and progesterone has been found to significantly reduce postmenopausal bone loss. Calcium intake must be between 1,000 to 1,500 mg per day to obtain a beneficial effect. A low-cholesterol diet may reduce serum cholesterol levels, but it frequently eliminates calcium-rich foods, such as milk, cheese, and ice cream, from the diet. Weight-bearing sports, such as walking, aerobics, and weight lifting, are effective in minimizing bone loss; swimming, cycling, and golfing are not considered weight-bearing sports unless the golfer walks the course instead of riding in a cart.

Nursing process step: Evaluation
Client needs category: Physiological integrity
Client needs subcategory: Reduction of risk potential
Taxonomic level: Application

13. *Correct answer:* C

While all of the studies listed will give information about bone appearance and condition, dual-energy X-ray absorptiometry is the best tool for determining bone mass.

Nursing process step: Assessment
Client needs category: Physiological integrity
Client needs subcategory: Reduction of risk potential
Taxonomic level: Knowledge

14. *Correct answer:* A

Osteoarthritis is a degenerative disease characterized by loss of cartilage from articular surfaces of weight-bearing joints and spur development. Rheumatoid arthritis is characterized by inflammation of synovial membranes and surrounding structures of the joints. Osteoarthritis may occur in one hip or knee and not the other. Rheumatoid arthritis commonly affects the same joints bilaterally. Rheumatoid arthritis is more common in women, and osteoarthritis affects both sexes equally.

Nursing process step: Assessment
Client needs category: Physiological integrity
Client needs subcategory: Reduction of risk potential
Taxonomic level: Knowledge

15. *Correct answer:* **B**

Because most hip replacement surgery is done on elderly patients, the risk of complications, such as pneumonia, hemorrhage, and wound infection, is high. However, thromboemboli caused by impaired circulation due to immobility is the most common complication and accounts for greater than 50% of all postoperative deaths in this patient population.

> *Nursing process step:* Planning
> *Client needs category:* Physiological integrity
> *Client needs subcategory:* Reduction of risk potential
> *Taxonomic level:* Application

16. *Correct answer:* **C**

Positioning the patient so that the head of the prosthesis remains within the acetabular cup is vital. The leg should be placed in abduction to prevent dislocation, and flexion should be limited to 90 degrees or less. Internal rotation and adduction should be avoided. Postoperatively, total hip replacement patients may be turned onto their unaffected side. Maintaining hip flexion is not necessary.

> *Nursing process step:* Implementation
> *Client needs category:* Physiological integrity
> *Client needs subcategory:* Reduction of risk potential
> *Taxonomic level:* Application

17. *Correct answer:* **D**

A stage 4 pressure ulcer involves full-thickness skin loss with exposure of muscle, bone, and surrounding support structures. A stage 1 pressure ulcer appears as an nonblanching erythema of intact skin. A stage 2 pressure ulcer involves an area of skin loss that extends to the dermis and has a shallow crater-like appearance. A stage 3 pressure ulcer involves an area of full-thickness skin loss with a deep crater that extends down through the subcutaneous tissue.

> *Nursing process step:* Assessment
> *Client needs category:* Physiological integrity
> *Client needs subcategory:* Physiological adaptation
> *Taxonomic level:* Knowledge

18. *Correct answer:* **B**

Osteomyelitis is a very serious infection of the bone that is difficult to treat. Long-term I.V. antibiotics are needed to eradicate this type of infection. Oral antibiotics are inadequate. Wound irrigations with an antibiotic solution are also inadequate to treat this type of infection; however, they may be used as an adjunct to I.V. therapy. Infected bone may need to be removed in advanced cases.

Nursing process step: Evaluation
Client needs category: Physiological integrity
Client needs subcategory: Reduction of risk potential
Taxonomic level: Analysis

19. *Correct answer:* **C**

A fracture straight across a bone is a transverse, or linear, fracture. A comminuted fracture produces more than one fracture line as well as displaced bone fragments. Colles' fractures and greenstick fractures do not extend through the entire diameter of the bone. Colles' fractures occur in the wrist and cause a "dinner fork" deformity (proximal depression and fullness in the distal aspect of the wrist). In a greenstick fracture, one side of the bone is broken while the other side is deformed.

Nursing process step: Assessment
Client needs category: Physiological integrity
Client needs subcategory: Physiological adaptation
Taxonomic level: Knowledge

20. *Correct answer:* **B**

A significant increase in pain that is unrelieved by analgesics and worsened by elevation of the extremity indicates compartment syndrome. This is a serious complication caused by bleeding and swelling that must be treated within 6 hours to prevent irreversible ischemia of the leg. The doctor must be notified immediately, and actions must be taken to relieve the pressure.

Nursing process step: Implementation
Client needs category: Physiological integrity
Client needs subcategory: Reduction of risk potential
Taxonomic level: Analysis

21. *Correct answer:* **C**

Skeletal traction is used to align the bone fracture before surgery. Surgical repair involves internal fixation with intramedullary nails and plates. Since surgical repair has become a treatment option it is no longer necessary to leave a patient in skeletal traction until a femoral fracture is completely healed. Nondisplaced or internally fixated femur fractures may be placed in a long leg cast until healing is complete.

Nursing process step: Implementation
Client needs category: Physiological integrity
Client needs subcategory: Reduction of risk potential
Taxonomic level: Comprehension

22. *Correct answer:* **D**

The symptoms described indicate that fat emboli have escaped from the bone fractures and are becoming lodged in the pulmonary circulation. Fat emboli can be fatal. Multiple long-bone fractures increase the risk of fat emboli. While some of the symptoms may indicate infection, pneumonia, or atelectasis, the combination of symptoms in this high-risk individual makes the diagnosis of fat embolism most likely.

> *Nursing process step:* Assessment
> *Client needs category:* Physiological integrity
> *Client needs subcategory:* Physiological adaptation
> *Taxonomic level:* Analysis

23. *Correct answer:* **C**

A thermal reaction is normal when a synthetic cast is applied. Once the cast has dried, the heat sensation should disappear. Normal drying time is about 20 minutes. A routine neurovascular assessment should be performed when the cast is applied and periodically after the cast has dried.

> *Nursing process step:* Implementation
> *Client needs category:* Physiological integrity
> *Client needs subcategory:* Reduction of risk potential
> *Taxonomic level:* Application

24. *Correct answer:* **A**

Compartment syndrome can be caused by swelling that occurs under a cast. The pressure may increase to the point of interfering with circulation. Elevating the extremity should help reduce the amount of swelling that develops. Wriggling the fingers will increase circulation to the fingers but will not decrease swelling. The patient should be instructed to take a mild analgesic, if necessary. Taking frequent deep breaths will do nothing to prevent compartment syndrome.

> *Nursing process step:* Implementation
> *Client needs category:* Physiological integrity
> *Client needs subcategory:* Reduction of risk potential
> *Taxonomic level:* Application

25. *Correct answer:* **A**

Physical therapy provided by a therapist or the patient should re-establish full range of motion of the wrist in 2 to 4 weeks. Continued stiffness or weakness may indicate an undiagnosed injury or ineffective physical therapy. Wrist weakness and stiffness, morning swelling, and red, dry, mottled skin are all normal sequelae of cast removal.

Nursing process step: Implementation
Client needs category: Physiological integrity
Client needs subcategory: Reduction of risk potential
Taxonomic level: Application

26. *Correct answer:* **D**

Crepitus is the grating sound and feeling of a joint that has irregular articular surfaces or a foreign body in the joint space. Fasciculation is muscle twitching. Kinesthesia is the ability to determine the position of an extremity. Claudication is pain felt in the calf muscles during exercise if there is impaired circulation of the lower extremity.

Nursing process step: Assessment
Client needs category: Physiological integrity
Client needs subcategory: Reduction of risk potential
Taxonomic level: Knowledge

27. *Correct answer:* **B**

Since the meniscus (internal structure of the knee) is composed of cartilage, an MRI will probably be ordered. MRIs are appropriate when diagnosing abnormalities of tendons, ligaments, and cartilage. Myelograms are specific for diagnosing spinal disorders. CT scans are helpful in diagnosing bone and soft tissue tumors and spinal fractures. Gallium scans provide imaging of bone abnormalities, such as malignancies, osteomyelitis, and osteoporosis.

Nursing process step: Planning
Client needs category: Physiological integrity
Client needs subcategory: Reduction of risk potential
Taxonomic level: Application

28. *Correct answer:* **C**

A limited amount of walking on the operated extremity is allowed during the immediate postoperative period. Excessive exercise should be avoided for several days to allow healing and decrease edema and hematoma formation.

Nursing process step: Planning
Client needs category: Physiological integrity
Client needs subcategory: Reduction of risk potential
Taxonomic level: Application

29. *Correct answer:* **B**

Numbness in the thumb, index, and middle fingers is considered a positive Phalen's sign. While the other reactions may also be abnormal, Phalen's test is

specific for nerve compression in the wrists that precipitates numbness in associated fingers.

> *Nursing process step:* Assessment
> *Client needs category:* Physiological integrity
> *Client needs subcategory:* Reduction of risk potential
> *Taxonomic level:* Comprehension

30. *Correct answer:* **D**

Occupations that require repetitive movements of the wrists such as typing or
keyboarding can precipitate the development of carpal tunnel syndrome.
Assessment of occupational tasks is an important part of diagnosing carpal tunnel syndrome.

> *Nursing process step:* Assessment
> *Client needs category:* Physiological integrity
> *Client needs subcategory:* Reduction of risk potential
> *Taxonomic level:* Comprehension

31. *Correct answer:* **C**

When the femur is fractured, the hip rotates externally and the leg shortens in
comparison to the unaffected side.

> *Nursing process step:* Assessment
> *Client needs category:* Physiological integrity
> *Client needs subcategory:* Physiological adaptation
> *Taxonomic level:* Knowledge

32. *Correct answer:* **B**

Early surgical intervention is necessary to encourage early mobilization and prevent complications of immobility. Buck's traction, sandbags, or trochanter rolls
may be used to reduce muscle spasm and pain until the fracture can be repaired;
crutch walking on an unrepaired fracture would be contraindicated.

> *Nursing process step:* Implementation
> *Client needs category:* Physiological integrity
> *Client needs subcategory:* Reduction of risk potential
> *Taxonomic level:* Knowledge

33. *Correct answer:* **A**

Fractures that occur within the capsule around the neck of the femur usually
cause damage to the blood supply and bone cells may die (necrose) from lack of
nutrients. Patients can be mobilized very soon after surgical repair of hip fractures. In elderly people, intertrochanteric fractures are more common than fractures of the neck of the femur. The length of surgery does not affect the ability of
the bone to heal.

Nursing process step: Assessment
Client needs category: Physiological integrity
Client needs subcategory: Reduction of risk potential
Taxonomic level: Knowledge

34. *Correct answer:* **B**

Foot flexion exercises should be done hourly, while awake, to avoid venous stasis and thromboembolism. Ambulation with a walker or crutches is encouraged to avoid complications of inactivity; adequate hydration is encouraged, and patients are taught to transfer to a commode or toilet to urinate.

Nursing process step: Planning
Client needs category: Physiological integrity
Client needs subcategory: Reduction of risk potential
Taxonomic level: Application

35. *Correct answer:* **B**

Underweight people place less load stress on bones than heavy people, which results in less bone mass. Blacks have a higher mineral content in their bones than whites. Replacing estrogen and participating in weight-bearing aerobic exercises help to prevent osteoporosis.

Nursing process step: Assessment
Client needs category: Health promotion and maintenance
Client needs subcategory: Prevention and early detection of disease
Taxonomic level: Knowledge

36. *Correct answer:* **D**

There are no clear signs and symptoms of early osteoporosis. Many people are not diagnosed until they sustain a fracture. Fractures from osteoporosis are increasing as life expectancy increases. Mineral content can be measured by bone densitometry studies, which are useful for people with multiple risk factors and to assess response to treatment.

Nursing process step: Assessment
Client needs category: Health promotion and maintenance
Client needs subcategory: Prevention and early detection of disease
Taxonomic level: Knowledge

37. *Correct answer:* **A**

Adequate calcium intake is essential during childhood, adolescence, and early adulthood to maximize bone density. Later in life, continued calcium intake can minimize bone loss. Dietary intake of calcium-rich foods and calcium-fortified foods is important for all age groups; supplementation may be necessary in some cases.

> *Nursing process step:* Planning
> *Client needs category:* Physiological integrity
> *Client needs subcategory:* Basic care and comfort
> *Taxonomic level:* Knowledge

38. *Correct answer:* **B**

Prior to surgery, the patient should begin exercises to strengthen the muscles of the upper extremities and shoulders, and he should learn crutch-walking. The home setting should be assessed and modified as needed for safety and mobility, and a discharge plan should be made. This positive attitude toward independent self-care should continue during the immediate postoperative period and rehabilitation process.

> *Nursing process step:* Planning
> *Client needs category:* Psychosocial integrity
> *Client needs subcategory:* Coping and adaptation
> *Taxonomic level:* Application

39. *Correct answer:* **B**

The nurse should assess the patient for excessive bleeding that may occur immediately after surgery. Pressure ulcers, flexion contracture, and neuroma are also complications that may occur after a below-the-knee amputation, but they do not occur immediately. Pressure ulcers on the stump would occur after ambulation with a prosthesis. Flexion contractures might develop because of prolonged hip flexion, either in bed or when crutch-walking. A neuroma sometimes develops at the site of an amputated nerve.

> *Nursing process step:* Assessment
> *Client needs category:* Physiological integrity
> *Client needs subcategory:* Reduction of risk potential
> *Taxonomic level:* Knowledge

40. *Correct answer:* **C**

Elastic bandages are commonly used to control edema and to shape the limb for a prosthesis. The patient should be taught how to wrap the stump. Patients are taught to massage the stump area to help desensitize it and to break down scar tissue. Elevating the stump on a pillow may cause flexion contraction of the hip and interfere with rehabilitation. The patient should be reassured that phantom limb sensations eventually disappear.

> *Nursing process step:* Planning
> *Client needs category:* Physiological integrity
> *Client needs subcategory:* Reduction of risk potential
> *Taxonomic level:* Knowledge

41. *Correct answer:* **D**

Autologous blood transfusion is the reinfusion of the patient's own blood. Allogeneic blood transfusion is the infusion of banked blood that has been tested to be compatible with the patient's blood. This is also called homologous blood transfusion. Leukocyte-poor red blood cells have been washed with saline to remove leukocytes and most of the plasma to reduce the risk of febrile, nonhemolytic reactions.

Nursing process step: Implementation
Client needs category: Physiological integrity
Client needs subcategory: Reduction of risk potential
Taxonomic level: Knowledge

42. *Correct answer:* **A**

Patients are instructed to discontinue — for 7 to 10 days prior to surgery — medications that may increase intraoperative and postoperative bleeding. Clotting factors should return to normal in that amount of time.

Nursing process step: Planning
Client needs category: Physiological integrity
Client needs subcategory: Reduction of risk potential
Taxonomic level: Application

43. *Correct answer:* **B**

Warfarin can have a variable dose response and requires close monitoring of PT. PTT is the laboratory study used to assess response to heparin. Warfarin is administered by mouth.

Nursing process step: Implementation
Client needs category: Physiological integrity
Client needs subcategory: Pharmacological and parenteral therapies
Taxonomic level: Knowledge

44. *Correct answer:* **A**

Hip dislocation precautions include not having the knees higher than the hips when sitting. Walk-in showers are recommended, but patients should not sit in a tub until the hip is healed. Rolling the knee inward puts the leg in adduction and could cause the hip to dislocate. Patients should not bend over past 90 degrees, so they are taught to use assistive devices to put on socks and shoes.

Nursing process step: Implementation
Client needs category: Physiological integrity
Client needs subcategory: Reduction of risk potential
Taxonomic level: Knowledge

45. *Correct answer:* **B**

Complex intra-articular fractures are repaired with external fixators because they have a better long-term outcome than those treated with casting. This is especially true in a young active patient. The incidence of complications, such as pin tract infections and neuritis, is 20 to 60%. Patients must be taught how to do pin care and assess for development of neurovascular complications.

> *Nursing process step:* Implementation
> *Client needs category:* Psychosocial integrity
> *Client needs subcategory:* Coping and adaptation
> *Taxonomic level:* Knowledge

46. *Correct answer:* **C**

Discharge instructions should include telling the patient to report drainage from the pin sites, which may indicate infection. Using the hand with the fixator in place will improve circulation and healing. The hand can be elevated for short periods above the heart to reduce mild edema, but it should not be elevated at all times. Swelling, redness, and pain are signs of infection and should be reported to the surgeon.

> *Nursing process step:* Planning
> *Client needs category:* Physiological integrity
> *Client needs subcategory:* Reduction of risk potential
> *Taxonomic level:* Knowledge

47. *Correct answer:* **C**

"RICE" is an acronym for Rest, Ice, Compression, Elevation. This is a conservative treatment for soft tissue injuries such as sprains.

> *Nursing process step:* Implementation
> *Client needs category:* Physiological integrity
> *Client needs subcategory:* Reduction of risk potential
> *Taxonomic level:* Knowledge

48. *Correct answer:* **C**

Arthroscopy is a surgical procedure that allows direct visualization inside the joint for diagnosis and treatment of tears, defects, or disease. It is usually done as an outpatient procedure.

> *Nursing process step:* Planning
> *Client needs category:* Physiological integrity
> *Client needs subcategory:* Reduction of risk potential
> *Taxonomic level:* Knowledge

49. *Correct answer:* **A**

Ligaments connect bone to bone and provide stability within a joint. Tendons connect muscle to bone.

> *Nursing process step:* Assessment
> *Client needs category:* Physiological integrity
> *Client needs subcategory:* Reduction of risk potential
> *Taxonomic level:* Knowledge

50. *Correct answer:* **A**

Decreased sensation would indicate the development of a problem affecting the nerves that travel through the knee and enervate the lower leg. Prompt intervention could minimize long-term deficits. Problems associated with anesthesia would be assessed before discharge. Insomnia and weight gain would not be directly related to the arthroscopic procedure.

> *Nursing process step:* Planning
> *Client needs category:* Physiological integrity
> *Client needs subcategory:* Reduction of risk potential
> *Taxonomic level:* Application

51. *Correct answer:* **D**

Elevating the leg on a pillow would reduce the effect of the traction in maintaining alignment of the fractured bone and reducing muscle spasm and pain. All pressure areas should be avoided, and the heel should be off the bed. Using an overhead trapeze will provide the patient with some independence. The head of the bed should not be elevated in Buck's traction.

> *Nursing process step:* Implementation
> *Client needs category:* Physiological integrity
> *Client needs subcategory:* Reduction of risk potential
> *Taxonomic level:* Knowledge

52. *Correct answer:* **B**

Immobility puts the patient at risk for the development of complications of all body systems.

> *Nursing process step:* Assessment
> *Client needs category:* Physiological integrity
> *Client needs subcategory:* Reduction of risk potential
> *Taxonomic level:* Application

53. *Correct answer:* **C**

Logrolling the patient maintains alignment of his hips and shoulders and eliminates spinal twisting in the operative area. The patient should sit up in a chair or with the head of the bed elevated only for short periods, because this puts pressure on the operative area. Range-of-motion exercises should be encouraged to maintain muscle strength.

> *Nursing process step:* Planning
> *Client needs category:* Physiological integrity
> *Client needs subcategory:* Reduction of risk potential
> *Taxonomic level:* Knowledge

54. *Correct answer:* A

Sensory and motor function of both lower extremities should be assessed by the nurse every 2 hours for the first 24 hours postoperatively and every 4 hours for the next 24 to 48 hours.

> *Nursing process step:* Assessment
> *Client needs category:* Physiological integrity
> *Client needs subcategory:* Reduction of risk potential
> *Taxonomic level:* Application

55. *Correct answer:* D

Healing of the paraspinal muscles takes up to 6 weeks. During that time activity should be increased gradually, as the patient tolerates. Driving an automobile produces flexion strain on the spine and should be delayed for about 4 to 6 weeks. Rest periods promote healing and decrease pain related to spasm.

> *Nursing process step:* Planning
> *Client needs category:* Physiological integrity
> *Client needs subcategory:* Reduction of risk potential
> *Taxonomic level:* Application

56. *Correct answer:* A

An unstable fracture would carry the risk of causing nerve damage and should be treated surgically with open reduction and fixation. A stable compression fracture, with damage limited to either the anterior or posterior structures, would be treated conservatively.

> *Nursing process step:* Planning
> *Client needs category:* Physiological integrity
> *Client needs subcategory:* Reduction of risk potential
> *Taxonomic level:* Knowledge

57. *Correct answer:* D

Pain increases with movement, coughing, or weight bearing. Bed rest until acute pain subsides will promote healing. Mrs. Myers will require analgesics for several weeks, although the frequency will decrease as healing takes place. Compression fracture is not an indication for placement in a long-term care facility.

Nursing process step: Planning
Client needs category: Physiological integrity
Client needs subcategory: Reduction of risk potential
Taxonomic level: Knowledge

58. *Correct answer:* **B**

Patients taking pain medication frequently for long periods should be warned of the risk of constipation. Increasing fluid intake, eating fiber-rich foods, and using a stool softener should be recommended.

Nursing process step: Planning
Client needs category: Physiological integrity
Client needs subcategory: Pharmacological and parenteral therapies
Taxonomic level: Knowledge

CHAPTER 7

ENDOCRINE AND REPRODUCTIVE SYSTEMS

QUESTIONS

1. Delores Rich, a 62-year-old patient, is diagnosed with pyelonephritis and possible septicemia. She had five urinary tract infections over the past 2 years. She's fatigued from lack of sleep; urinates frequently, even overnight; and has lost weight recently. Tests reveal the following: a sodium level of 152 mEq/L, osmolality of 340 mOsm/L, a blood glucose level of 125 mg/dl, and a potassium level of 3.8 mEq/L. Which diagnosis is appropriate for this patient?

    A. Fluid volume deficit related to inability to conserve water
    B. Altered nutrition: less than body requirements related to hypermetabolic state
    C. Fluid volume deficit related to osmotic diuresis induced by hyponatremia
    D. Altered nutrition: less than body requirements related to catabolic effects of insulin deficiency

SITUATION: *Sheila O'Brien is admitted to the hospital with a serum glucose level of 618 mg/dl. She's awake and oriented, with hot, dry skin; a temperature of 100.6° F (38.1° C); a heart rate of 116 beats/minute, and a blood pressure of 108/70 mm Hg.*

Questions 2 to 5 refer to this situation.

2. Based on Ms. O'Brien's assessment findings, which nursing diagnosis takes highest priority?

    A. Fluid volume deficit related to osmotic diuresis
    B. Decreased cardiac output related to elevated heart rate
    C. Altered nutrition: less than body requirements related to insulin deficiency
    D. Ineffective thermoregulation related to dehydration

3. The nurse should include which instruction when teaching Ms. O'Brien about insulin administration?

    A. "Administer insulin after the first meal of the day."
    B. "Administer insulin at a 45-degree angle into the deltoid muscle."
    C. "Shake the vial of insulin vigorously before withdrawing the medication."
    D. "Draw up clear insulin first when mixing two types of insulin in one syringe."

4. When teaching Ms. O'Brien about insulin therapy, the nurse should instruct her to avoid which over-the-counter preparation that can interact with insulin?

    A. Antacids

    B. Acetaminophen preparations

    C. Vitamins with iron

    D. Salicylate preparations

5. Ms. O'Brien's family should be taught to recognize which signs and symptoms of hypoglycemia?

    A. Polyuria, headache, and fatigue

    B. Polyphagia and flushed, dry skin

    C. Polydipsia, pallor, and irritability

    D. Nervousness, diaphoresis, and confusion

SITUATION: *Claire Mullen, age 63, has type 2 diabetes mellitus. Diet and exercise fail to control her blood glucose level, so she has started taking an oral antidiabetic drug.*

Questions 6 to 8 refer to this situation.

6. Glipizide (Glucotrol) is prescribed for Mrs. Mullen. After oral administration, glipizide acts in:

    A. 20 to 30 minutes.

    B. 30 to 60 minutes.

    C. 1 to 1½ hours.

    D. 2 to 3 hours.

7. The nurse teaches Mrs. Mullen to recognize and report adverse drug reactions. Mrs. Mullen is most likely to experience which adverse reaction to glipizide?

    A. Headache

    B. Constipation

    C. Hypotension

    D. Photosensitivity

8. After taking glipizide for 9 months, Mrs. Mullen experiences secondary failure. Her doctor will most likely:

    A. initiate insulin therapy.

    B. switch her to a different oral antidiabetic drug.

    C. prescribe an additional oral antidiabetic drug.

    D. restrict her carbohydrate intake to less than 30% of the total caloric intake.

SITUATION: *Nancy Nesbit, age 68, is admitted with a tentative diagnosis of hyperosmolar hyperglycemic nonketotic syndrome. Her medical history reveals that she has type 2 diabetes that is being controlled with the oral antidiabetic drug tolazamide.*

Questions 9 to 11 refer to this situation.

9. The nurse anticipates that the most important laboratory test for confirming a diagnosis of hyperosmolar hyperglycemic nonketotic syndrome (HHNS) is:

    A. serum potassium level.
    B. serum sodium level.
    C. arterial blood gas (ABG) values.
    D. serum osmolarity.

10. Ms. Nesbit requires fluid resuscitation. Which statement about fluid replacement is true for the patient with hyperosmolar hyperglycemic nonketotic syndrome?

    A. Administer 2 to 3 L of I.V. fluid rapidly.
    B. Administer 6 L of I.V. fluid over the first 24 hours.
    C. Administer a dextrose solution containing normal saline solution.
    D. Administer I.V. fluid slowly to prevent circulatory overload and collapse.

11. Ms. Nesbit's condition is stabilized, and she's prepared for discharge. The nurse develops a teaching plan to prepare her for discharge and home management. Which statement indicates that the patient understands her condition and the preventive measures to control it?

    A. "I can avoid getting sick by not becoming dehydrated and by paying attention to my need to urinate, drink, or eat more than usual."
    B. "If I experience trembling, weakness, and headache, I should drink a glass of soda that contains sugar."
    C. "I'll have to monitor my blood glucose level closely and notify the doctor if it's constantly elevated."
    D. "If I begin to feel especially hungry and thirsty, I'll eat a snack high in carbohydrates."

SITUATION: *Barbara Bellet, age 35, was admitted to the hospital to have a pituitary tumor removed. After surgery, she developed diabetes insipidus, a common complication of this surgery.*

Questions 12 to 14 refer to this situation.

12. The nurse should expect to administer which drug to treat Ms. Bellet's diabetes insipidus?

    A. Vasopressin (Pitressin)
    B. Furosemide (Lasix)
    C. Regular insulin (Humulin R)
    D. Dextrose 10% in water

13. Which outcome indicates that treatment for Ms. Bellet's diabetes insipidus has been effective?

    A. Fluid intake of less than 2,500 ml in 24 hours
    B. Urine output of more than 200 ml/hour
    C. Blood pressure of 90/50 mm Hg
    D. Pulse rate of 126 beats/minute

14. A nursing diagnosis of risk for fluid volume excess related to aggressive fluid resuscitation is appropriate for Ms. Bellet because she requires water replacement. When the nurse evaluates her response to water replacement, which signs and symptoms would indicate water intoxication?

    A. Confusion and seizures
    B. Sunken eyeballs and spasticity
    C. Flaccidity and thirst
    D. Tetany and increased blood urea nitrogen levels

SITUATION: *Julie Kramer is a 36-year-old mother of three children, ages 4, 7, and 10. During her last breast self-examination, which she only does sporadically, she noticed a lump in the upper outer quadrant of her left breast. Her family medical history indicates that her mother and her oldest sister had breast cancer. Her personal history includes menarche at age 15, para 4, gravida 3, with one pregnancy ending in spontaneous abortion at 7 weeks. Mammography and fine-needle biopsy confirm medullary carcinoma of the breast.*

Questions 15 to 19 refer to this situation.

15. Which factor in Mrs. Kramer's history indicates that she's at increased risk for breast cancer?

    A. Spontaneous abortion
    B. Breast cancer in her mother and sister
    C. Late menarche
    D. Her age during pregnancies

16. The cancer is measured at 3.5 cm. After discussion with the health care team and her husband, Mrs. Kramer decides to have a modified radical mastectomy, which includes axillary node removal, and immediate reconstruction. The axillary nodes will be removed in order to:

    A. prevent metastases.
    B. facilitate postoperative recovery.
    C. facilitate breast reconstruction.
    D. provide prognostic information.

17. Postoperatively, blood pressure should be measured from the right arm, and Mrs. Kramer should keep her left arm and hand elevated as much as possible to prevent:

    A. lymphedema.
    B. Trousseau's sign.
    C. I.V. infusion infiltration.
    D. muscle atrophy related to immobility.

18. On discharge, Mrs. Kramer expresses relief that "the cancer" has been treated. When discussing this issue with Mrs. Kramer, the nurse should stress that she:

    A. should continue to perform breast self-examination (BSE) on her right breast.
    B. is lucky that the cancer was caught in time.
    C. should schedule a follow-up appointment in 6 months.
    D. will have irregular menstrual periods.

19. Mrs. Kramer's most effective coping mechanism is meditation and walking. The nurse encourages her to continue these activities and suggests that she contact:

    A. Reach to Recovery.
    B. a psychiatrist.
    C. a dietitian.
    D. an aerobic-exercise instructor.

SITUATION: *Ana Cruz is a 76-year-old retired widow who has been diagnosed with breast cancer. Hormone therapy, specifically tamoxifen citrate (Nolvadex), is being considered.*

Questions 20 to 22 refer to this situation.

20. For tamoxifen therapy to be considered, Mrs. Cruz must:

    A. be a premenopausal female.
    B. have a tumor that is progesterone-receptor positive.
    C. have a tumor that is estrogen-receptor positive.
    D. not have axillary nodal involvement.

21. Mrs. Cruz is dating a man from her bridge group, and they're considering marriage. She asks if tamoxifen will affect her sex life. The nurse should counsel her that tamoxifen will:

    A. have no effect on her sex life.
    B. most likely cause vaginal dryness.
    C. cause menstruation to restart.
    D. not have any adverse effects.

22. Mrs. Cruz should be counseled to have an annual Papanicolaou (Pap) test and pelvic examination because she:

    A. will have vaginal dryness.
    B. is planning to resume sexual relations.
    C. is at higher risk for endometrial cancer.
    D. is at higher risk for vaginal cancer.

SITUATION: *Eva Lamont, a 58-year-old female computer programmer, complains of anxiety, insomnia, weight loss, and the inability to concentrate. She also complains that her eyes feel "gritty." Thyroid function tests show the following levels: thyroid stimulating hormone, 0.02 µU/ml; thyroxine, 20 µg/dl; and triiodothyronine, 253 ng/dl. A 6-hour radioactive iodine uptake showed a diffuse uptake of 85%.*

    Questions 23 to 26 refer to this situation.

23. Mrs. Lamont's symptoms and laboratory findings are consistent with which diagnosis?

    A. Thyroiditis
    B. Grave's disease
    C. Hashimoto's disease
    D. Multinodular goiter

24. Mrs. Lamont requires a subtotal thyroidectomy. Before surgery she's given potassium iodide (Lugol's solution) and propylthiouracil (PTU). She should be instructed that these drugs will relieve her symptoms:

    A. in a few days.
    B. in 3 to 4 months.
    C. immediately.
    D. in 1 to 2 weeks.

25. For the first 72 hours after a thyroidectomy, the nurse should use Chvostek's and Trousseau's signs to assess Mrs. Lamont for:

A. hypocalcemia.
B. hypercalcemia.
C. hypokalemia.
D. hyperkalemia.

26. Discharge teaching for Mrs. Lamont must include which instruction?

A. How to keep an accurate record of her intake and output
B. How to use nasal desmopressin acetate (DDAVP)
C. Importance of regular follow-up care
D. Importance of exercise to improve cardiovascular fitness

SITUATION: *Mary Lynne Anderson, a 73-year-old patient, has been diagnosed with Hashimoto's disease, an autoimmune disorder.*

Questions 27 to 31 refer to this situation.

27. Mrs. Anderson exhibited which signs and symptoms that lead to the diagnosis of Hashimoto's disease?

A. Weight loss, increased appetite, and hyperdefecation
B. Weight loss, increased urination, and increased thirst
C. Weight gain, decreased appetite, and constipation
D. Weight gain, increased urination, and purplish red striae

28. Ms. Anderson probably exhibited which of the following laboratory test values for thyroxine (T_4), triiodothyronine (T_3), and thyroid stimulating hormone (TSH)?

A. T_4, 22 μg/dl; T_3, 320 ng/dl; TSH, undetectable
B. T_4, 22 μg/dl; T_3, 15 ng/dl; TSH 45 μU/ml
C. T_4, 2μ/dl, T_3, 35 ng/dl; TSH undetectable
D. T_4, 2μ/dl; T_3, 35 ng/dl; TSH, 45 μU/ml

29. Mrs. Anderson has a history of two myocardial infarctions and coronary artery disease. Because of her cardiac history, the nurse should instruct Mrs. Anderson that her thyroid replacement dose of levothyroxine (Synthroid) will be:

A. 25 g/day, initially.
B. 100 g/day, initially.
C. delayed until after thyroid surgery.
D. initiated prior to thyroid surgery.

30. Mrs. Anderson develops flulike symptoms and forgets to take her thyroid replacement medicine. Skipping her medication will put her at risk for which life-threatening complication?

A. Exophthalmos
B. Thyroid storm
C. Myxedema coma
D. Tibial myxedema

31. Mrs. Anderson is admitted to the hospital with myxedema coma. The most critical nursing intervention for the patient at this time is:

A. administering an oral dose of levothyroxine (Synthroid).
B. warming the patient with a warming blanket.
C. measuring and recording intake and output accurately.
D. maintaining a patent airway.

SITUATION: *Ruth Hunsberger is a 68-year-old patient who has been complaining of sleeping more and having anorexia, weakness, irritability, depression, bone pain, and increased urination. Because of her pain, she rarely goes outdoors.*

Questions 32 to 36 refer to this situation.

32. Based on these signs and symptoms, Ms. Hunsberger most likely has:

A. diabetes mellitus.
B. diabetes insipidus.
C. hypoparathyroidism.
D. hyperparathyroidism.

33. While preparing to teach Ms. Hunsberger about hyperparathyroidism, the nurse knows that parathyroid hormone (PTH) has what effect in the kidney?

A. PTH stimulates calcium reabsorption and phosphate excretion.
B. PTH stimulates phosphate reabsorption and calcium excretion.
C. PTH increases absorption of vitamin D and excretion of vitamin E.
D. PTH increases absorption of vitamin E and excretion of vitamin D.

34. Ms. Hunsberger's laboratory findings would include which finding?

A. Hypocalcemia
B. Hypercalcemia
C. Hyperphosphatemia
D. Hypophosphaturia

35. When instructing Ms. Hunsberger about her diet, the nurse should stress the importance of:

A. restricting fluids.
B. restricting sodium.
C. forcing fluids.
D. restricting potassium.

36. Ms. Hunsberger decides against parathyroid surgery at this time. Her medical management will include hormone replacement therapy with estrogen and progesterone. In addition to forcing fluids, the nurse should encourage her to:

A. develop and maintain a moderate exercise program.
B. rest as much as possible.
C. lose weight.
D. develop and maintain a vigorous exercise program.

SITUATION: *Heather Gibson, a 35-year-old patient, complains of weight gain, facial hair, absent menstruation, frequent bruising, and acne. The doctor's diagnosis is Cushing's syndrome.*

Questions 37 to 40 refer to this situation.

37. Mrs. Gibson's Cushing's syndrome was most likely caused by:

A. an ectopic corticotropin-secreting tumor.
B. adrenal carcinoma.
C. a corticotropin-secreting pituitary adenoma.
D. an inborn error of metabolism.

38. Mrs. Gibson is diagnosed with a corticotropin-secreting pituitary adenoma. Which laboratory results lead to this conclusion?

A. High corticotropin levels and low cortisol levels
B. Low corticotropin levels and high cortisol levels
C. High corticotropin levels and high cortisol levels
D. Low corticotropin levels and low cortisol levels

39. Mrs. Gibson will undergo a transsphenoidal hypophysectomy to remove the pituitary tumor. Preoperatively, the nurse should assess the patient for potential complications by:

A. testing for ketones in her urine.
B. testing her urine specific gravity.
C. checking her temperature every 4 hours.
D. performing capillary glucose testing every 4 hours.

40. In the immediate postoperative period following transsphenoidal hypophysectomy, the nurse should carefully assess Mrs. Gibson for:

    A. hypocortisolism.
    B. hypoglycemia.
    C. hyperglycemia.
    D. hypercalcemia.

SITUATION: *Victor Abbot, age 52, was admitted to the hospital with acute adrenal insufficiency. He has a history of Addison's disease for which he has been taking hydrocortisone. Over the past week, he has had flulike symptoms accompanied by nausea and vomiting. When he awoke this morning, his wife noticed that he was confused and extremely weak, so she brought him to the hospital for evaluation.*

Questions 41 to 43 refer to this situation.

41. Mr. Abbot's blood pressure is 90/58 mm Hg, his heart rate is 116 beats/minute, and his temperature is 101° F (38.3° C). The nurse should expect to start an I.V. infusion of:

    A. insulin.
    B. hydrocortisone.
    C. potassium.
    D. hypotonic saline.

42. During the initial 24 hours after admission, the nurse should frequently:

    A. weigh the patient.
    B. test the patient's urine for ketones.
    C. assess vital signs.
    D. administer oral hydrocortisone.

43. The patient in addisonian crisis is unable to respond to stress. Before discharge, the nurse should instruct Mr. Abbot and his family that during stress it'll be necessary to:

    A. administer cortisone I.M.
    B. drink 8 oz (237 ml) of fluids.
    C. perform capillary blood glucose monitoring four times daily.
    D. continue to take his usual dose of hydrocortisone.

SITUATION: *Clifford Haven, a 58-year-old mail carrier, had a severe exacerbation of asthma for which he was prescribed prednisone (Deltasone). He tells the nurse that he doesn't like taking this drug because of its adverse effects.*

Questions 44 and 45 refer to this situation.

44. Mr. Haven probably complains of which of prednisone's adverse effects?

A. Throat irritation and a bad taste in his mouth
B. Tachycardia and tremors
C. Headache and dizziness
D. Weight gain and bruising

45. Although Mr. Haven doesn't like prednisone's adverse effects, he agrees to continue taking it. When teaching him about his drug, the nurse should stress the importance of:

A. not stopping the drug abruptly.
B. stopping the drug as soon as he feels better.
C. taking the drug at night.
D. not using his bronchodilator.

SITUATION: *Karen Hughes, age 37, has a history of hypertension. Her laboratory tests reveal chronic hypokalemia. She has been diagnosed with primary hyperaldosteronism.*

Questions 46 to 49 refer to this situation.

46. The diagnosis of primary hyperaldosteronism indicates that Mrs. Hughes's hypertension is caused by excessive hormone secretion by the:

A. adrenal cortex.
B. pancreas.
C. adrenal medulla.
D. parathyroid glands.

47. The most common cause of hyperaldosteronism is:

A. excessive sodium intake.
B. a pituitary adenoma.
C. deficient potassium intake.
D. an adrenal adenoma.

48. Mrs. Hughes was diagnosed with a unilateral aldosteronoma for which she undergoes a unilateral adrenalectomy. Postoperatively, the nurse can identify hyperkalemia by assessing the patient for:

A. muscle weakness.
B. tremors.
C. diaphoresis.
D. constipation.

49. After surgery, Mrs. Hughes is treated with spironolactone, a potassium-sparing diuretic. The nurse should inform her that an adverse effect of this medication is:

A. breast tenderness.
B. menstrual irregularities.
C. increased facial hair.
D. hair loss.

SITUATION: *Roseanna Vega, age 52, weighs 210 lb (95 kg) and has been diagnosed with hyperglycemia. The nurse notices that she has large hands and a hoarse voice. She tells the nurse that her husband sleeps in another room because her snoring keeps him awake.*

Questions 50 to 52 refer to this situation.

50. A possible cause of Mrs. Vega's hyperglycemia is:

    A. acromegaly.
    B. type 1 diabetes mellitus.
    C. hypothyroidism.
    D. deficient growth hormone.

51. Pharmacologic treatment for Mrs. Vega's acromegaly might include:

    A. radioactive iodine.
    B. octreotide.
    C. somatomedin C.
    D. vasopressin.

52. Mrs. Vega is scheduled for surgery to remove a pituitary adenoma that is causing her acromegaly. Preoperative teaching should include telling her that:

    A. she'll have an I.V. insulin infusion when she returns from surgery.
    B. she'll be able to brush her teeth right after the surgery.
    C. her bed will be kept flat after surgery.
    D. she should avoid bending over, straining, and blowing her nose after surgery.

SITUATION: *James Higgins, an unrestrained driver, was admitted to the hospital after a motor vehicle accident. His head hit the windshield, and he's very sleepy. His serum sodium level is 132 mEq/L, his serum osmolality is 270 mOsm/L, and his urine specific gravity is 1.007. He's being observed for syndrome of inappropriate antidiuretic hormone.*

Questions 53 and 54 refer to this situation.

53. Which would alert the nurse that Mr. Higgins's hyponatremia is worsening?

    A. Chvostek's sign
    B. Vomiting and abdominal cramps
    C. Diaphoresis and tremors
    D. Hyporeflexia and paresthesia

54. Mr. Higgins is thirsty and frequently asks the nurse for water. The most appropriate response would be to:

    A. keep adequate water at his bedside.
    B. give him extra fluids with his medications.
    C. explain that his fluid intake must be restricted to 27 to 34 oz (800 to 1,000 ml)/day.
    D. prepare an I.V. infusion of hypotonic saline.

SITUATION: *Christian Delgato, age 32, is recovering from cranial surgery. The nurse notices that his urine output is greater than his intake and his urine specific gravity is 1.003.*

Questions 55 and 56 refer to this situation.

55. The nurse knows that these signs indicate that Mr. Delgato most likely has:

    A. diabetes mellitus.
    B. syndrome of inappropriate antidiuretic hormone (SIADH).
    C. hypercalcemia.
    D. diabetes insipidus.

56. Which of the following should take top priority when caring for Mr. Delgato?

    A. Administering an I.V. insulin infusion
    B. Restricting fluids
    C. Instructing the patient about vasopressin (Pitressin) administration
    D. Measuring and recording intake and output accurately

SITUATION: *Anita Rich, age 26, sees her doctor for an oral contraceptive. He prescribes a progestin-only oral contraceptive, or minipill.*

Questions 57 to 59 refer to this situation.

57. The nurse is teaching the patient about this contraceptive agent. Progestin use can increase her risk of:

    A. endometriosis.
    B. female hypogonadism.
    C. ectopic pregnancy.
    D. premenstrual syndrome.

58. Ms. Rich would need to use an alternative contraceptive method during concomitant use of which of the following drugs?

    A. Cyclosporine
    B. Primidone
    C. Erythromycin
    D. Hydrocortisone

59. While taking the oral contraceptive, Ms. Rich is most likely to experience which adverse GI reaction?

    A. Nausea
    B. Abdominal cramps
    C. Diarrhea
    D. Epigastric burning

SITUATION: *Charlotte Serling, age 28, is diagnosed with female hypogonadism. Her doctor prescribes conjugated estrogenic substances.*

Questions 60 to 63 refer to this situation.

60. When teaching Mrs. Serling about conjugated estrogenic substances, the nurse includes information about potential drug interactions. Which drug may decrease estrogenic activity?

    A. Ampicillin (Omnipen)
    B. Phenytoin (Dilantin)
    C. Propranolol (Inderal)
    D. Acetaminophen (Tylenol)

61. The nurse should inform Mrs. Serling that estrogens might interfere with the absorption of which of the following nutrients?

    A. Folic acid
    B. Calcium
    C. Vitamin K
    D. Iron

62. The nurse should advise Mrs. Serling that estrogen therapy places her at risk for which types of cancer?

    A. Cervical cancer
    B. Endometrial cancer
    C. Vaginal cancer
    D. Colon cancer

63. At a follow-up visit, the nurse should assess Mrs. Serling for which of the following adverse cardiovascular reactions to estrogen?

    A. Myocardial ischemia
    B. Cardiac arrhythmias
    C. Pericarditis
    D. Hypertension

SITUATION: *After an alleged sexual assault, a female patient is brought to the hospital. She's tearful and withdrawn. No external injuries are found.*

Question 64 and 65 refer to this situation.

64. Which of the following test results provides information for treatment that is important immediately postassault?

    A. Negative serologic test for syphilis
    B. Normal complete blood count (CBC)
    C. Positive rhesus (Rh) factor
    D. Negative pregnancy test

65. When evidence is collected, the patient's clothing should be?

    A. Shaken out carefully to look for hidden evidence
    B. Returned to the patient after determining no evidence is present
    C. Placed in a plastic bag and labeled with the patient's name
    D. Placed in a paper bag and sealed with evidence tape

SITUATION: *Theresa Hershey is a 20-year-old woman with type 1 diabetes mellitus. She was admitted to the hospital after 3 days of lethargy, polyuria, and polydipsia. She began vomiting 2 days prior to admission and decided not to use her insulin. She was diagnosed with diabetic ketoacidosis.*

Questions 66 to 68 refer to this situation.

66. Ms. Hershey's diagnosis of diabetic ketoacidosis (DKA) was based on which of the following laboratory values?

A. Serum glucose level, 350 mg/dl; pH, 7.4; creatinine level, 1.6 mEq/L; hematocrit, 60%
B. Serum glucose level, 800 mg/dl; pH 7.4; creatinine level, 1.0 mEq/L; hematocrit, 43%
C. Serum glucose level, 350 mg/dl; pH, 7.0; creatinine level, 1.6 mEq/L; hematocrit, 60%
D. Serum glucose level, 100 mg/dl; pH, 7.0; creatinine level, 1.0 mEq/L; hematocrit, 43%

67. Ms. Hershey's serum potassium level was 4.8 mEq/L on admission. During infusion of saline and insulin, Ms. Hershey's serum potassium level dropped to 3.2 mEq/L. This hypokalemia represents:

A. inaccurate laboratory testing.
B. inadequate insulinization.
C. adequate hydration.
D. depletion of intercellular potassium.

68. Because Ms. Hershey is of childbearing age, she should be counseled about:

A. avoiding pregnancy.
B. the effect of pregnancy on neuropathy.
C. the importance of controlling blood glucose levels before conception.
D. the importance of birth control.

ANSWER SHEET

	A B C D		A B C D		A B C D
1	○ ○ ○ ○	24	○ ○ ○ ○	47	○ ○ ○ ○
2	○ ○ ○ ○	25	○ ○ ○ ○	48	○ ○ ○ ○
3	○ ○ ○ ○	26	○ ○ ○ ○	49	○ ○ ○ ○
4	○ ○ ○ ○	27	○ ○ ○ ○	50	○ ○ ○ ○
5	○ ○ ○ ○	28	○ ○ ○ ○	51	○ ○ ○ ○
6	○ ○ ○ ○	29	○ ○ ○ ○	52	○ ○ ○ ○
7	○ ○ ○ ○	30	○ ○ ○ ○	53	○ ○ ○ ○
8	○ ○ ○ ○	31	○ ○ ○ ○	54	○ ○ ○ ○
9	○ ○ ○ ○	32	○ ○ ○ ○	55	○ ○ ○ ○
10	○ ○ ○ ○	33	○ ○ ○ ○	56	○ ○ ○ ○
11	○ ○ ○ ○	34	○ ○ ○ ○	57	○ ○ ○ ○
12	○ ○ ○ ○	35	○ ○ ○ ○	58	○ ○ ○ ○
13	○ ○ ○ ○	36	○ ○ ○ ○	59	○ ○ ○ ○
14	○ ○ ○ ○	37	○ ○ ○ ○	60	○ ○ ○ ○
15	○ ○ ○ ○	38	○ ○ ○ ○	61	○ ○ ○ ○
16	○ ○ ○ ○	39	○ ○ ○ ○	62	○ ○ ○ ○
17	○ ○ ○ ○	40	○ ○ ○ ○	63	○ ○ ○ ○
18	○ ○ ○ ○	41	○ ○ ○ ○	64	○ ○ ○ ○
19	○ ○ ○ ○	42	○ ○ ○ ○	65	○ ○ ○ ○
20	○ ○ ○ ○	43	○ ○ ○ ○	66	○ ○ ○ ○
21	○ ○ ○ ○	44	○ ○ ○ ○	67	○ ○ ○ ○
22	○ ○ ○ ○	45	○ ○ ○ ○	68	○ ○ ○ ○
23	○ ○ ○ ○	46	○ ○ ○ ○		

ANSWERS AND RATIONALES

1. *Correct answer:* **A**

The patient has signs and symptoms of diabetes insipidus, probably caused by failure of her renal tubules to respond to antidiuretic hormone as a consequence of pyelonephritis. The hypernatremia is secondary to her water loss. Altered nutrition related to hypermetabolic state or catabolic effect of insulin deficiency is an inappropriate nursing diagnosis for the patient.

> *Nursing process step:* Analysis
> *Client needs category:* Physiological integrity
> *Client needs subcategory:* Reduction of risk potential
> *Taxonomic level:* Application

2. *Correct answer:* **A**

A serum glucose level of 618 mg/dl indicates hyperglycemia, which causes polyuria and fluid volume deficit. In this patient, tachycardia is more likely to result from fluid volume deficit than decreased cardiac output because the blood pressure is normal. Although the patient's serum glucose level is elevated, food isn't a priority because fluids and insulin should be administered to lower the level. Therefore, *altered nutrition: less than body requirements* isn't an appropriate nursing diagnosis. A temperature of 100.6° F (38.1° C) isn't life-threatening, eliminating ineffective thermoregulation as the top priority.

> *Nursing process step:* Analysis
> *Client needs category:* Physiological integrity
> *Client needs subcategory:* Reduction of risk potential
> *Taxonomic level:* Analysis

3. *Correct answer:* **D**

When mixing insulins, the patient should draw the clear (regular) insulin into the syringe first. The daily insulin dose typically is administered to fatty tissue at a 90-degree angle, before the first meal of the day. If cloudy (Humulin NPH or Humulin N) insulin must be administered, the patient should gently roll the vial between the palms before withdrawing the medication.

> *Nursing process step:* Implementation
> *Client needs category:* Physiological integrity
> *Client needs subcategory:* Pharmacological and parenteral therapies
> *Taxonomic level:* Knowledge

4. *Correct answer:* **D**

Salicylates may interact with insulin to cause hypoglycemia. Antacids, acetaminophen preparations, and vitamins with iron don't interact with insulin.

Nursing process step: Planning
Client needs category: Physiological integrity
Client needs subcategory: Pharmacological and parenteral therapies
Taxonomic level: Knowledge

5. *Correct answer:* **D**

Signs and symptoms of hypoglycemia include nervousness, diaphoresis, weakness, light-headedness, confusion, paresthesia, irritability, headache, hunger, tachycardia, and changes in speech, hearing, and vision. If untreated, signs and symptoms may progress to unconsciousness, seizures, coma, and death. Polydipsia, polyuria, and polyphagia are signs of hyperglycemia.

Nursing process step: Assessment
Client needs category: Physiological integrity
Client needs subcategory: Reduction of risk potential
Taxonomic level: Comprehension

6. *Correct answer:* **C**

Glipizide acts in 1 to 1½ hours. The oral antidiabetic drug tolbutamide acts in 30 to 60 minutes.

Nursing process step: Implementation
Client needs category: Physiological integrity
Client needs subcategory: Pharmacological and parenteral therapies
Taxonomic level: Comprehension

7. *Correct answer:* **D**

Glipizide may cause adverse skin reactions, such as rash, pruritus, and photosensitivity. It doesn't cause headache, constipation, or hypotension.

Nursing process step: Implementation
Client needs category: Physiological integrity
Client needs subcategory: Pharmacological and parenteral therapies
Taxonomic level: Comprehension

8. *Correct answer:* **B**

From 25% to 60% of patients with secondary failure respond to a different oral antidiabetic drug. Therefore, it isn't appropriate to initiate insulin therapy at this time. However, if a new antidiabetic drug doesn't keep blood glucose levels at an acceptable level, insulin may be used with the antidiabetic drug.

Nursing process step: Planning
Client needs category: Physiological integrity
Client needs subcategory: Pharmacological and parenteral therapies
Taxonomic level: Knowledge

9. *Correct answer:* **D**

Serum osmolarity is the most important test for confirming HHNS; it's also used to guide treatment strategies and determine evaluation criteria. A patient with HHNS typically has a serum osmolarity of above 350 mOsm/L. Serum potassium and serum sodium levels and ABG values are also measured, but they aren't as important as serum osmolarity in confirming the diagnosis of HHNS. A patient with HHNS typically has hypernatremia and osmotic diuresis. ABG values reveal acidosis, and the potassium level is variable.

> *Nursing process step:* Assessment
> *Client needs category:* Physiological integrity
> *Client needs subcategory:* Reduction of risk potential
> *Taxonomic level:* Comprehension

10. *Correct answer:* **A**

Regardless of the patient's medical history, rapid fluid resuscitation is critical for cardiovascular integrity. Profound intravascular depletion requires aggressive fluid replacement. A typical fluid resuscitation protocol is 6 L of fluid over the first 12 hours, with more fluid to follow over the next 24 hours. Various fluids can be used, depending on the degree of hypovolemia. Commonly prescribed fluids include dextran (in cases of hypovolemic shock), isotonic normal saline solution and, when the patient's condition is stabilized, hypotonic half-normal saline solution.

> *Nursing process step:* Implementation
> *Client needs category:* Physiological integrity
> *Client needs subcategory:* Pharmacological and parenteral therapies
> *Taxonomic level:* Application

11. *Correct answer:* **A**

Inadequate fluid intake during hyperglycemic episodes commonly leads to hyperosmolar hyperglycemic nonketotic syndrome (HHNS). By recognizing the signs of hyperglycemia (polyuria, polydipsia, and polyphagia) and increasing her fluid intake, the patient may prevent HHNS. Drinking a glass of nondiet soda would be appropriate for hypoglycemia. A patient whose diabetes is controlled with oral antidiabetic drugs usually need not monitor the blood glucose level. A high-carbohydrate diet would exacerbate the patient's condition, particularly if her fluid intake were low.

> *Nursing process step:* Evaluation
> *Client needs category:* Physiological integrity
> *Client needs subcategory:* Reduction of risk potential
> *Taxonomic level:* Analysis

12. *Correct answer:* **A**

Because diabetes insipidus results from decreased antidiuretic hormone (vasopressin) production, the nurse should expect hormone replacement therapy with synthetic vasopressin. The diuretic furosemide is contraindicated because the patient experiences polyuria in this disorder. Insulin and dextrose are used to treat diabetes mellitus and its complications — not diabetes insipidus.

> *Nursing process step:* Implementation
> *Client needs category:* Physiological integrity
> *Client needs subcategory:* Pharmacological and parenteral therapies
> *Taxonomic level:* Knowledge

13. *Correct answer:* **A**

Diabetes insipidus is characterized by polyuria (up to 8 L/day), constant thirst, and an unusually high oral intake of fluids. Treatment with the appropriate drug should decrease urine output and oral fluid intake. A urine output of 200 ml/hour indicates continuing polyuria. A blood pressure of 90/50 mm Hg and a pulse rate of 126 beats/minute are signs of compensation for continued fluid deficit, suggesting that treatment hasn't been effective.

> *Nursing process step:* Evaluation
> *Client needs category:* Physiological integrity
> *Client needs subcategory:* Physiological adaptation
> *Taxonomic level:* Analysis

14. *Correct answer:* **A**

Classic signs of water intoxication include confusion and seizures, both of which are caused by cerebral edema. Weight gain will also occur. Sunken eyeballs, thirst, and increased blood urea nitrogen levels indicate fluid volume deficit. Spasticity, flaccidity, and tetany are unrelated to water intoxication.

> *Nursing process step:* Evaluation
> *Client needs category:* Physiological integrity
> *Client needs subcategory:* Reduction of risk potential
> *Taxonomic level:* Analysis

15. *Correct answer:* **B**

Breast cancer in first-degree relatives, especially on the maternal side, is a risk factor for breast cancer, particularly breast cancer that develops in women younger than age 40. Breast cancer is also associated with early menarche, late menopause, never having had children, or having children after age 30.

> *Nursing process step:* Assessment
> *Client needs category:* Physiological integrity
> *Client needs subcategory:* Reduction of risk potential
> *Taxonomic level:* Comprehension

16. *Correct answer:* **D**

Lymph node dissection helps determine if chemotherapy is indicated. Although removal of lymph nodes may assist in prevention of metastases, lymph node dissection isn't a guarantee that metastases won't occur. This procedure doesn't affect breast reconstruction and may actually make postoperative recovery more difficult.

Nursing process step: Implementation
Client needs category: Physiological integrity
Client needs subcategory: Reduction of risk potential
Taxonomic level: Knowledge

17. *Correct answer:* **A**

Lymphedema is a common adverse effect of modified radical mastectomy and lymph node dissection. Elevation will allow gravity to assist lymph drainage. Other preventive measures include exercises in which the arms are elevated. Trousseau's sign is an indication of hypocalcemia and wouldn't be expected in this situation. Neither I.V. infusions nor venipunctures should be given in the left arm. Although muscle atrophy is a potential adverse effect if the patient doesn't exercise her left arm, it wouldn't be prevented by elevation.

Nursing process step: Implementation
Client needs category: Physiological integrity
Client needs subcategory: Reduction of risk potential
Taxonomic level: Application

18. *Correct answer:* **A**

Having breast cancer on her left side puts her at increased risk for cancer on the contralateral side and chest wall. Therefore, the nurse should stress the importance of monthly BSE and annual mammograms. Although the tumor was found, its size placed the patient at risk for metastasis. Follow-up appointments should be monthly for the first few months and then at the direction of her doctor. Modified radical mastectomy shouldn't affect the menstrual cycle.

Nursing process step: Implementation
Client needs category: Physiological integrity
Client needs subcategory: Reduction of risk potential
Taxonomic level: Application

19. *Correct answer:* **A**

The nurse should suggest that the patient contact Reach to Recovery, a rehabilitation program of the American Cancer Society designed for women recovering from breast surgery. This organization helps with psychological, physical, and cosmetic needs. If Reach to Recovery isn't available, the nurse can contact the American Cancer Society or the National Cancer Institute to find local resources.

Because initial coping mechanisms may begin to lose their effectiveness after 3 months, the patient may be at risk for depression. Ongoing support should be encouraged. A psychiatrist may be necessary if the patient shows severely ineffective coping, but it would inappropriate for the nurse to make a referral. A dietitian is usually not indicated postoperatively if the patient is in otherwise good health. Mrs. Kramer is already walking, but she should also exercise her arm to prevent lymphedema and help maintain the function of her left arm and hand. Arm exercises should be done four times per day and should be increased as tolerated, but they should be stopped if pain results.

> *Nursing process step:* Implementation
> *Client needs category:* Psychosocial integrity
> *Client needs subcategory:* Coping and adaptation
> *Taxonomic level:* Application

20. *Correct answer:* **C**

Tamoxifen, an antiestrogen drug that blocks the estrogen receptor of estrogen-receptor-positive cancerous cells, is generally the treatment choice for postmenopausal women. Tamoxifen can cause tumor regression and prevent recurrence of cancer as well as occurrence of new tumors. It's effective regardless of whether the patient has axillary node involvement. Postmenopausal women are most apt to have estrogen-receptor-positive tumors. Progesterone-receptor-positive tumors aren't treated with tamoxifen.

> *Nursing process step:* Assessment
> *Client needs category:* Physiological integrity
> *Client needs subcategory:* Reduction of risk potential
> *Taxonomic level:* Knowledge

21. *Correct answer:* **B**

Because tamoxifen is an antiestrogen drug, it can cause vaginal dryness. The patient should be counseled to use vaginal lubricants when she has sexual intercourse. It won't cause her menstrual cycle to resume. Adverse effects of tamoxifen are mainly caused by the loss of estrogen and include dry skin, hot flashes, vaginal bleeding, nausea, and vomiting.

> *Nursing process step:* Planning
> *Client needs category:* Physiological integrity
> *Client needs subcategory:* Pharmacological and parenteral therapies
> *Taxonomic level:* Knowledge

22. *Correct answer:* **C**

Women treated with tamoxifen are at higher risk for developing endometrial cancer. Therefore, an annual Pap test and pelvic examination are indicated for early detection. Although she may have vaginal dryness and may be planning to resume sexual relations, these aren't the major reasons for an annual Pap test and pelvic examination. She isn't at higher risk for vaginal cancer.

Nursing process step: Planning
Client needs category: Physiological integrity
Client needs subcategory: Reduction of risk potential
Taxonomic level: Knowledge

23. *Correct answer:* **B**

Grave's disease, an autoimmune disease causing hyperthyroidism, is most prevalent in middle-aged women. In Hashimoto's disease, the most common form of hypothyroidism, thyroid stimulating hormone levels are high and thyroid hormone levels low. In thyroiditis, there's a low ($\leq 2\%$) radioactive iodine uptake, and nodular goiter will show an uptake in the high normal range (3% to 10%).

Nursing process step: Assessment
Client needs category: Physiological integrity
Client needs subcategory: Reduction of risk potential
Taxonomic level: Analysis

24. *Correct answer:* **D**

Potassium iodide reduces the vascularity of the thyroid gland and is used to prepare the gland for surgery. Potassium iodide reaches its maximum effect in 1 to 2 weeks. PTU blocks the conversion of thyroxine to triiodothyronine, the more biologically active thyroid hormone. PTU effects are also seen in 1 to 2 weeks. To relieve symptoms of hyperthyroidism in the interim, patients are usually given a beta-adrenergic blocker such as propranolol.

Nursing process step: Implementation
Client needs category: Physiological integrity
Client needs subcategory: Pharmacological and parenteral therapies
Taxonomic level: Comprehension

25. *Correct answer:* **A**

The patient who has undergone a thyroidectomy is at risk for hypocalcemia from inadvertent removal or damage to the parathyroid gland. The patient with hypocalcemia will exhibit a positive Chvostek's sign (facial muscle contraction when the facial nerve in front of the ear is tapped) and a positive Trousseau's sign (carpal spasm when a blood pressure cuff is inflated for a few minutes). These signs aren't present with hypokalemia or hyperkalemia.

Nursing process step: Assessment
Client needs category: Physiological integrity
Client needs subcategory: Reduction of risk potential
Taxonomic level: Comprehension

26. *Correct answer:* **C**

Regular follow-up care for the patient with Grave's disease is critical because most cases eventually result in hypothyroidism. Annual tests for thyroid stimulating hormone and the patient's ability to recognize signs and symptoms of thyroid dysfunction will help detect thyroid abnormalities early. Intake and output is important for patients with fluid and electrolyte imbalances but not thyroid disorders. DDAVP is used to treat diabetes insipidus. Although exercise to improve cardiovascular fitness is important, for this particular patient, the importance of regular follow-up is critical.

> *Nursing process step:* Planning
> *Client needs category:* Physiological integrity
> *Client needs subcategory:* Reduction of risk potential
> *Taxonomic level:* Application

27. *Correct answer:* **C**

Hashimoto's disease is the most common cause of hypothyroidism. It's common in women older than age 40. Weight gain, decreased appetite, constipation, lethargy, brittle nails, coarse hair, muscle cramps, weakness, sleep apnea, and dry, cool skin are signs and symptoms of Hashimoto's disease. Weight loss, increased appetite, and hyperdefecation are characteristic of hyperthyroidism. Weight loss, increased urination, and thirst are characteristic of uncontrolled diabetes mellitus. Weight gain, increased urination, and purplish red striae are characteristic of hypercortisolism.

> *Nursing process step:* Assessment
> *Client needs category:* Physiological integrity
> *Client needs subcategory:* Reduction of risk potential
> *Taxonomic level:* Knowledge

28. *Correct answer:* **D**

Normal thyroid function test results are as follows: T_4, 5 to 12 µ/dl; T_3, 65 to 195 ng/dl; TSH 0.3 to 5.4 µU/ml. Hashimoto's disease is a primary thyroid disorder; therefore, thyroid hormone levels (T_4 and T_3) are below normal. These low levels continually stimulate the pituitary gland to secrete TSH to stimulate the thyroid to secrete an adequate amount of thyroid hormone. The TSH level is the most sensitive test to diagnose hypothyroidism. Elevated thyroid hormone levels and low TSH levels indicates primary hyperthyroidism. Elevated thyroid hormone and TSH levels indicate secondary hyperthyroidism. Low thyroid hormone and TSH levels indicate secondary hypothyroidism (pituitary failure).

> *Nursing process step:* Assessment
> *Client needs category:* Physiological integrity
> *Client needs subcategory:* Reduction of risk potential
> *Taxonomic level:* Comprehension

29. *Correct answer:* **A**

Elderly patients or those with cardiac disease should begin with low-dose levothyroxine, increased at 2- to 4-week intervals until 100 g/day is reached. This slow dosage adjustment prevents further cardiac stress. Younger patients are started on the usual maintenance dose of 100 g/day. Patients with Hashimoto's disease don't require surgical intervention.

> *Nursing process step:* Planning
> *Client needs category:* Physiological integrity
> *Client needs subcategory:* Pharmacological and parenteral therapies
> *Taxonomic level:* Application

30. *Correct answer:* **C**

Myxedema coma, or severe hypothyroidism, is a life-threatening condition that may develop if thyroid replacement medication isn't taken. Exophthalmos, or protrusion of the eyeballs, is seen with hyperthyroidism. Thyroid storm is life-threatening, but it's caused by severe hyperthyroidism. Tibial myxedema, or peripheral mucinous edema involving the lower leg, is associated with hypothyroidism but isn't life-threatening.

> *Nursing process step:* Assessment
> *Client needs category:* Physiological integrity
> *Client needs subcategory:* Reduction of risk potential
> *Taxonomic level:* Knowledge

31. *Correct answer:* **D**

Because respirations are depressed in myxedema coma, maintaining a patent airway is the most critical nursing intervention. Ventilatory support is usually needed. Although myxedema coma is associated with severe hypothermia, a warming blanket shouldn't be used because it may cause vasodilation and shock. Gradual warming with blankets would be appropriate. Thyroid replacement will be administered I.V., and although intake and input is important, it isn't critical at this time.

> *Nursing process step:* Implementation
> *Client needs category:* Physiological integrity
> *Client needs subcategory:* Reduction of risk potential
> *Taxonomic level:* Application

32. *Correct answer:* **D**

Hyperparathyroidism is most common in older women and is characterized by bone pain and weakness from excess parathyroid hormone (PTH). Patients also exhibit hypercalciuria-causing polyuria. Although patients with diabetes mellitus and diabetes insipidus also exhibit polyuria, they don't exhibit bone pain or increased sleeping. Hypoparathyroidism is characterized by urinary frequency rather than polyuria.

Nursing process step: Assessment
Client needs category: Physiological integrity
Client needs subcategory: Reduction of risk potential
Taxonomic level: Analysis

33. *Correct answer:* **A**

PTH stimulates the kidneys to reabsorb calcium and excrete phosphate. PTH converts vitamin D to its active form, 1,25-dihydroxyvitamin D. PTH doesn't have a role in the metabolism of vitamin E.

Nursing process step: Planning
Client needs category: Physiological integrity
Client needs subcategory: Reduction of risk potential
Taxonomic level: Application

34. *Correct answer:* **B**

Hypercalcemia is the hallmark of excess parathyroid hormone levels. Serum phosphate levels will be low, and there will be increased urinary phosphate levels because phosphate excretion is increased.

Nursing process step: Assessment
Client needs category: Physiological integrity
Client needs subcategory: Reduction of risk potential
Taxonomic level: Knowledge

35. *Correct answer:* **C**

The patient should be encouraged to force fluids to prevent renal calculi formation. Restricting potassium and sodium isn't necessary in hyperparathyroidism.

Nursing process step: Implementation
Client needs category: Physiological integrity
Client needs subcategory: Basic care and comfort
Taxonomic level: Application

36. *Correct answer:* **A**

A moderate exercise program will help strengthen the patient's bones and prevent bone loss that occurs from excess parathyroid hormone. Walking or swimming provides the most beneficial exercise. Because of the patient's weakened bones, a rigorous exercise program such as jogging would be contraindicated. Weight loss might be beneficial, but it isn't as important as developing a moderate exercise program.

Nursing process step: Implementation
Client needs category: Physiological integrity
Client needs subcategory: Reduction of risk potential
Taxonomic level: Application

37. *Correct answer:* **C**

A corticotropin-secreting pituitary adenoma is the most common cause of Cushing's syndrome in women between ages 20 and 40. Mrs. Gibson's diagnosis is Cushing's *syndrome,* because Cushing's *syndrome* refers to excess cortisol secretion, resulting from neoplasms of the adrenal cortex or prolonged and excessive intake of glucocorticoids. Cushing's disease is Cushing's syndrome secondary to excessive corticotropin secretion with or without a pituitary adenoma. Ectopic corticotropin-secreting tumors are more common in older men and generally associated with weight loss. Adrenal carcinoma usually isn't accompanied by hirsutism. A female with an inborn error of metabolism wouldn't be menstruating.

Nursing process step: Assessment
Client needs category: Physiological integrity
Client needs subcategory: Reduction of risk potential
Taxonomic level: Knowledge

38. *Correct answer:* **C**

A corticotropin-secreting pituitary tumor would cause high corticotropin and high cortisol levels. A high corticotropin level with a low cortisol level and a low corticotropin with a low cortisol level would be associated with hypocortisolism. Low corticotropin levels and high cortisol levels would be seen if there was a primary defect in the adrenal glands.

Nursing process step: Assessment
Client needs category: Physiological integrity
Client needs subcategory: Reduction of risk potential
Taxonomic level: Knowledge

39. *Correct answer:* **D**

The nurse should perform capillary glucose testing every 4 hours because excess cortisol may cause insulin resistance, placing the patient at risk for hyperglycemia. Urine ketone testing isn't indicated because she does secrete insulin and therefore isn't at risk for ketosis. Urine specific gravity isn't indicated because, although fluid balance may be compromised, it usually isn't dangerously imbalanced. Temperature regulation may be affected by excess cortisol; it doesn't accurately indicate infection.

Nursing process step: Implementation
Client needs category: Physiological integrity
Client needs subcategory: Reduction of risk potential
Taxonomic level: Application

40. *Correct answer:* **A**

The nurse should assess Mrs. Gibson for hypocortisolism. Abrupt withdrawal of endogenous cortisol may lead to severe adrenal insufficiency. Corticosteroids are given during surgery to prevent hypocortisolism from occurring. Signs and symptoms of hypocortisolism are vomiting, increased weakness, dehydration, and hypotension. Once the corticotropin-secreting tumor is removed, the patient shouldn't be at risk for hyperglycemia. Calcium imbalance shouldn't occur in this situation.

> *Nursing process step:* Assessment
> *Client needs category:* Physiological integrity
> *Client needs subcategory:* Reduction of risk potential
> *Taxonomic level:* Application

41. *Correct answer:* **B**

Emergency treatment for acute adrenal insufficiency (addisonian crisis) is I.V. infusion of hydrocortisone and saline solution. Insulin isn't indicated in this situation because adrenal insufficiency is usually associated with hypoglycemia. Potassium isn't indicated because these patients are usually hyperkalemic. Mr. Abbot needs normal saline, not hypotonic saline.

> *Nursing process step:* Planning
> *Client needs category:* Physiological integrity
> *Client needs subcategory:* Pharmacological and parenteral therapies
> *Taxonomic level:* Application

42. *Correct answer:* **C**

Because the patient in addisonian crisis has an unstable condition, vital signs and fluid and electrolyte balance should be assessed every 30 minutes until the patient's condition is stable. Daily weights are sufficient when assessing the patient's condition. The patient shouldn't have ketones in his urine, so there is no need to assess the urine for their presence. Oral hydrocortisone isn't administered during the first 24 hours in severe adrenal insufficiency.

> *Nursing process step:* Implementation
> *Client needs category:* Physiological integrity
> *Client needs subcategory:* Reduction of risk potential
> *Taxonomic level:* Application

43. *Correct answer:* **A**

Patients with Addison's disease and their family members should know how to administer I.M. hydrocortisone during periods of stress. It's important to keep well hydrated during stress, but the critical component of discharge planning in this situation is to know how and when to administer hydrocortisone I.M.

Capillary blood glucose monitoring isn't indicated in this situation because the patient doesn't have diabetes mellitus and cortisol replacement doesn't cause insulin resistance.

Nursing process step: Implementation
Client needs category: Physiological integrity
Client needs subcategory: Reduction of risk potential
Taxonomic level: Application

44. *Correct answer:* **D**

Prednisone, which is used to decrease bronchial edema and mucus production in asthma, is associated with adverse effects, such as weight gain, bruising, epigastric distress, hypertension, cataracts, and muscle weakness. Female patients may also experience menstrual irregularities. Tachycardia, tremors, headache, and dizziness are adverse effects of beta-adrenergic agonists. Throat irritation and a bad taste in the mouth are associated with mast cell stabilizers.

Nursing process step: Assessment
Client needs category: Physiological integrity
Client needs subcategory: Pharmacological and parenteral therapies
Taxonomic level: Knowledge

45. *Correct answer:* **A**

Prednisone should never be stopped abruptly because the patient may suffer severe adrenal insufficiency. Prednisone turns off corticotropin secretion, making the adrenal gland unable to produce cortisol. Prednisone doses should always be tapered gradually. Prednisone usually isn't taken at night because it causes insomnia. If prednisone is ordered twice a day, the larger dose should be taken in the morning to mimic the physiologic circadian rhythm of endogenous cortisol secretion. Prednisone may be taken with bronchodilators.

Nursing process step: Implementation
Client needs category: Physiological integrity
Client needs subcategory: Pharmacological and parenteral therapies
Taxonomic level: Application

46. *Correct answer:* **A**

Excessive secretion of aldosterone in the adrenal cortex is responsible for the patient's hypertension. This hormone acts on the renal tubule, where it promotes reabsorption of sodium and excretion of potassium and hydrogen ions. The adrenal medulla secretes the catecholamines, epinephrine, and norepinephrine. The pancreas mainly secretes hormones involved in fuel metabolism, and the parathyroids secrete parathyroid hormone.

Nursing process step: Assessment
Client needs category: Physiological integrity
Client needs subcategory: Reduction of risk potential
Taxonomic level: Application

47. *Correct answer:* **D**

An autonomous aldosterone-producing adenoma is the most common cause of hyperaldosteronism. Hyperplasia is the second most common cause. Aldosterone secretion is independent of sodium and potassium intake and of pituitary stimulation.

Nursing process step: Assessment
Client needs category: Physiological integrity
Client needs subcategory: Reduction of risk potential
Taxonomic level: Knowledge

48. *Correct answer:* **A**

Muscle weakness, bradycardia, nausea, diarrhea, and paresthesia of the hands, feet, tongue, and face are common with hyperkalemia. The hyperkalemia is transient and occurs from transient hypoaldosteronism when the adenoma is removed. Tremors, diaphoresis, and constipation aren't seen in hyperkalemia.

Nursing process step: Assessment
Client needs category: Physiological integrity
Client needs subcategory: Reduction of risk potential
Taxonomic level: Application

49. *Correct answer:* **B**

Menstrual irregularities and decreased libido are adverse effects of spironolactone. Men may also experience gynecomastia and impotence. Breast tenderness, increased facial hair, and hair loss aren't among spironolactone's adverse effects.

Nursing process step: Planning
Client needs category: Physiological integrity
Client needs subcategory: Pharmacological and parenteral therapies
Taxonomic level: Knowledge

50. *Correct answer:* **A**

Acromegaly, which is caused by a pituitary tumor that releases excessive growth hormone, is associated with hyperglycemia, hypertension, diaphoresis, peripheral neuropathy, and joint pain. Enlarged hands and feet are related to lateral bone growth, which is seen in adults with this disorder. The accompanying soft-tissue swelling causes hoarseness and, in many cases, sleep apnea. Type 1 diabetes is usually seen in children, and newly diagnosed persons are usually very ill and thin. Hypothyroidism and growth hormone deficiency aren't associated with hyperglycemia.

Nursing process step: Assessment
Client needs category: Physiological integrity
Client needs subcategory: Reduction of risk potential
Taxonomic level: Analysis

51. *Correct answer:* B

Octreotide is a somatostatin analogue that in many cases reduces growth hormone levels to normal. It's frequently used to reduce tumor size before surgery. Radioactive iodine is used to treat thyroid disorders. Somatomedin C (insulin-like growth factor) levels are used to diagnose acromegaly, with high levels indicating growth hormone excess. Vasopressin is used to treat diabetes insipidus, an abnormality of the posterior pituitary.

Nursing process step: Planning
Client needs category: Physiological integrity
Client needs subcategory: Pharmacological and parenteral therapies
Taxonomic level: Knowledge

52. *Correct answer:* D

Because the incision is made in the inner aspect of the upper lip and gingivae, the patient should avoid pressure on this area, which can occur with bending over, straining, and blowing her nose. Stool softeners may be prescribed to prevent constipation. To protect the suture line, mouth care must be done with soft cotton-tipped swabs, and tooth brushing is avoided for at least 10 days postoperatively. She won't need an insulin infusion because her hyperglycemia will resolve postoperatively. The head of her bed should be elevated at least 30 degrees to promote drainage and relieve headache.

Nursing process step: Implementation
Client needs category: Physiological integrity
Client needs subcategory: Reduction of risk potential
Taxonomic level: Application

53. *Correct answer:* B

Vomiting and abdominal cramps indicate that the patient's hyponatremia and, therefore, his syndrome of inappropriate antidiuretic hormone (SIADH) are worsening. Head trauma is a common cause of SIADH. Other possible causes are pulmonary conditions, meningitis, subarachnoid hemorrhage, acquired immunodeficiency syndrome, delirium tremens, or a variety of medications. Chvostek's sign, facial muscle contraction when the facial nerve in front of the ear is tapped, indicates hypocalcemia. Diaphoresis and tremors may indicate hypoglycemia, not hyponatremia. Hyporeflexia and paresthesia are seen in hypokalemia.

Nursing process step: Assessment
Client needs category: Physiological integrity
Client needs subcategory: Reduction of risk potential
Taxonomic level: Knowledge

54. *Correct answer:* C

Along with meticulous intake and output, fluid restriction is an important nursing intervention in syndrome of inappropriate antidiuretic hormone to prevent further dilutional hyponatremia. Ice chips may be offered for severe thirst. A hypotonic saline infusion would cause further fluid retention. If I.V. fluids are given because of severe hyponatremia, hypertonic (3% to 5%) saline is used.

Nursing process step: Implementation
Client needs category: Physiological integrity
Client needs subcategory: Reduction of risk potential
Taxonomic level: Knowledge

55. *Correct answer:* D

Many patients develop diabetes insipidus after head trauma or brain surgery. Signs of diabetes insipidus include polyuria (which can reach 10 L/day) and a urine specific gravity of ≤ 1.005. Polyuria is also a symptom of diabetes mellitus, SIADH, and hypercalcemia, but urine specific gravity is high in these conditions.

Nursing process step: Assessment
Client needs category: Physiological integrity
Client needs subcategory: Reduction of risk potential
Taxonomic level: Analysis

56. *Correct answer:* D

Measuring and recording intake and output accurately is essential in the patient with diabetes insipidus. If urine output is allowed to exceed the patient's intake over time, the patient can quickly become dehydrated. Insulin isn't indicated in diabetes insipidus, and fluids must be forced, not restricted, to prevent dehydration. Subcutaneous vasopressin isn't used for long-term treatment of diabetes insipidus. If the condition persists, which is unlikely, he should be instructed to administer vasopressin by intranasal insufflation.

Nursing process step: Implementation
Client needs category: Physiological integrity
Client needs subcategory: Reduction of risk potential
Taxonomic level: Application

57. *Correct answer:* **C**

Women taking the minipill have a higher incidence of ectopic pregnancies, possibly because of the progestin's effects on the female reproductive system. Progestin use doesn't put the patient at risk for endometriosis, female hypogonadism, or premenstrual syndrome.

> *Nursing process step:* Implementation
> *Client needs category:* Physiological integrity
> *Client needs subcategory:* Pharmacological and parenteral therapies
> *Taxonomic level:* Knowledge

58. *Correct answer:* **B**

Primidone and certain other drugs can decrease the efficacy of oral contraceptives, requiring the use of an alternative contraceptive. Cyclosporine, erythromycin, and hydrocortisone don't affect the efficacy of oral contraceptives.

> *Nursing process step:* Assessment
> *Client needs category:* Physiological integrity
> *Client needs subcategory:* Pharmacological and parenteral therapies
> *Taxonomic level:* Knowledge

59. *Correct answer:* **A**

The most common adverse reaction to oral contraceptives is nausea. Abdominal cramps, diarrhea, and epigastric burning aren't commonly experienced with oral contraceptives.

> *Nursing process step:* Assessment
> *Client needs category:* Physiological integrity
> *Client needs subcategory:* Pharmacological and parenteral therapies
> *Taxonomic level:* Knowledge

60. *Correct answer:* **B**

Phenytoin, rifampin, and other drugs that interact with estrogens typically result in decreased estrogenic activity. Ampicillin, propranolol, and acetaminophen don't interact with estrogens.

> *Nursing process step:* Implementation
> *Client needs category:* Physiological integrity
> *Client needs subcategory:* Pharmacological and parenteral therapies
> *Taxonomic level:* Comprehension

61. *Correct answer:* **A**

Estrogens interfere with the absorption of dietary folic acid, which may lead to folic acid deficiency. Estrogens don't interfere with the absorption of calcium, vitamin K, or iron.

Nursing process step: Planning
Client needs category: Physiological integrity
Client needs subcategory: Pharmacological and parenteral therapies
Taxonomic level: Knowledge

62. *Correct answer:* **B**

The risk of endometrial cancer increases fourfold to eightfold in women taking estrogens. Estrogens don't increase the risk of cervical, vaginal, or colon cancer.

Nursing process step: Planning
Client needs category: Physiological integrity
Client needs subcategory: Pharmacological and parenteral therapies
Taxonomic level: Knowledge

63. *Correct answer:* **D**

Hypertension may occur during estrogen therapy. Myocardial ischemia, cardiac arrhythmias, and pericarditis aren't adverse cardiovascular reactions to estrogen therapy.

Nursing process step: Planning
Client needs category: Physiological integrity
Client needs subcategory: Pharmacological and parenteral therapies
Taxonomic level: Knowledge

64. *Correct answer:* **D**

It's important to know if the client was pregnant before the attack so that pregnancy prevention medication can be started, if appropriate. Treatment for patients who've been sexually assaulted also includes the use of prophylactic antibiotic therapy. Cultures and tests for syphilis won't be finished for several days, so antibiotics may be routinely given before receiving test results. A CBC doesn't provide vital information for this patient. The positive Rh factor doesn't require treatment.

Nursing process step: Planning
Client needs category: Safe, effective care environment
Client needs subcategory: Safety and infection control
Taxonomic level: Comprehension

65. *Correct answer:* **D**

Evidence obtained in a rape examination, including the clothing, should be placed in a paper bag and secured with evidence tape to ensure no tampering occurs. The patient's clothing should be carefully removed but not shaken out; microscopic evidence may be lost. All clothing should be given to the police; it's their responsibility to determine if evidence is present. Clothing shouldn't be placed in plastic bags, which cause mildew and moisture retention. Both conditions can cause loss of evidence. All evidence collected should be labeled with the patient's name, site of collection, date and time of collection, and the name of the person collecting the evidence.

Nursing process step: Implementation
Client needs category: Safe, effective care environment
Client needs subcategory: Management of care
Taxonomic level: Comprehension

66. *Correct answer:* C

The hallmark of DKA is a low pH, usually less than 7.2. The glucose level is 250 mg/dl or greater. Creatinine and blood urea nitrogen levels and hematocrit are elevated because of associated dehydration. In addition, white blood cell count and liver function studies usually show elevated levels.

Nursing process step: Assessment
Client needs category: Physiological integrity
Client needs subcategory: Reduction of risk potential
Taxonomic level: Analysis

67. *Correct answer:* D

Intercellular potassium is always depleted in diabetic ketoacidosis (DKA) because of inadequate insulinization. As insulin is replaced, potassium moves from the circulation into the cells to replace intercellular potassium, resulting in hypokalemia. Although it's possible that the laboratory test is inaccurate, this is most likely not the case in this situation. If insulinization were still inadequate, the potassium wouldn't move back into the cells. Insulinization, not hydration, is the major determinant of potassium balance in DKA.

Nursing process step: Assessment
Client needs category: Physiological integrity
Client needs subcategory: Reduction of risk potential
Taxonomic level: Application

68. *Correct answer:* C

Diabetic women should be counseled about the importance of normalizing their blood glucose levels before conceiving. Doing so decreases the risk of congenital anomalies in the neonate. Pregnancy doesn't affect neuropathy, and birth control need not be discussed at this time.

Nursing process step: Planning
Client needs category: Health promotion and maintenance
Client needs subcategory: Prevention and early detection of disease
Taxonomic level: Application

HEMATOLOGIC AND IMMUNOLOGIC SYSTEMS

QUESTIONS

SITUATION: *Jan Lyons, age 34, comes to the clinic complaining of joint pain, fever, weight loss, knee swelling, and ulnar deviation of the hands. She takes aspirin for pain. Rheumatoid arthritis is diagnosed.*

Questions 1 to 7 refer to this situation.

1. Which would the nurse expect in a patient with rheumatoid arthritis?

    A. Warm, swollen joints

    B. Butterfly rash over the cheeks and nose

    C. Pain and stiffness that increases as the day progresses

    D. Unilateral leg swelling and calf pain

2. Mrs. Lyons complains of stiffness in the morning. The nurse should suggest that the patient:

    A. splint or brace the joint at all times.

    B. take a hot bath or shower each morning.

    C. apply ice packs for 1 hour each morning.

    D. retire later at night and rise later in the morning.

3. Mrs. Lyons is scheduled for a paraffin hand bath. The nurse would use extreme caution with a paraffin bath if the patient had a history of:

    A. kidney stones.

    B. myocardial infarction.

    C. diabetes mellitus.

    D. seizure disorder.

4. Mrs. Lyons is measured for a cane. When properly used, the cane:

    A. should advance with the unaffected leg for better balance.

    B. is held opposite the affected leg and advanced with the affected leg.

    C. allows for 90-degree elbow flexion with the elbow's xiphoid process level during use.

    D. should be avoided if the joint is hot and swollen.

5. Mrs. Lyons is prescribed prednisone (Deltasone) to:

    A. improve her glucose tolerance.

    B. relieve stress on painful joints.

    C. limit depression associated with chronic illness.

    D. mediate immune response and prevent further joint destruction.

6. Mrs. Lyons' left knee becomes hot, extremely swollen, and tender to touch. Arthrocentesis is planned. While teaching the patient about the procedure, the nurse explains that it involves:

    A. inserting a scope into the affected joint to visualize and repair damaged tissue or tendons.

    B. removing synovial fluid under local anesthesia to evaluate fluid and relieve tissue pressure.

    C. injecting medication into the joint to reduce inflammation and pain.

    D. fusing painful joints to eliminate motion and stress on the joint.

7. Mrs. Lyons takes large doses of aspirin for joint pain. She asks the nurse the difference between plain aspirin and enteric-coated aspirin. The nurse explains that:

    A. high doses of enteric-coated aspirin may lead to liver damage, but plain aspirin doesn't.

    B. the enteric coating prevents toxic reaction to aspirin and stomach ulcers, but plain aspirin doesn't.

    C. enteric-coated aspirin may be used safely in children with chickenpox, but plain aspirin can't.

    D. the onset of action of enteric-coated aspirin may be slower because absorption is delayed.

SITUATION: *Michael Rodriguez is a 45-year-old patient with a history of human immunodeficiency virus who is hospitalized with fever, chills, and cough that has lasted for 5 days. The doctor suspects* Pneumocystis carinii *pneumonia.*

Questions 8 to 12 refer to this situation.

8. Which of the following isolation precautions should be instituted with Mr. Rodriguez?

    A. standard precautions

    B. blood and body fluid precautions

    C. enteric precautions

    D. no isolation precautions are needed at this time

9. Mr. Rodriguez has started taking zidovudine (AZT). The nurse teaches the patient about the drug and its potential drug-drug interactions. Teaching is effective when the patient states:

A. "I know I should avoid taking Tylenol because it could affect my liver."
B. "I know I should avoid taking antacids because they could affect the drug's absorption."
C. "I know I should avoid ascorbic acid because it can make my drug levels too high."
D. "I know I should avoid stool softeners because they could decrease the drug's effectiveness.

10. The nurse notes dime-size, purple, nonblanching macules on Mr. Rodriguez's legs and notifies the doctor. These macules may indicate:

A. petechiae from platelet destruction.
B. cutaneous acquired immunodeficiency syndrome (AIDS).
C. telangiectasia.
D. Kaposi's sarcoma.

11. Mr. Rodriguez begins alpha-interferon therapy for Kaposi's sarcoma. The nurse discusses adverse effects of interferon therapy, which typically include:

A. bradycardia.
B. thromboembolism.
C. influenza-like symptoms.
D. hypertension.

12. The nurse documents successful teaching when Mr. Rodriguez's partner states:

A. "I should avoid using the same drinking glass as my partner."
B. "A condom should be used during sexual relations."
C. "As long as my partner doesn't develop full-blown acquired immunodeficiency syndrome (AIDS), I can't get the disease."
D. "Zidovudine (AZT) will keep the disease from spreading to me."

SITUATION: *Kimberly Watkins was working on the medical-surgical floor when she stuck herself with a needle from a patient infected with acquired immunodeficiency syndrome. She's very upset and reports to employee health services immediately.*

Questions 13 to 15 refer to this situation.

13. The employee health nurse attempts to make Ms. Watkins feel more at ease by:

A. telling her that everything will be all right.
B. providing her with information about the services available for employees who experience needlesticks.
C. telling her that it's unlikely she'll get acquired immunodeficiency syndrome (AIDS).
D. reassuring her that staff will be available if she becomes upset.

14. The nurse has blood drawn for an enzyme-linked immunosorbent assay (ELISA) test. The test results are positive, indicating previous exposure to the human immunodeficiency virus (HIV). Which test would be performed next to confirm the presence of HIV antibodies in her blood?

A. Western blot
B. $CD4^+$ lymphocyte count
C. Hepatitis B surface antigen (HBsAg)
D. Anti-Smith antibody

15. The nurse is prescribed zidovudine. After receiving therapy for several weeks, she complains of fatigue and shortness of breath. Which should she have evaluated?

A. Her serum albumin level
B. Her hemoglobin level and hematocrit
C. Her serum potassium level
D. Her mental status

SITUATION: *Kendra Adams is a 22-year-old woman with a history of idiopathic thrombocytopenic purpura. She's admitted to the medical-surgical floor with recurrent epistaxis. Her hemoglobin level is 9.3 g/dl; her hematocrit, 27.7%; and her platelet count, 18,000/µl. Posterior nasal packing is placed, and she begins taking methylprednisolone (Solu-Medrol).*

Questions 16 to 19 refer to this situation.

16. When teaching Ms. Adams about idiopathic thrombocytopenic purpura (ITP), the nurse should instruct her to avoid:

A. aspirin.
B. acetaminophen (Tylenol).
C. diazepam (Valium).
D. famotidine (Pepcid).

17. When questioning Ms. Adams about her condition, the nurse would expect her to report:

    A. myalgia.
    B. joint pain.
    C. a smooth, beefy tongue.
    D. heavy menses.

18. The nurse notes that Ms. Adams has red dotlike areas on her trunk and documents these as:

    A. papules.
    B. petechiae.
    C. ecchymoses.
    D. hematomas.

19. Ms. Adams asks the nurse what causes idiopathic thrombocytopenic purpura (ITP). The nurse explains:

    A. "Your body makes antibodies that destroy your platelets, which causes you to bleed."
    B. "ITP is caused by a recent bacterial infection."
    C. "Your excessive intake of aspirin has caused this problem."
    D. "This form of anemia will improve with iron supplements."

SITUATION: *Raul Shahid, a 48-year-old business executive, is admitted to the hospital with upper GI bleeding . He recently injured his back and has been taking ibuprofen (Motrin) every 4 hours around the clock. On admission, his hemoglobin level is 8.2 g/dl, his hematocrit is 23.4%, his pulse rate is 106 beats/minute, and his blood pressure is 110/74 mm Hg. The doctor prescribes two units of packed red blood cells to be infused as soon as possible.*

Questions 20 to 23 refer to this situation.

20. Which of the following is important when transfusing packed red blood cells?

    A. Begin the infusion at 50 drops/minute for the first 15 minutes.
    B. Infuse the blood through an I.V. catheter that's 20G or larger.
    C. Warm the blood to body temperature before infusing.
    D. Piggyback the blood through an infusion of 5% dextrose and water.

21. Which of the following statements are true concerning packed red blood cells (RBCs)?

    A. A unit of packed RBCs contains red cells, white cells, and platelets.
    B. A unit of packed RBCs doesn't require typing and crossmatching.
    C. A unit of packed RBCs has 70% to 80% of the plasma removed.
    D. A unit of packed RBCs usually contains more fluid than a unit of whole blood.

22. About 2 hours after the transfusion begins, Mr. Shahid develops a cough that produces frothy sputum. The nurse auscultates his lungs and notices crackles in the lower half of his lung fields. These assessment findings indicate:

    A. a hemolytic transfusion reaction.
    B. a febrile reaction.
    C. that the blood was mismatched.
    D. that the patient is overloaded with fluid.

23. The nurse knows that Mr. Shahid's transfusion is effective when she:

    A. observes a decreased urine output.
    B. auscultates a normal heart rate.
    C. performs a stool test for occult blood and gets a negative result.
    D. assesses a normal temperature.

SITUATION: *Edna Miller is an 86-year-old patient admitted to the hospital for diabetes mellitus management and iron-deficiency anemia.*

Questions 24 to 26 refer to this situation.

24. Mrs. Miller is started on ferrous sulfate orally three times a day. The nurse should instruct her to take the iron supplement with which of the following to enhance supplement absorption?

    A. vitamin D
    B. aluminum hydroxide gel
    C. pyridoxine
    D. ascorbic acid

25. The nurse suggests that Mrs. Miller increase her intake of which of the following iron-rich foods?

    A. fortified wheat products and red meat
    B. fish and white rice
    C. dairy products and sardines
    D. eggs and cheese

26. Because iron supplements can cause gastric distress, Mrs. Miller should be instructed to take them:

    A. at bedtime.
    B. before meals.
    C. with meals.
    D. until she feels better.

SITUATION: *June Summers, age 46, is admitted to the medical-surgical floor with anemia, shortness of breath, weakness, pallor, and bone pain. She'll soon undergo bone marrow aspiration. Her white blood cell count is 90,000/μl.*

Questions 27 to 36 refer to this situation.

27. Mrs. Summers is very anxious about the procedure. To help allay her anxiety, the nurse describes the procedure. How is a bone marrow aspiration best described?

    A. "A blood sample is analyzed for elements normally found in the bone marrow."

    B. "A small amount of marrow is taken from the posterior iliac crest and analyzed."

    C. "You will receive a transfusion of red blood cells into an I.V. catheter in your arm."

    D. "Donor bone marrow will be injected into your circulation through an I.V. catheter."

28. Acute myeloblastic leukemia is diagnosed. Which abnormal test result would the nurse anticipate in patients with leukemia?

    A. CD4+ lymphocyte count of less than 200

    B. Leukocyte count of 90,000/μl

    C. Serum potassium level greater than 5 mEq/L

    D. Calcium level of 10.5 mEq/L

29. Mrs. Summers begins chemotherapy treatment that includes methotrexate (Folex). Allopurinol (Zyloprim) is also prescribed to:

    A. relieve gout-associated pain in her great toe and other joints.

    B. inhibit uric acid synthesis that is caused by tissue destruction from chemotherapy.

    C. decrease nausea and vomiting associated with chemotherapy.

    D. shrink swollen lymphoid tissue.

30. During Mrs. Summers's chemotherapy regimen, which is important to include in her plan of care?

    A. Instruct her to consume plenty of raw fruits and vegetables.

    B. Take rectal temperatures for greater accuracy.

    C. Tell her to avoid crowds and infected individuals.

    D. Ask friends and relatives not to visit during the course of chemotherapy.

31. When caring for Mrs. Summers, the nurse would anticipate transfusing packed red blood cells (RBCs) for:

A. frequent sore throats.
B. complaints of feeling chilly all the time.
C. chest pain.
D. petechiae and bruising.

32. During the course of chemotherapy, Mrs. Summers complains of mouth soreness and painful swallowing. The nurse instructs the patient to:

A. floss after meals and visit the dentist every 3 months.
B. use a soft swab to clean her teeth and eat foods that are moist and cool.
C. use an acetic-acid mouthwash to neutralize the saliva.
D. take only liquids until her mouth ulcers heal.

33. Mrs. Summers's hair begins to fall out as a result of chemotherapy. The nurse suggests that she:

A. use a dandruff shampoo daily.
B. buy a wig.
C. sleep on a satin pillowcase.
D. take folic acid supplements.

34. The nurse realizes the dose-limiting factor for Mrs. Summers's chemotherapy will be:

A. uric acid levels.
B. hypercalcemia.
C. xerostomia.
D. bone marrow suppression.

35. Filgrastim (Neupogen) is prescribed for Mrs. Summers to:

A. stimulate bone marrow production of erythropoietin.
B. provide immunosuppression and decrease white blood cell destruction.
C. synthesize prothrombin and decrease the risk of bleeding.
D. stimulate bone marrow production of granulocytes.

36. Mrs. Summers complains of severe abdominal and bone pain. The doctor prescribes patient-controlled analgesia with morphine. The nurse should monitor the patient for which of morphine's adverse effects?

A. sedation, hypotension, and constipation
B. headache, dizziness, and dry mouth
C. ataxia, slurred speech, and confusion
D. drowsiness, rash, and hepatitis

SITUATION: *Jeanette Woodrow, age 35, is admitted to the medical-surgical floor with fatigue, malaise, pallor, and oliguria. She has a 10-year history of systemic lupus erythematosus for which she receives prednisone (Deltasone), hydroxychloroquine (Plaquenil), and sulindac (Clinoril).*

Questions 37 to 41 refer to this situation.

37. Because Mrs. Woodrow is receiving prednisone, she should be assessed for:

    A. hypotension.
    B. polyuria.
    C. hypocalcemia.
    D. hyperglycemia.

38. The nurse enters the room and finds Mrs. Woodrow crying. She states, "My face is fat and ugly. I can't stand it anymore." The nurse's best response would be:

    A. "You've been sick a long time. It must be very difficult."
    B. "You can't stop taking prednisone abruptly because you'll become quite ill."
    C. "Obviously, you're experiencing an adverse effect of prednisone; it will go away soon."
    D. "If you'd like your privacy now, I'll leave."

39. Which of the following laboratory reports should the nurse evaluate when assessing Mrs. Woodrow for complications of systemic lupus erythematosus (SLE)?

    A. Antinuclear antibody (ANA) level
    B. Vitamin B_6 level
    C. Creatinine level
    D. Enzyme-linked immunosorbent assay (ELISA)

40. Which statement by Mrs. Woodrow indicates successful teaching about hydroxychloroquine (Plaquenil)?

    A. "I should rise slowly from a supine position."
    B. "I should eat a banana every day with my Plaquenil."
    C. "This medication is reserved for when my joint pain becomes severe."
    D. "I must see the eye doctor every 6 months."

41. Which of the following could trigger an exacerbation of Mrs. Woodrow's systemic lupus erythematosus (SLE)?

A. Sun exposure
B. Change in body temperature
C. Dietary salt intake
D. Exercise

SITUATION: *James Cutler, a 32-year-old black man, is admitted to the hospital in vaso-occlusive sickle cell crisis. He complains of chest pain, shortness of breath, severe myalgia, and arthralgia.*

Questions 42 to 48 refer to this situation.

42. Which of the following may have triggered Mr. Cutler's vaso-occlusive crisis?

A. Aspirin use
B. Recent chest cold
C. Jaundice
D. Spicy foods

43. During vaso-occlusive crisis, the nurse should encourage Mr. Cutler to:

A. change his position frequently.
B. restrict his fluid intake.
C. decrease his protein intake.
D. drink 5 qt (5 L) of fluid each day.

44. Which of the following may be effective in relieving Mr. Cutler's joint pain?

A. Applying ice packs to the joints.
B. Performing active resistive range-of-motion exercises.
C. Applying warm compresses to the joints.
D. Applying transcutaneous electrical nerve stimulation (TENS).

45. On the 3rd day of treatment, Mr. Cutler complains that meperidine (Demerol) isn't relieving his pain. The nurse interprets this as:

A. drug addiction.
B. drug tolerance.
C. attention-seeking behavior.
D. drug abuse.

46. Unrelieved abdominal pain that occurs during vaso-occlusive crisis may indicate:

A. fecal impaction.
B. mesenteric infarction.
C. attention-seeking behavior.
D. pancreatitis.

47. Mr. Cutler complains of chest pain. The nurse should:

    A. notify the doctor.
    B. offer emotional support.
    C. massage the affected area.
    D. distract the patient.

48. Mr. Cutler complains of priapism during vaso-occlusive crisis. The nurse suggests that:

    A. taking a warm bath may alleviate the problem.
    B. taking folic acid supplements can prevent priapism.
    C. he should stop thinking sexually arousing thoughts.
    D. he should stand to void.

SITUATION: *Gary Smith, age 68, is admitted to the hospital with shaking chills and fever. His red blood cell count is abnormally low, causing the doctor to suspect aplastic anemia.*

Questions 49 to 52 refer to this situation.

49. Mr. Smith is at greater risk for infection with aplastic anemia because:

    A. a large amount of immature red blood cells (RBCs) are produced.
    B. granulocyte production is depressed.
    C. an excessive number of thrombocytes are present.
    D. vitamin B_{12} isn't being absorbed by the stomach.

50. Which of the following should be included in Mr. Smith's plan of care?

    A. Avoiding I.M. injections
    B. Maintaining strict bed rest
    C. Measuring and recording hourly intake and output
    D. Checking pedal pulses every 4 hours

51. Which of the following drugs that Mr. Smith has taken may be responsible for causing aplastic anemia?

    A. Ibuprofen (Motrin)
    B. Sulfamethoxazole-trimethoprim (Bactrim)
    C. Levothyroxine (Synthroid)
    D. Heparin (Liquaeim)

52. Mr. Smith has severe granulocytopenia. The nurse should teach him to:

    A. avoid raw fruits and vegetables.
    B. take vitamin C to ward off the common cold.
    C. observe for polydipsia and polyuria.
    D. restrict sodium in the diet.

SITUATION: *William Painter, age 60, is admitted to the hospital with shortness of breath, chest pain, and numbness and tingling in his hands. His hemoglobin level is 6.4 mg/dl and his hematocrit 19.2%. A Schilling test is ordered to rule out the diagnosis of pernicious anemia.*

    Questions 53 to 56 refer to this situation.

53. When teaching Mr. Painter about a Schilling test, the nurse explains that:

    A. this test studies vitamin B_{12} absorption from the stomach.
    B. after an iron injection he'll need to produce a urine sample.
    C. his urine will be collected for 24 hours to determine the folic acid content.
    D. a blood sample will be taken from his arm, and his red blood cell distribution width will be measured.

54. The nurse begins the 24-hour urine collection for the Shilling test at 7 a.m. Mr. Painter is instructed:

    A. to collect all of his urine from 7 a.m. today until 7 a.m. tomorrow.
    B. to discard the first voided specimen at 7 a.m. today and save all urine, including that from 7 a.m. the next day.
    C. to discard the first voided specimen today and tomorrow but save all urine in between.
    D. that an indwelling urinary catheter will be inserted to ensure no urine is lost during the 24-hour period.

55. Mr. Painter states, "The doctor says if I have pernicious anemia, I'll need shots the rest of my life. Why can't I just take a pill?" A nurse's best response would be, "When you have pernicious anemia:

    A. vitamin B_{12} can't be absorbed in your stomach because you lack the intrinsic factor needed for absorption."
    B. the B vitamins are destroyed by the gastric mucosa before absorption."
    C. an overproduction of erythropoietin inactivates vitamin B_{12} in your stomach."
    D. your bone marrow is incapable of producing red blood cells (RBCs)."

56. Anemia that results from vitamin B_{12} deficiency differs from other anemias because:

    A. death from sepsis is likely with vitamin B_{12} deficiency.
    B. neurologic dysfunction may result from vitamin B_{12} deficiency.
    C. bruising, bleeding, and ecchymosis are common with vitamin B_{12} deficiency.
    D. shortness of breath and tachycardia result from vitamin B_{12} deficiency.

SITUATION: *Harry Graham, a 59-year-old patient with pancreatic cancer, is admitted to the hospital with gram-negative sepsis. Mr. Graham is anxious and restless. He has petechiae all over his body and blood oozing from a venipuncture site. Disseminated intravascular coagulation is suspected.*

Question 57 to 59 refer to this situation.

57. For treatment of DIC, the nurse should expect to administer:

    A. albumin.
    B. fresh frozen plasma.
    C. packed red blood cells.
    D. tissue plasminogen activator (tPA).

58. Mr. Graham's toes on his left foot are cyanotic, mottled, and cool to the touch. The nurse suspects:

    A. hematoma formation.
    B. cancer metastasis.
    C. a thromboembolism.
    D. petechiae.

59. Mr. Graham becomes restless and anxious. His heart rate increases to 125 beats/minute, and his blood pressure drops to 78/42 mm Hg. The nurse notifies the doctor because she suspects the patient may have:

    A. an internal hemorrhage.
    B. oliguria.
    C. oxygen toxicity.
    D. brain metastasis.

SITUATION: *Susan Adams, age 36, is admitted to the medical-surgical floor with intractable vomiting. She has been receiving chemotherapy for acute leukemia. Her treatment regimen includes intrathecal methotrexate; I.V. daunorubicin (Cerubidine), cytarabine (Cytosar-U), and vincristine (Oncovin); and oral prednisone (Deltasone).*

Questions 60 to 67 refer to this situation.

60. Intrathecal methotrexate is administered into the:

    A. peritoneal cavity.
    B. bone marrow.
    C. spinal canal.
    D. peripherally inserted central venous catheter (PICC).

61. Mrs. Adams develops severe anemia from methotrexate therapy. The nurse anticipates administration of which drug?

    A. Leucovorin (Wellcovorin)
    B. Erythropoietin (Epogen)
    C. Prednisone (Deltasone)
    D. Ferrous sulfate

62. While Mrs. Adams is receiving daunorubicin (Cerubidine), the nurse should assess her for:

    A. visual disturbances.
    B. heart failure.
    C. polycythemia.
    D. hyperglycemia.

63. Mrs. Adams complains of numbness in her feet. The nurse recognizes that this is an adverse effect of:

    A. methotrexate.
    B. prednisone (Deltasone).
    C. vincristine (Oncovin).
    D. doxorubicin (Adriamycin).

64. Mrs. Adams is to receive a bone marrow transplant. When teaching the patient about bone marrow transplantation, the nurse should include which of the following in her teaching plan?

    A. Bone marrow transplantation is performed before chemotherapy to reduce complications.
    B. Bone marrow from a cadaver may be used if the patient has no living related donor.
    C. Donor bone marrow is administered through a central venous catheter.
    D. A small amount of bone marrow is removed from multiple donors, processed, and returned to the client.

65. Mrs. Adams develops graft-versus-host (GVH) disease 7 days after transplantation. GVH disease is best described as:

    A. an infection transferred from donor to recipient.
    B. bone marrow rejection.
    C. immunosuppression caused by bone marrow failure.
    D. an adverse effect of alpha interferon therapy.

66. The nurse should recognize which signs and symptoms of graft-versus-host (GVH) disease?

    A. Polyuria, polydipsia, and polyphagia
    B. Hyperglycemia, polyuria, and polydipsia
    C. Depression, dermatitis, and aplastic anemia
    D. Hepatitis, dermatitis, and hemolytic anemia

67. Mrs. Adams requires a blood transfusion. While the blood is infusing, she complains of low back pain. In addition to calling the doctor, the most appropriate intervention is to:

    A. administer the ordered analgesic and massage the area.
    B. slow the infusion rate of the blood and infuse normal saline solution.
    C. stop the transfusion and obtain urine and blood samples.
    D. draw blood to evaluate the patient's prothrombin time and activated partial thromboplastin time.

ANSWER SHEET

	A B C D		A B C D		A B C D
1	○ ○ ○ ○	24	○ ○ ○ ○	47	○ ○ ○ ○
2	○ ○ ○ ○	25	○ ○ ○ ○	48	○ ○ ○ ○
3	○ ○ ○ ○	26	○ ○ ○ ○	49	○ ○ ○ ○
4	○ ○ ○ ○	27	○ ○ ○ ○	50	○ ○ ○ ○
5	○ ○ ○ ○	28	○ ○ ○ ○	51	○ ○ ○ ○
6	○ ○ ○ ○	29	○ ○ ○ ○	52	○ ○ ○ ○
7	○ ○ ○ ○	30	○ ○ ○ ○	53	○ ○ ○ ○
8	○ ○ ○ ○	31	○ ○ ○ ○	54	○ ○ ○ ○
9	○ ○ ○ ○	32	○ ○ ○ ○	55	○ ○ ○ ○
10	○ ○ ○ ○	33	○ ○ ○ ○	56	○ ○ ○ ○
11	○ ○ ○ ○	34	○ ○ ○ ○	57	○ ○ ○ ○
12	○ ○ ○ ○	35	○ ○ ○ ○	58	○ ○ ○ ○
13	○ ○ ○ ○	36	○ ○ ○ ○	59	○ ○ ○ ○
14	○ ○ ○ ○	37	○ ○ ○ ○	60	○ ○ ○ ○
15	○ ○ ○ ○	38	○ ○ ○ ○	61	○ ○ ○ ○
16	○ ○ ○ ○	39	○ ○ ○ ○	62	○ ○ ○ ○
17	○ ○ ○ ○	40	○ ○ ○ ○	63	○ ○ ○ ○
18	○ ○ ○ ○	41	○ ○ ○ ○	64	○ ○ ○ ○
19	○ ○ ○ ○	42	○ ○ ○ ○	65	○ ○ ○ ○
20	○ ○ ○ ○	43	○ ○ ○ ○	66	○ ○ ○ ○
21	○ ○ ○ ○	44	○ ○ ○ ○	67	○ ○ ○ ○
22	○ ○ ○ ○	45	○ ○ ○ ○		
23	○ ○ ○ ○	46	○ ○ ○ ○		

ANSWERS AND RATIONALES

1. *Correct answer:* **A**

Symptoms associated with rheumatoid arthritis include bilateral pain, swelling, erythema, and warm joints. A butterfly rash is typical in patients with systemic lupus erythematosus. Pain and stiffness in rheumatoid arthritis is worse in the morning or after periods of immobility. Unilateral leg swelling and pain are typical of deep vein thrombosis.

> *Nursing process step:* Assessment
> *Client needs category:* Physiological integrity
> *Client needs subcategory:* Physiological adaptation
> *Taxonomic level:* Knowledge

2. *Correct answer:* **B**

Moist heat reduces pain and muscle spasm by relaxing muscles and increasing blood flow. Movement and exercise will be less painful following heat applications. Splinting joints is reserved for periods of acute inflammation or to prevent deformities and their progression. Ice (used for 20 minutes) relieves pain by desensitizing nerve endings. Usually reserved for acute inflammation, ice also decreases cellular activity and edema. Rising later in the morning won't relieve stiffness.

> *Nursing process step:* Implementation
> *Client needs category:* Physiological integrity
> *Client needs subcategory:* Basic care and comfort
> *Taxonomic level:* Application

3. *Correct answer:* **C**

Paraffin baths involve applying melted wax to joints to relieve stiffness and pain. Patients with diabetes are prone to neuropathy and decreased sensation, which would place the patient at risk for a thermal injury if the paraffin is too hot. Individuals with the other disorders wouldn't be at risk for thermal injury.

> *Nursing process step:* Planning
> *Client needs category:* Physiological integrity
> *Client needs subcategory:* Reduction of risk potential
> *Taxonomic level:* Application

4. *Correct answer:* **B**

The cane is held by the hand on the unaffected side with the elbow at hip level for proper support and balance. Advancing the cane with the affected leg and same hand will throw the patient off balance. The cane will relieve pressure on joints and prevent further injury, so the cane should be used if the joint is hot and swollen.

Nursing process step: Assessment
Client needs category: Physiological integrity
Client needs subcategory: Reduction of risk potential
Taxonomic level: Application

5. *Correct answer:* **D**

Rheumatoid arthritis is an autoimmune disorder. Corticosteroids, such as prednisone, will mediate the immune response and decrease inflammation in patients not responding to nonsteroidal anti-inflammatory drugs. Corticosteroids may cause glucose intolerance and mood changes, including depression. They don't relieve stress on joints.

Nursing process step: Implementation
Client needs category: Physiological integrity
Client needs subcategory: Pharmacological and parenteral therapies
Taxonomic level: Knowledge

6. *Correct answer:* **B**

Arthrocentesis involves removing synovial fluid under local anesthesia to evaluate fluid and relieve pressure caused by the fluid. Arthroscopy involves inserting a scope into the affected joint to visualize and repair damaged tissues or tendons. An intra-articular injection involves injecting medication into the joint to reduce pain and inflammation. Arthrodesis involves fusing joints to eliminate motion and stress on a joint.

Nursing process step: Implementation
Client needs category: Physiological integrity
Client needs subcategory: Reduction of risk potential
Taxonomic level: Knowledge

7. *Correct answer:* **D**

Enteric coating delays the absorption of the drug, delaying the onset of action. Large doses of enteric-coated aspirin will be absorbed and may cause a toxic reaction. Acetaminophen, not enteric-coated aspirin, in high doses may cause hepatic damage. Aspirin must not be used in children with viral illnesses because of the risk of Reye's syndrome.

Nursing process step: Implementation
Client needs category: Physiological integrity
Client needs subcategory: Pharmacological and parenteral therapies
Taxonomic level: Comprehension

8. *Correct answer:* **A**

Standard precautions should be instituted for this patient and should also be used routinely for any patient who doesn't require specific isolation precautions. There is no indication that the patient has infected stool, so enteric precautions aren't necessary. Blood and body fluid precautions are part of standard precautions.

> *Nursing process step:* Planning
> *Client needs category:* Safe, effective care environment
> *Client needs subcategory:* Safety and infection control
> *Taxonomic level:* Application

9. *Correct answer:* **A**

Acetaminophen (Tylenol) shouldn't be taken concomitantly with zidovudine because of the risk of liver damage. Antacids, ascorbic acid, and stool softeners can be taken with zidovudine.

> *Nursing process step:* Evaluation
> *Client needs category:* Physiological integrity
> *Client needs subcategory:* Pharmacological and parenteral therapies
> *Taxonomic level:* Comprehension

10. *Correct answer:* **D**

Kaposi's sarcoma, a neoplastic disorder, is commonly found on the skin and internal organs of patients with AIDS. Petechiae are dotlike hemorrhages less than 1 mm in size, indicating a low platelet level. AIDS doesn't produce a cutaneous reaction. In telangiectasia, ruptured superficial arterioles appear with pinpoint red centers with fine spidery veins emanating from the center. They occur as a result of portal hypertension that occurs with cirrhosis.

> *Nursing process step:* Assessment
> *Client needs category:* Physiological integrity
> *Client needs subcategory:* Reduction of risk potential
> *Taxonomic level:* Analysis

11. *Correct answer:* **C**

Adverse effects of interferon therapy include flulike symptoms, dizziness, confusion, somnolence, fatigue, diarrhea, thrombocytopenia, anemia, leukopenia, and hypotension.

> *Nursing process step:* Implementation
> *Client needs category:* Physiological integrity
> *Client needs subcategory:* Pharmacological and parenteral therapies
> *Taxonomic level:* Knowledge

12. *Correct answer:* **B**

Transmission of the human immunodeficiency virus occurs through contact with blood and such body fluids as semen or vaginal secretions. Therefore, the partner should wear a condom during sexual relations. Using the same drinking glass, if blood isn't present, doesn't put the partner at risk for AIDS. Zidovudine is an antiviral drug that inhibits viral replication but doesn't cure AIDS or prevent the disease from spreading to others.

> *Nursing process step:* Evaluation
> *Client needs category:* Safe, effective care environment
> *Client needs subcategory:* Safety and infection control
> *Taxonomic level:* Analysis

13. *Correct answer:* **B**

Providing the employee with information about available services will help her to feel more at ease. Telling her everything will be all right and telling her she isn't likely to get AIDS is offering her false reassurance. There is no guarantee that everything will be all right. Reassuring her that staff will be available if she becomes upset implies that staff is only available to her when she's upset.

> *Nursing process step:* Implementation
> *Client needs category:* Psychosocial integrity
> *Client needs subcategory:* Coping and adaptation
> *Taxonomic level:* Knowledge

14. *Correct answer:* **A**

ELISA is used to detect HIV antibodies. A reactive ELISA test alone can't be used to diagnose acquired immunodeficiency syndrome (AIDS). Western blot, or indirect fluorescent antibody, is specific and confirms the presence of HIV antibody. Although a low CD4+ lymphocyte count indicates AIDS progression, it isn't diagnostic for HIV. HBsAg confirms the presence of hepatitis B. Anti-Smith antibodies are present in systemic lupus erythematosus.

> *Nursing process step:* Planning
> *Client needs category:* Physiological integrity
> *Client needs subcategory:* Physiological adaptation
> *Taxonomic level:* Knowledge

15. *Correct answer:* **B**

Because zidovudine may cause anemia and bone marrow suppression, the nurse should have her hemoglobin levels and hematocrit evaluated. Serum albumin and potassium levels may be abnormal and the patient's mental status may change with acquired immunodeficiency syndrome, but these don't result from zidovudine therapy.

> *Nursing process step:* Planning
> *Client needs category:* Physiological integrity
> *Client needs subcategory:* Pharmacological and parenteral therapies
> *Taxonomic level:* Comprehension

16. *Correct answer:* **A**

Aspirin inhibits platelet aggregation and is contraindicated in patients with bleeding disorders such as ITP. Acetaminophen, diazepam, and famotidine aren't contraindicated in clients with ITP.

> *Nursing process step:* Planning
> *Client needs category:* Physiological integrity
> *Client needs subcategory:* Pharmacological and parenteral therapies
> *Taxonomic level:* Application

17. *Correct answer:* **D**

Thrombocytopenia that results from immunologic platelet destruction is known as idiopathic thrombocytopenic purpura (ITP). Antibodies that reduce the life span of platelets have been found in nearly all patients. Signs and symptoms of ITP include epistaxis, oral bleeding, purpura, and petechiae. A female patient may complain of menorrhagia. Myalgia and arthralgia aren't associated with ITP. The tongue has a smooth, beefy appearance in patients with macrocytic anemia.

> *Nursing process step:* Assessment
> *Client needs category:* Physiological integrity
> *Client needs subcategory:* Physiological adaptation
> *Taxonomic level:* Comprehension

18. *Correct answer:* **B**

Petechiae are small dotlike skin hemorrhages associated with thrombocytopenia. Papules are raised pustules. Ecchymosis refers to bruising. A hematoma is a collection of blood.

> *Nursing process step:* Assessment
> *Client needs category:* Physiological integrity
> *Client needs subcategory:* Physiological adaptation
> *Taxonomic level:* Comprehension

19. *Correct answer:* **A**

In ITP, the body forms antibodies that destroy platelets causing the patient to bleed. ITP in the acute form usually follows a viral infection, such as rubella or chickenpox, and can result from immunization with a live vaccine. The chronic form seldom follows infection and is commonly linked with other immunologic disorders such as systemic lupus erythematosus. Excessive aspirin intake can cause bleeding but not ITP. Iron-deficiency anemia, not ITP, will improve with iron supplements.

> *Nursing process step:* Implementation
> *Client needs category:* Physiological integrity
> *Client needs subcategory:* Reduction of risk potential
> *Taxonomic level:* Knowledge

20. *Correct answer:* **B**

Blood must be transfused through a catheter that has a lumen size of 20G or larger because a smaller lumen size will destroy blood cells. Initially, blood should be infused at a rate of 1 ml/kg/hour to monitor the patient for a transfusion reaction. The drip factor of blood tubing is 10 gtt/ml, so an infusion rate of 50 gtt/minute would be too rapid. Blood isn't warmed unless the patient is hypothermic or multiple units are transfused. Blood products should be administered with normal saline solution only because other fluids will cause blood cell hemolysis.

> *Nursing process step:* Planning
> *Client needs category:* Physiological integrity
> *Client needs subcategory:* Pharmacological and parenteral therapies
> *Taxonomic level:* Application

21. *Correct answer:* **C**

A unit of packed RBCs contains RBCs that have been separated from plasma and platelets. Typing and crossmatching is necessary whenever RBCs are infused. A unit of whole blood contains both plasma and RBCs and each unit contains about 500 ml. A unit of packed RBCs contains approximately 250 ml.

> *Nursing process step:* Implementation
> *Client needs category:* Physiological integrity
> *Client needs subcategory:* Reduction of risk potential
> *Taxonomic level:* Comprehension

22. *Correct answer:* **D**

Dyspnea, orthopnea, tachycardia, jugular vein distention, sudden anxiety, and the presence of crackles on auscultation are classic signs and symptoms of fluid overload. Hemolytic reactions occur within the first 15 minutes after the transfusion is begun; symptoms include chills, low back pain, headache, nausea, and chest tightness. Febrile reactions result from sensitivity to the donor's white cells, platelets, or plasma proteins; the patient doesn't have a fever.

> *Nursing process step:* Assessment
> *Client needs category:* Physiological integrity
> *Client needs subcategory:* Physiological adaptation
> *Taxonomic level:* Analysis

23. *Correct answer:* **B**

Symptoms of anemia include fatigue, weakness, pallor, tachycardia, and dyspnea. The heart rate returns to normal when enough blood has been transfused to restore the oxygen-carrying capacity of the blood. Oliguria is a sign of acute hypovolemia, which was not present in this patient. Blood transfusions should increase urine output in the patient with acute hypovolemia. Depending on the source of bleeding, the stools may contain blood after the blood is transfused. A normal temperature indicates that a febrile transfusion reaction hasn't occurred.

> *Nursing process step:* Evaluation
> *Client needs category:* Physiological integrity
> *Client needs subcategory:* Physiological adaptation
> *Taxonomic level:* Analysis

24. *Correct answer:* **D**

Ascorbic acid, found in orange juice, enhances the GI tract's absorption of iron. Aluminum hydroxide gel decreases the absorption of iron supplements. Vitamin D and pyridoxine don't affect iron supplement absorption.

> *Nursing process step:* Planning
> *Client needs category:* Physiological integrity
> *Client needs subcategory:* Pharmacological and parenteral therapies
> *Taxonomic level:* Application

25. *Correct answer:* **A**

Eating green leafy vegetables, fortified and whole grains, and organ and red meats and using cast iron cookware will increase dietary intake of iron. Fish and white rice are suggested for a low-residue diet. Dairy products and sardines add calcium to the diet. Eggs and cheese are dietary sources of vitamin B_{12}.

> *Nursing process step:* Implementation
> *Client needs category:* Physiological integrity
> *Client needs subcategory:* Basic care and comfort
> *Taxonomic level:* Knowledge

26. *Correct answer:* **C**

The patient should be instructed to take iron supplements with meals because the presence of food in the stomach decreases gastric distress. Iron must be taken for the prescribed time — to ensure that iron stores are replaced — and shouldn't be discontinued when the patient feels better.

> *Nursing process step:* Planning
> *Client needs category:* Physiological integrity
> *Client needs subcategory:* Pharmacological and parenteral therapies
> *Taxonomic level:* Comprehension

27. *Correct answer:* **B**

During a bone marrow aspiration, a small amount of bone marrow is taken from the posterior iliac crest, under local anesthesia, and analyzed. A blood sample isn't analyzed as part of the bone marrow aspiration. A transfusion of blood into an I.V. catheter in the patient's arm is a blood transfusion. Injecting bone marrow into the circulation through an I.V. catheter describes a bone marrow transplant.

> *Nursing process step:* Implementation
> *Client needs category:* Psychosocial integrity
> *Client needs subcategory:* Coping and adaptation
> *Taxonomic level:* Knowledge

28. *Correct answer:* **B**

Acute leukemia begins as a malignant proliferation of white blood cell precursors, or blasts, in the bone marrow or lymph tissue, resulting in an accumulation of these cells in peripheral blood, bone marrow, and body tissues. CD4+ lymphocyte count is used to determine human immunodeficiency virus progression. A serum potassium level greater than 5 mEq/L is high normal and not typical in leukemia. Hypercalcemia may occur with leukemia.

> *Nursing process step:* Assessment
> *Client needs category:* Physiological integrity
> *Client needs subcategory:* Reduction of risk potential
> *Taxonomic level:* Knowledge

29. *Correct answer:* **B**

Chemotherapy accelerates malignant and nonmalignant tissue destruction, leading to increased uric acid production. Allopurinol combats uric acid synthesis. Allopurinol doesn't decrease nausea or vomiting or shrink swollen lymphoid tissue. There is no indication that this patient has gout in her great toe.

> *Nursing process step:* Implementation
> *Client needs category:* Physiological integrity
> *Client needs subcategory:* Pharmacological and parenteral therapies
> *Taxonomic level:* Analysis

30. *Correct answer:* **C**

The patient receiving chemotherapy is susceptible to infection from bone marrow suppression and granulocytopenia. Patients should be instructed to avoid malls, movie theaters, and infected individuals. Raw fruits and vegetables may be contaminated by pathogens and should be avoided during severe neutropenia or washed in hot soapy water. Although rectal temperatures may be more accurate, they aren't appropriate for the neutropenic patient. Rectal temperatures increase the risk of rectal abscess due to rectal trauma. Meticulous hand washing by staff and visitors will prevent the spread of infection; there is no need for sterile garb and no need to avoid visiting; the patient will need emotional support from family at this time.

Nursing process step: Planning
Client needs category: Safe, effective care environment
Client needs subcategory: Safety and infection control
Taxonomic level: Application

31. *Correct answer:* **C**

The nurse should anticipate transfusing packed RBCs if the patient with leukemia experiences chest pain. Chest pain, a symptom of ischemia, results from inadequate oxygen-carrying capacity of the blood. Although feeling chilly may be a symptom of anemia, it isn't an indication for transfusion. Frequent sore throats indicate an inadequate number or functioning of WBCs. Petechiae indicate thrombocytopenia.

Nursing process step: Planning
Client needs category: Physiological integrity
Client needs subcategory: Reduction of risk potential
Taxonomic level: Analysis

32. *Correct answer:* **B**

Meticulous mouth care is necessary during chemotherapy because rapidly dividing cells in the mouth may be destroyed, causing stomatitis, xerostomia, and pain. Soft swabs should be used for mouth and gum care to avoid tissue trauma. Moistening foods with gravy or broth or eating cool foods may be helpful. Flossing and using harsh mouthwashes that contain alcohol or vinegar should be avoided. Visiting the dentist every 3 months isn't a substitute for daily mouth care. Eliminating nutrition will impair tissue healing.

Nursing process step: Implementation
Client needs category: Physiological integrity
Client needs subcategory: Pharmacological and parenteral therapies
Taxonomic level: Application

33. *Correct answer:* **C**

The nurse should suggest that the patient use a satin pillowcase because it will tug at hair less than a cotton pillowcase. Dandruff shampoo and other harsh shampoos should be replaced with protein or gentle shampoo. There is no indication that the patient is disturbed by the hair loss, so suggesting a wig would be inappropriate. Nurses don't prescribe drugs, so suggesting a folic acid supplement would also be inappropriate.

Nursing process step: Implementation
Client needs category: Physiological integrity
Client needs subcategory: Pharmacological and parenteral therapies
Taxonomic level: Comprehension

34. *Correct answer:* **D**

Bone marrow suppression that leads to severe granulocytopenia, thrombocytopenia, and anemia will limit the chemotherapy dose. Hypercalcemia and hyperuricemia are treated with medications and fluids. Xerostomia doesn't limit chemotherapy doses.

> *Nursing process step:* Evaluation
> *Client needs category:* Physiological integrity
> *Client needs subcategory:* Pharmacological and parenteral therapies
> *Taxonomic level:* Analysis

35. *Correct answer:* **D**

Filgrastim, or granulocyte colony-stimulating factor, stimulates bone marrow production of granulocytes for fighting infection. It also stimulates platelet and red blood cell production, but to a lesser degree. Erythropoietin (Epogen) stimulates the bone marrow to produce red blood cells. Filgrastim doesn't cause immunosuppression or synthesize prothrombin.

> *Nursing process step:* Implementation
> *Client needs category:* Physiological integrity
> *Client needs subcategory:* Pharmacological and parenteral therapies
> *Taxonomic level:* Knowledge

36. *Correct answer:* **A**

Sedation, hypotension, constipation, vomiting, pupillary constriction, and respiratory depression are adverse effects of morphine. Headache, dizziness, and dry mouth are adverse effects of nalbuphine (Nubain). Ataxia, slurred speech, and confusion are adverse effects of phenytoin (Dilantin). Drowsiness, rash, and hepatitis are adverse effects of allopurinol (Zyloprim).

> *Nursing process step:* Assessment
> *Client needs category:* Physiological integrity
> *Client needs subcategory:* Pharmacological and parenteral therapies
> *Taxonomic level:* Comprehension

37. *Correct answer:* **D**

Prednisone, a corticosteroid, impairs glucose tolerance, causing hyperglycemia. Other adverse effects of corticosteroids include hypertension, mood swings, hypokalemia, and ulcers. Hypotension, polyuria, and hypocalcemia aren't adverse effects of prednisone.

> *Nursing process step:* Assessment
> *Client needs category:* Physiological integrity
> *Client needs subcategory:* Pharmacological and parenteral therapies
> *Taxonomic level:* Comprehension

38. *Correct answer:* **A**

Telling the patient that it must be very difficult being sick validates her feelings and shows respect. The "moon face" the patient is experiencing is an adverse effect of prednisone; saying that this effect will go away soon ignores the patient's feelings. Leaving the room without the patient's request may leave the patient feeling abandoned when she needs emotional support.

> *Nursing process step:* Implementation
> *Client needs category:* Psychosocial integrity
> *Client needs subcategory:* Coping and adaptation
> *Taxonomic level:* Application

39. *Correct answer:* **C**

Renal failure is a complication that occurs in 20% or more of those with SLE, so the patient's creatinine level should be checked at regular intervals. The ANA level is elevated in SLE, rheumatoid arthritis, and arteritis. ELISA tests for human immunodeficiency virus antibodies. Vitamin B_6 level is incorrect.

> *Nursing process step:* Assessment
> *Client needs category:* Physiological integrity
> *Client needs subcategory:* Reduction of risk potential
> *Taxonomic level:* Analysis

40. *Correct answer:* **D**

Hydroxychloroquine may cause retinopathy; the patient should have an eye examination every 6 months. The drug must be taken continually to be effective, not just when joint pain is severe. Hydroxychloroquine doesn't cause orthostatic hypotension, so the patient doesn't have to rise slowly from a supine position. A patient doesn't have to eat bananas with hydroxychloroquine.

> *Nursing process step:* Evaluation
> *Client needs category:* Physiological integrity
> *Client needs subcategory:* Pharmacological and parenteral therapies
> *Taxonomic level:* Application

41. *Correct answer:* **A**

Exposure to sunlight may trigger skin eruptions. The patient with SLE may have a low-grade fever, but it doesn't exacerbate the patient's condition. Sodium doesn't exacerbate SLE either. Exercise should be encouraged during periods of remission.

> *Nursing process step:* Planning
> *Client needs category:* Physiological integrity
> *Client needs subcategory:* Reduction of risk potential
> *Taxonomic level:* Knowledge

42. *Correct answer:* **B**

Dehydration, infection, or hypoxemia may trigger vaso-occlusive crisis. Jaundice may occur as a result of hemolytic crisis. Aspirin and spicy foods don't trigger vaso-occlusive crisis.

> *Nursing process step:* Assessment
> *Client needs category:* Physiological integrity
> *Client needs subcategory:* Reduction of risk potential
> *Taxonomic level:* Comprehension

43. *Correct answer:* **D**

Encouraging increased fluid intake decreases blood viscosity and prevents dehydration. The nurse should help the patient conserve energy by encouraging rest and limiting activities. The nurse should reposition the patient frequently and encourage a diet high in protein and vitamins.

> *Nursing process step:* Planning
> *Client needs category:* Physiological integrity
> *Client needs subcategory:* Reduction of risk potential
> *Taxonomic level:* Application

44. *Correct answer:* **C**

Warm compresses increase blood flow to the affected joint, relieving pain. Ice causes decreased blood flow to the affected joint, increasing pain. The nurse should turn the patient frequently to prevent skin breakdown and conserve the patient's energy. TENS application is reserved for chronic pain.

> *Nursing process step:* Planning
> *Client needs category:* Physiological integrity
> *Client needs subcategory:* Basic care and comfort
> *Taxonomic level:* Application

45. *Correct answer:* **B**

Tolerance to narcotics may occur, requiring increased dosages to relieve pain. Drug addiction is the physical and psychological need for a drug. Withdrawal of the drug will cause physical effects. Patients who are experiencing pain aren't exhibiting attention-seeking behavior. Drug abuse is the constant craving that causes the individual to seek the drug regardless of the consequences.

> *Nursing process step:* Assessment
> *Client needs category:* Physiological integrity
> *Client needs subcategory:* Pharmacological and parenteral therapies
> *Taxonomic level:* Knowledge

46. Correct answer: **B**

During vaso-occlusive crisis, hemoglobin S becomes rigid and crescent-shaped, obstructing blood flow. Mesenteric artery blood flow obstruction is responsible for the patient's abdominal pain. The patient isn't exhibiting attention-seeking behavior. Fecal impaction and pancreatitis don't result from vaso-occlusive crisis.

Nursing process step: Assessment
Client needs category: Physiological integrity
Client needs subcategory: Reduction of risk potential
Taxonomic level: Analysis

47. *Correct answer:* **A**

The nurse should notify the doctor for prompt recognition and treatment of the patient's chest pain. The nurse can offer emotional support after the doctor is notified and treatment has begun. Massaging the affected area and distracting the patient won't treat the pain.

Nursing process step: Implementation
Client needs category: Physiological integrity
Client needs subcategory: Reduction of risk potential
Taxonomic level: Application

48. *Correct answer:* **A**

Priapism, painful sustained erection, can be treated by emptying the bladder at onset. Taking folic acid supplements and standing to void won't alleviate the problem. Priapism isn't brought on by sexual arousal.

Nursing process step: Implementation
Client needs category: Physiological integrity
Client needs subcategory: Reduction of risk potential
Taxonomic level: Application

49. *Correct answer:* **B**

Aplastic anemia results when the bone marrow produces insufficient quantities of RBCs, white blood cells, and platelets. Granulocytes, a type of white blood cell, are needed to fight infection. The quantity of blood cells is affected, but not the quality; immature RBCs aren't produced. Thrombocyte production affects blood clotting, and vitamin B_{12} deficiency leads to pernicious anemia.

Nursing process step: Planning
Client needs category: Physiological integrity
Client needs subcategory: Reduction of risk potential
Taxonomic level: Comprehension

50. *Correct answer:* **A**

As the bone marrow fails, thrombocytopenia develops, leaving the patient with aplastic anemia at risk for bleeding. I.M injections should be avoided. Activities are permitted as tolerated. Measuring and recording intake and output every hour and checking pedal pulses every 4 hours aren't necessary.

> *Nursing process step:* Planning
> *Client needs category:* Physiological integrity
> *Client needs subcategory:* Reduction of risk potential
> *Taxonomic level:* Application

51. Correct answer: **B**

Sulfa drugs such as sulfamethoxazole-trimethoprim are occasionally linked to aplastic anemia. Ibuprofen, levothyroxine, and heparin don't cause aplastic anemia.

> *Nursing process step:* Assessment
> *Client needs category:* Physiological integrity
> *Client needs subcategory:* Pharmacological and parenteral therapies
> *Taxonomic level:* Application

52. *Correct answer:* **A**

The nurse should teach the patient to avoid raw fruits and vegetables because they may harbor pathogens, putting him at risk for infection. It's inappropriate for the nurse to suggest that the patient take vitamin C because she doesn't prescribe medications. Polyuria and polydipsia are present with diabetes mellitus, not granulocytopenia. A patient with granulocytopenia doesn't need to restrict sodium intake.

> *Nursing process step:* Planning
> *Client needs category:* Physiological integrity
> *Client needs subcategory:* Basic care and comfort
> *Taxonomic level:* Application

53. *Correct answer:* **A**

During the first phase of a Schilling test, radioactive B_{12} is ingested and given I.M. If radioactive B_{12} is absorbed by the stomach, it will be present in the urine, indicating that pernicious anemia isn't present. A 24-hour urine specimen is then collected. If radioactive B_{12} doesn't appear in the urine, the test is repeated in several days using an oral dose of intrinsic factor. The presence of radioactive B_{12} in the urine after administration of intrinsic factor confirms pernicious anemia.

> *Nursing process step:* Implementation
> *Client needs category:* Physiological integrity
> *Client needs subcategory:* Reduction of risk potential
> *Taxonomic level:* Knowledge

54. *Correct answer:* **B**

The proper procedure for 24-hour urine collection is to discard the first voided urine specimen on the 1st day regardless of time, to collect urine for 24 hours, and to include the first voided specimen on the 2nd day. There is no indication that the patient is incontinent or unable to follow directions, so an indwelling urinary catheter isn't necessary.

> *Nursing process step:* Implementation
> *Client needs category:* Physiological integrity
> *Client needs subcategory:* Reduction of risk potential
> *Taxonomic level:* Knowledge

55. *Correct answer:* **A**

Vitamin B_{12} can't be absorbed by the stomach in the patient with pernicious anemia because intrinsic factor is lacking. The remaining B vitamins are absorbed in the gastric mucosa because they don't require intrinsic factor for absorption. Overproduction of erythropoietin would affect RBC production. A decreased production of RBCs in bone marrow leads to hemolytic anemia.

> *Nursing process step:* Implementation
> *Client needs category:* Physiological integrity
> *Client needs subcategory:* Pharmacological and parenteral therapies
> *Taxonomic level:* Application

56. *Correct answer:* **B**

Because vitamin B_{12} is necessary for myelin sheath production, paresthesia, proprioception, and balance problems may result from deficiency. Death from sepsis and bruising and bleeding may occur with aplastic anemia. Shortness of breath and tachycardia are common in anemias when there is a reduction in the red blood cell count and the hemoglobin level, diminishing the blood's oxygen-carrying capacity.

> *Nursing process step:* Assessment
> *Client needs category:* Physiological integrity
> *Client needs subcategory:* Reduction of risk potential
> *Taxonomic level:* Comprehension

57. *Correct answer:* **B**

The nurse should expect to administer fresh frozen plasma to the patient with DIC. Fresh frozen plasma supplies the patient with clotting factors absent in DIC. Albumin is given to restore intravascular fluid volume. Red blood cells replace oxygen-carrying capacity of the blood and may be used in hemorrhage. The thrombolytic agent tPA isn't indicated for DIC.

Nursing process step: Planning
Client needs category: Physiological integrity
Client needs subcategory: Physiological adaptation
Taxonomic level: Application

58. *Correct answer:* **C**

Disseminated intravascular coagulation results from widespread clotting in the microcirculation. Cool, mottled feet and diminished peripheral pulses are signs of arterial occlusion. Hematoma wouldn't involve all the toes on his left foot; it would be limited to one area. Metastasis to the foot isn't likely and wouldn't present with cyanosis, mottling, and coolness to touch. Petechiae are small dotlike hemorrhages smaller than 1 mm.

Nursing process step: Assessment
Client needs category: Physiological integrity
Client needs subcategory: Reduction of risk potential
Taxonomic level: Analysis

59. *Correct answer:* **A**

A change in mental status, tachycardia, hypotension, and cool, clammy skin are signs of hypovolemic shock. Because the patient has disseminated intravascular coagulation, the nurse should suspect an internal hemorrhage. Oliguria is a urine output of less than 30 ml/hour, which may also be present in hypovolemic shock. Oxygen toxicity occurs from administration of high concentrations of oxygen over an extended time. The patient with brain metastasis won't have these signs.

Nursing process step: Assessment
Client needs category: Physiological integrity
Client needs subcategory: Physiological adaptation
Taxonomic level: Analysis

60. *Correct answer:* **C**

Intrathecal drug administration involves injecting a drug into the intrathecal space of the spinal canal. Intrathecal administration doesn't involve administering a drug into the peritoneal cavity or bone marrow or through a PICC.

Nursing process step: Implementation
Client needs category: Physiological integrity
Client needs subcategory: Pharmacological and parenteral therapies
Taxonomic level: Comprehension

61. *Correct answer:* **A**

Leucovorin is administered to restore bone marrow function. Erythropoietin is used to stimulate red blood cell production when adequate iron stores are present and bone marrow is functioning. Prednisone is used to treat autoimmune anemias and suppress white blood cell production in leukemia. Ferrous sulfate is used to treat iron deficiency anemia.

Nursing process step: Planning
Client needs category: Physiological integrity
Client needs subcategory: Pharmacological and parenteral therapies
Taxonomic level: Application

62. *Correct answer:* **B**

Daunorubicin may cause irreversible cardiomyopathy, leading to heart failure. Visual disturbances, hyperglycemia, and polycythemia aren't adverse effects of daunorubicin administration.

Nursing process step: Assessment
Client needs category: Physiological integrity
Client needs subcategory: Pharmacological and parenteral therapies
Taxonomic level: Comprehension

63. *Correct answer:* **C**

Vincristine may cause peripheral neuropathy, or numbness, in her feet. Methotrexate, prednisone, and doxorubicin don't cause this adverse effect.

Nursing process step: Assessment
Client needs category: Physiological integrity
Client needs subcategory: Pharmacological and parenteral therapies
Taxonomic level: Knowledge

64. *Correct answer:* **C**

Bone marrow transplantation is performed after chemotherapy and radiation destroys all the recipient's existing bone marrow and malignant cells. The bone marrow is taken from a single donor and infused I.V. through a central venous catheter. Bone marrow from a cadaver isn't used.

Nursing process step: Planning
Client needs category: Physiological integrity
Client needs subcategory: Physiological adaptation
Taxonomic level: Application

65. *Correct answer:* **B**

GVH disease occurs when T lymphocytes view the recipient's tissues as foreign and cause an immune response against the recipient's tissues. GVH disease isn't an infectious process, immunosuppression, or an adverse effect of alpha interferon therapy.

Nursing process step: Assessment
Client needs category: Physiological integrity
Client needs subcategory: Physiological adaptation
Taxonomic level: Knowledge

66. *Correct answer:* **D**

On the 7th day after bone marrow transplantation, the nurse should begin to watch for signs of GVH disease, such as hepatitis, dermatitis, hemolytic anemia, and thrombocytopenia. Polyuria, polydipsia, polyphagia, and hyperglycemia are signs and symptoms of diabetes mellitus.

Nursing process step: Assessment
Client needs category: Physiological integrity
Client needs subcategory: Reduction of risk potential
Taxonomic level: Knowledge

67. *Correct answer:* **C**

If the patient receiving a blood transfusion complains of low back pain, chills, headache, nausea, or chest tightness, she's experiencing a hemolytic transfusion reaction. The nurse should immediately stop the blood transfusion, assess the patient's vital signs, and obtain urine and blood samples according to facility policy. Ordering an analgesic and massaging the area will delay appropriate treatment. To evaluate bleeding potential, blood may be drawn at a later time.

Nursing process step: Implementation
Client needs category: Physiological integrity
Client needs subcategory: Physiological adaptation
Taxonomic level: Application

COMPREHENSIVE EXAMINATION

1. Which sign suggests that a patient with syndrome of inappropriate antidiuretic hormone (SIADH) has developed complications?

    A. Tetanic contractions
    B. Neck vein distention
    C. Weight loss
    D. Polyuria

2. Maria Leoni, age 27, comes in for an appointment 6 months after delivering her child. She states she was unable to breast-feed her baby and is concerned that she hasn't menstruated. The best action by the nurse would be to:

    A. reassure her that this is normal and her menses should return soon.
    B. ask if she had any hemorrhaging during or after her delivery.
    C. refer her to a support group.
    D. ask her if she had gestational diabetes mellitus.

3. George Whelan, age 75, is admitted to the medical-surgical floor with weakness and left-sided chest pain. The symptoms have been present for several weeks after a viral illness. Which assessment finding is most symptomatic of pericarditis?

    A. Pericardial friction rub
    B. Bilateral crackles auscultated at the lung bases
    C. Pain unrelieved by a change in position
    D. Third heart sound (S_3)

4. When the nurse attempts to ventilate a patient during cardiopulmonary resuscitation, she notices an airway obstruction. In an unresponsive adult, the most common cause of airway obstruction is:

    A. the patient's dentures.
    B. a foreign body.
    C. the tongue.
    D. the epiglottis.

5. Ron Black is admitted to the hospital with right-sided heart failure. When assessing him for jugular vein distention, the nurse should position him:

    A. lying on his side with the head of the bed flat.
    B. sitting upright.
    C. flat on his back.
    D. lying on his back with the head of the bed elevated 30 to 45 degrees.

6. Drainage on a craniotomy dressing must be measured and marked. Which of the following should be reported immediately to the doctor?

    A. Bloody drainage
    B. Yellowish drainage
    C. Greenish drainage
    D. Foul-smelling drainage

7. Judy Peterson was diagnosed with asthma and is receiving albuterol (Proventil) inhalation treatments. The nurse should assess the patient for which adverse effects?

    A. Tachycardia
    B. Bradycardia
    C. Hypotension
    D. Lethargy

8. A nurse has just finished teaching a group of new patient care aides about the spread of tuberculosis (TB). She knows her teaching has been effective when one of the aides states:

    A. "I could get TB by coming in contact with the patient's stool."
    B. "I could get TB if I become contaminated with the patient's blood."
    C. "I could get TB if I inhale infected droplets when the patient coughs."
    D. "I could get TB if I handle the patient's urine without wearing gloves."

9. The nurse is interviewing a slightly overweight 43-year-old man with mild emphysema and borderline hypertension. He admits to smoking a pack of cigarettes per day. When developing a teaching plan, which of the following should receive highest priority to help decrease respiratory complications?

    A. Weight reduction
    B. Decreasing salt intake
    C. Smoking cessation
    D. Decreasing caffeine intake

10. When assessing breath sounds, the nurse would anticipate hearing bronchoalveolar sounds:

    A. over the trachea only.
    B. over the central airways.
    C. throughout the entire lung fields.
    D. throughout the peripheral lung fields only.

11. A patient admitted to the hospital with a pneumothorax has the following arterial blood gas (ABG) analysis: pH, 7.19; $Paco_2$, 63 mm Hg; and HCO_3^-, 22 mEq/L. A chest tube was inserted and oxygen administered at 4 L/minute by nasal cannula. An hour after the initiation of treatment, ABG analysis reveals: pH, 7.28; $Paco_2$, 52 mm Hg; and HCO_3^-, 22 mEq/L. This change in ABG analysis indicates:

    A. respiratory alkalosis.
    B. impending respiratory arrest.
    C. the need for intubation.
    D. improved respiratory status.

12. A patient complains to the nurse that his sputum is thick and he has difficulty expectorating. The nurse should:

    A. offer him milk.
    B. offer him water.
    C. start I.V. fluids immediately.
    D. tell him to avoid drinking apple juice.

13. What is the ratio of chest compressions to ventilations when one rescuer performs cardiopulmonary resuscitation (CPR) on an adult?

    A. 15:1
    B. 15:2
    C. 12:1
    D. 12:2

14. Which nursing diagnosis takes priority for the patient with Bell's palsy?

    A. Risk for dysfunctional grieving
    B. Risk for injury related to corneal laceration
    C. Risk for chronic low self-esteem
    D. Risk for impaired physical mobility

15. When assessing a patient for fluid and electrolyte balance, the nurse is aware that the organs most important in maintaining this balance are the:

    A. pituitary gland and pancreas.
    B. liver and gallbladder.
    C. brain stem and heart.
    D. lungs and kidneys.

16. When the nurse performs a neurologic assessment on Anne Jones, her pupils are dilated and don't respond to light. Ms. Jones most likely has:

A. glaucoma.

B. damage to the third cranial nerve.

C. damage to the lumbar spine.

D. Bell's palsy.

17. When the doctor obtains a cerebrospinal fluid (CSF) specimen during a lumbar puncture, it's important that the nurse:

A. number all of the specimens in the order that they were drawn.

B. dispose of the first specimen drawn.

C. dispose of the last specimen drawn.

D. combine all fluid into one sterile container.

18. In a comatose patient, hearing is the last sense to be lost. Therefore, the nurse should always:

A. talk loudly in case the patient can hear.

B. speak softly before gently touching the patient.

C. tell others in the room not to talk to the patient.

D. tell family members that the patient probably can't hear.

19. The least serious form of brain trauma, characterized by a brief loss of consciousness and period of confusion, is called:

A. contusion.

B. concussion.

C. coup.

D. contrecoup.

20. Capillary refill time is normally:

A. 1 to 2 seconds.

B. 3 to 5 seconds.

C. 6 to 8 seconds.

D. 9 to 10 seconds.

21. Increased intracranial pressure (ICP) usually occurs as a result of:

A. cerebral edema.

B. spinal cord trauma.

C. cerebral herniation.

D. seizures.

22. Mrs. Krane experiences orthostatic hypotension while receiving furosemide (Lasix). The nurse should:

A. administer I.V. fluids as ordered.
B. administer a vasodilator as prescribed.
C. instruct her to sit up for several minutes before standing.
D. insert an indwelling urinary catheter to track output.

23. Digoxin (Lanoxin) therapy is effective when the patient with atrial fibrillation has an electrocardiogram (ECG) showing:

A. a heart rate of 70 beats/minute.
B. supraventricular tachycardia.
C. Mobitz II heart block.
D. a heart rate of 50 beats/minute.

24. Signs and symptoms of retinal detachment include:

A. painless decrease in vision, veil over the visual field, and flashing lights.
B. veil over the visual field, increased intraocular pressure, and yellow-green halos around visual images.
C. photophobia, yellow-green halos around visual images, and blurred vision.
D. unilateral eye inflammation, cloudy cornea, and moderately dilated pupil.

25. Treatment for Raynaud's disease includes:

A. avoiding cold and stress.
B. vasodilator drug therapy.
C. amputating the affected hand.
D. removing the blood clot.

26. Which signs and symptoms are associated with an acoustic neuroma?

A. Amenorrhea and obesity
B. Acromegaly
C. Ataxia and intention tremor
D. Unilateral hearing loss and tinnitus

27. When administering the patient's sucralfate (Carafate), the nurse should give the drug:

A. with meals.
B. 30 minutes after meals.
C. between meals with a snack.
D. 1 hour before meals.

28. Audrey Winters complains of a severe, throbbing headache following a lumbar puncture. The priority nursing intervention for this patient is to:

    A. restrict fluid intake.
    B. increase fluid intake.
    C. raise the head of the bed.
    D. assess vital signs.

29. Ida Weller, age 59, is transferred to the medical-surgical floor after being treated with nitroglycerin for an angina attack. To prevent further chest pain, the doctor prescribes the beta-adrenergic blocker propranolol (Inderal). The nurse assesses Mrs. Weller before administering each dose. Which finding should prompt the nurse to withhold the drug and notify the doctor?

    A. Complaints of chest pain
    B. Pulse rate greater than 90 beats/minute
    C. Systolic blood pressure less than 90 mm Hg
    D. Diastolic blood pressure more than 80 mm Hg

30. Vagal stimulation on the heart primarily causes:

    A. increased parasympathetic tone.
    B. increased sympathetic tone.
    C. decreased parasympathetic tone.
    D. decreased sympathetic tone.

31. The nurse should instruct the patient taking antacids to:

    A. stagger them with other medications.
    B. take them with all other medications.
    C. take them only at night.
    D. drink a glass of water immediately after taking them.

32. Following a total gastrectomy, the patient should receive which supplement to prevent pernicious anemia?

    A. Calcium
    B. Phosphorus
    C. Vitamin D
    D. Vitamin B_{12}

33. The nurse should instruct the patient suspected of having postpolio syndrome to:

    A. perform strenuous exercise three times a week.
    B. run, not walk.
    C. swim in warm water.
    D. swim in cold water.

34. A patient with appendicitis is at risk for developing:

    A. peritonitis.
    B. hemorrhage.
    C. bowel obstruction.
    D. renal failure.

35. Anne Dougherty must learn how to reduce risk factors and manage the acute pain of angina. When developing the plan of care, the nurse should include the expected outcome "The patient should verbalize the need to:

    A. call the doctor if acute pain lasts more than 2 hours."
    B. avoid exercise."
    C. stop smoking."
    D. restrict dietary fat, fiber, and cholesterol."

36. A patient with tuberculosis is taking isoniazid (Laniazid) and rifampin (Rifadin). What additional medication typically is given to minimize the adverse effects of isoniazid?

    A. Pyridoxine (vitamin B_6)
    B. Ethambutol hydrochloride (Myambutol)
    C. Magnesium sulfate
    D. Cyanocobalamin (vitamin B_{12})

37. The patient with myasthenia gravis is experiencing a sudden increase in weakness. He's unable to clear his secretions and breathe easily. These observations suggest the patient is experiencing:

    A. a hypertensive crisis.
    B. a hypo-osmolar state.
    C. an allergic reaction to immunosuppressants.
    D. myasthenic crisis.

38. A patient with a bowel obstruction located high in the intestinal tract will have:

    A. pain relief with defecation.
    B. a fecal breath odor.
    C. respiratory difficulty.
    D. pain relief with vomiting.

39. If the intestinal obstruction is located high in the small intestine, the nurse would expect vomitus that:

    A. has a fecal odor.
    B. is light green.
    C. is dark green.
    D. is bright red.

40. Which of the following dosage forms can be crushed, dissolved in water, and administered through a nasogastric (NG) tube?

    A. Simple compressed tablets
    B. Enteric-coated tablets
    C. Time-release capsules
    D. Controlled-delivery capsules

41. The patient asks the nurse what he can do to prevent exacerbations of myasthenia gravis. What is the most appropriate response?

    A. "There is nothing you can do to prevent exacerbations except take your medication on schedule."
    B. "Avoid exposure to excessive heat, crowds, and emotional extremes."
    C. "Take you medication, get plenty of rest, and participate in frequent hard, physical exercise."
    D. "Exposure to sunlight has beneficial effects and will cause your medication dosage to be decreased."

42. The doctor writes an order for the nurse to discontinue a patient's nasogastric (NG) tube. Before removing the tube, the nurse should:

    A. make sure the patient is able to chew food.
    B. assess the patient for bowel sounds.
    C. determine if the patient is hungry and wants to eat.
    D. aspirate gastric contents to make sure that the residual volume is less than 100 ml.

43. The most common cause of cardiac arrest in an adult is:

    A. electrolyte disturbance.
    B. respiratory arrest.
    C. ventricular fibrillation.
    D. drug toxicity.

44. The nurse is evaluating a patient's ventilation and perfusion. Which of the following statements should the nurse use to support the outcome?

    A. Normally, ventilation and perfusion are equally balanced throughout the lung.
    B. The normal ventilation-perfusion ratio is 0.8:1.
    C. Perfusion scans are performed by having the patient inhale a radioactive substance.
    D. A low ventilation-perfusion ratio occurs in pulmonary embolism.

45. A 32-year-old man with chronic renal failure is admitted to the hospital with bilateral infiltrates of the lungs. His first arterial blood gas analysis reveals: pH, 7.24; $Paco_2$, 40 mm Hg; Pao_2, 64 mm Hg; and HCO_3^-, 13 mEq/L. His respiratory rate is 22 breaths/minute. What is the patient's acid-base status?

    A. Uncompensated respiratory alkalosis with hypoxia
    B. Uncompensated respiratory acidosis with hypoxia
    C. Uncompensated respiratory acidosis with mixed metabolic alkalosis
    D. Uncompensated metabolic acidosis with hypoxia

46. The patient with neuropathy affecting the legs and feet should be instructed to:

    A. avoid walking barefoot.
    B. keep his feet warm with heating pads or heavy wool socks.
    C. take vasoconstricting drugs on schedule.
    D. include foods high in vitamin K in his diet.

47. When assessing the patient with a new ileostomy, the nurse knows that the effluent from the ileostomy should be:

    A. well-formed stool.
    B. soft stool.
    C. pasty to soft stool.
    D. liquid to pasty stool.

48. Dietary planning for a patient with an ileostomy should include:

    A. telling the patient to restrict his fluid intake.
    B. instructing the patient to limit potassium-rich foods.
    C. explaining that he should limit his calorie intake.
    D. telling the patient to avoid high-fiber foods.

49. Stridor is described as a:

    A. continuous, high-pitched sound that has musical quality.
    B. very loud musical sound that's usually heard without a stethoscope.
    C. short, explosive or popping sound usually heard during inspiration.
    D. loud, grating sound caused by inflamed or damaged pleurae.

50. Neomycin (Neo-Tabs) is administered before bowel surgery to:

    A. decrease the risk of wound infection.
    B. increase the body's immunologic response to surgery.
    C. decrease the incidence of postoperative atelectasis.
    D. prevent postoperative bladder atony.

51. Which nursing diagnosis is most appropriate for a patient with syndrome of inappropriate antidiuretic hormone (SIADH) and hyponatremia?

    A. Risk for injury related to seizure activity
    B. Impaired skin integrity related to peripheral edema
    C. Fluid volume excess related to increased thyrotropin secretion
    D. Impaired gas exchange related to pulmonary edema

52. Cardiomyopathy may lead to heart failure. When assessing a patient with left-sided heart failure, the nurse should expect to see:

    A. air hunger and tachypnea.
    B. ascites.
    C. jugular vein distention.
    D. pitting edema of the legs.

53. Which event may trigger pain in the patient with trigeminal neuralgia?

    A. Walking in the mall
    B. Sitting in the sun
    C. Eating lunch
    D. Sleeping

54. Brad Carlson returns from surgery with a sigmoid colostomy. An ostomy appliance is attached. The priority nursing diagnosis for daily observation and care is:

    A. alteration in bowel elimination related to diarrhea.
    B. alteration in skin integrity related to seepage.
    C. alteration in nutrition related to high-fat diet.
    D. risk for immobility related to surgical procedure.

55. What is the most common portal of entry for microorganisms associated with sepsis?

    A. Skin
    B. GI tract
    C. Respiratory tract
    D. Urinary tract

56. The nurse prepares discharge instructions for a patient with chronic syndrome of inappropriate antidiuretic hormone (SIADH). Which statement indicates that the patient understands these instructions?

A. "I'll check all food labels to make sure that I restrict my sodium intake."

B. "I'll keep a log of my daily weight and call the doctor if I gain 2 lb (0.90 kg) or more in a day without changing my eating habits."

C. "I'll check my pulse every morning and will contact my doctor if it's irregular or rapid."

D. "I'll measure my urine and check the specific gravity with a refractometer. If it begins to gradually rise, I'll tell my doctor."

57. The doctor inserts a chest tube and attaches it to a water-seal drainage device set at 20 cm of suction. The doctor orders a chest X-ray to:

A. check the position of the chest tube.

B. advance the tube 1 cm further.

C. visualize a single layer of the lungs.

D. record sound waves that penetrate the lungs.

58. Otorrhea and rhinorrhea are most commonly seen with which type of skull fracture?

A. basilar

B. temporal

C. occipital

D. parietal

59. Mrs. Bryant has prosopagnosia. The nurse can help the patient and her family cope by suggesting the family:

A. involve the patient in hygiene and grooming activities.

B. bring in familiar photographs that include the patient.

C. assist the patient in frequent exercise that includes walking.

D. remind the patient to sing songs that encourage facial exercise.

60. The nurse is caring for Zelda Zimmerman, who had a right total-knee replacement yesterday. Her leg has been placed in a continuous passive motion (CPM) exerciser, or CPM machine. The nurse's role with the client requiring CPM therapy is to:

A. ensure proper placement of the knee as well as degree of extension and flexion.

B. assist with active range of motion at least four times daily.

C. maintain bed rest without complications until a flexion of 90 degrees can be tolerated.

D. remove the leg from the machine three times daily and thoroughly massage the extremity.

61. Nonhormonal drugs, such as calcitonin (Calcimar) and alendronate (Fosamax), are used for treating osteoporosis because they:

    A. inhibit the activity of osteoblasts.
    B. inhibit the activity of osteoclasts.
    C. increase the production of estrogen.
    D. increase vitamin D metabolism.

62. Pericardiocentesis is performed on a patient with cardiac tamponade. This procedure would be deemed effective if:

    A. aspirated blood clots rapidly.
    B. blood pressure decreases.
    C. blood pressure increases.
    D. heart sounds become muffled.

63. Pain from osteoarthritis is described as mechanical pain, which means:

    A. the pain responds to mechanical device use.
    B. the pain is relieved by rest and worsened by activity.
    C. the pain is worse at the beginning of the day and improves with activity.
    D. rest and activity have no effect on the pain.

64. Nursing care immediately after a supratentorial craniotomy includes:

    A. lying flat in bed.
    B. neurologic checks and vital signs every 4 hours.
    C. limiting fluids to 1½ qt (1.5 L) in 24 hours.
    D. allowing no pillows under the head.

65. When listening to heart sounds, the nurse can best hear the first heart sound (S_1) at the:

    A. base of the heart.
    B. apex of the heart.
    C. mitral valve area of the heart.
    D. tricuspid area of the heart.

66. Which intervention is critical in managing a patient with chronic syndrome of inappropriate antidiuretic hormone (SIADH)?

    A. Administering diuretics
    B. Infusing hypotonic sodium chloride replacement solution
    C. Restricting fluid intake
    D. Administering potassium supplements

67. A Glasgow Coma Scale score of 8 in a patient with a new head injury indicates:

> **A.** a mild head injury.
> **B.** a brief loss of consciousness.
> **C.** a severe head injury.
> **D.** death will occur within minutes.

68. Leonard Frizzle's medical history reveals that he has several preexisting conditions. Which of the following conditions requires cautious use of promethazine (Phenergan)?

> **A.** Diabetes mellitus
> **B.** Prostatic hyperplasia
> **C.** Hypercalcemia
> **D.** Renal insufficiency

69. To help prevent superinfection during loracarbef (Lorabid) therapy, the nurse should teach the patient to eat which of the following foods?

> **A.** Yogurt and buttermilk
> **B.** Green leafy vegetables
> **C.** High-fiber cereals
> **D.** Citrus fruits

70. Which functional losses contraindicate vancomycin (Vancocin) use?

> **A.** Visual loss
> **B.** Hearing loss
> **C.** Perceptual loss
> **D.** Kinesthetic loss

71. Which is the priority nursing diagnosis for a patient experiencing angina?

> **A.** Decreased cardiac output
> **B.** Pain
> **C.** Anxiety
> **D.** Altered tissue perfusion

72. Hepatitis A is least likely to be transmitted through:

> **A.** sexual contact.
> **B.** the oral-fecal route.
> **C.** contaminated food, shellfish, or milk products.
> **D.** blood.

73. Which respiratory sound is most commonly associated with laryngotracheobronchitis (croup)?

    A. Crackles
    B. Barky cough
    C. Wheezing during inhalation
    D. Wheezing during exhalation

74. The patient with acute bronchitis requires careful monitoring when receiving:

    A. oxygen therapy.
    B. fluid resuscitation.
    C. humidified air.
    D. postural drainage.

75. An indwelling urinary catheter has been inserted in an adult patient who was dehydrated from vomiting. Which urine output indicates that the patient has received adequate fluid replacement?

    A. 15 ml/hour
    B. 25 ml/hour
    C. 30 ml/hour
    D. 5 ml/hour

76. When implementing initial treatment of a patient in anaphylactic shock, the priority is:

    A. administering antihistamines.
    B. maintaining airway patency.
    C. establishing I.V. access.
    D. infusing a bolus of 200 ml of lactated Ringer's solution.

77. One early sign associated with Lyme disease is:

    A. synovitis.
    B. arthritic pain.
    C. reddened lesion with central clearing.
    D. myocarditis.

78. A repeat clean-catch urine specimen may need to be collected if which of the following is present in the urinalysis?

    A. Bacteria
    B. Increased epithelial cells
    C. Increased white blood cells (WBCs)
    D. Pus

79. Which laboratory finding supports a diagnosis of pyelonephritis?

A. Myoglobinuria
B. Ketonuria
C. Pyuria
D. Low white blood cell count

80. What is an appropriate intervention for a patient with a kidney stone?

A. I.V. fluids at a keep-vein-open rate
B. Narcotic analgesics, preferably I.V.
C. Indwelling urinary catheter
D. Nasogastric (NG) tube to low suction

81. Stephanie Walters is a 24-year-old prostitute infected with the human immunodeficiency virus who is now presenting with symptoms of acquired immunodeficiency syndrome. Ms. Walters is prescribed didanosine (Videx). The nurse instructs her to:

A. take the medication with an antacid to prevent GI upset.
B. dissolve the powder in orange juice to replace potassium.
C. take the medication on an empty stomach with water.
D. avoid lying down for 1/2 hour after taking the medication.

82. Which vaginal infection doesn't require treatment for sexual partners?

A. *Neisseria gonorrhoeae*
B. *Candida albicans*
C. *Trichomonas vaginalis*
D. *Chlamydia trachomatis*

83. Which individuals are at risk for developing pernicious anemia?

A. Those with a history of gastrectomy surgery
B. I.V. drug users
C. Patients with colostomies
D. Alcoholics

84. Nancy Draver is recovering from mitral valve replacement surgery without incident and actively participates in discharge teaching. Teaching is effective when Mrs. Draver states:

A. "I don't have any new prescriptions."
B. "I'll need to take Coumadin for a while."
C. "I'll need to take one aspirin a day."
D. "I'll need to take an iron supplement."

SITUATION: *Evelyn Tracy, a 56-year-old school teacher, has been using a cane to ambulate and has been taking large doses of anti-inflammatory medications. The* *pain from osteoarthritis in her left knee has become the focus of her life, and she has finally agreed to surgical joint replacement.*

Questions 85 to 87 refer to this situation.

85. After speaking with her doctor, Mrs. Tracy agrees to continuous epidural analgesia with opiates for postoperative pain control. The most common adverse effects associated with epidural analgesia are:

    A. hypertension and respiratory depression.
    B. confusion and lethargy.
    C. inadequate pain control and excessive sedation.
    D. itching, nausea, vomiting, and urine retention.

86. Preoperatively, Mrs. Tracy is told about the continuous passive motion (CPM) machine that her leg will be placed in immediately after the surgery. The purpose of CPM is to:

    A. improve mobility.
    B. decrease bleeding.
    C. decrease pain.
    D. decrease clot formation.

87. Mrs. Tracy is taught how to avoid infection of the prosthesis. What must she do for the rest of her life?

    A. avoid swimming in public pools
    B. take antibiotics before dental procedures
    C. take antibiotics only before major surgical procedures
    D. take her temperature on a regular schedule

SITUATION: *Thomas Rogers, a 77-year-old retired man, was admitted to the intensive care unit after a motor vehicle accident. He has a chest tube to treat a pneumothorax secondary to rib fractures. A fracture of his right radius was reduced in the emergency department and a cast applied. Several hours after arriving in the intensive care unit, he complains of increased pain in his right arm, which isn't relieved by the I.V. narcotic ordered.*

Questions 88 and 89 refer to this situation.

88. Mr. Rogers is diagnosed with compartment syndrome of his right arm. To decrease tissue pressure and maintain arterial perfusion to the lower arm, the nurse would prepare to assist the doctor in:

    A. giving vasodilators I.V.
    B. splitting or removing the cast.
    C. taking Mr. Rogers to the operating room.
    D. elevating the arm on a pole.

89. The nurse reinforces the doctor's description of a fasciotomy for the patient. When a fasciotomy is performed to alleviate compartment syndrome, the fascia is opened along the length of the muscle compartment and:

    A. the skin is sutured loosely.
    B. a pressure dressing is applied.
    C. the skin is left open.
    D. a skin graft is placed.

SITUATION: *For the past 2 years, Reginald Anderson has been treated for left-sided heart failure; he's now taking hydrochlorothiazide (HydroDIURIL). He comes to his doctor's office complaining of the inability to bear weight on his right foot. Assessment reveals swelling and tenderness of the right great toe. The diagnosis of gout is made.*

    Questions 90 to 92 refer to this situation.

90. Mr. Anderson has blood tests done to confirm the diagnosis of gout. The tests should include:

    A. complete blood count (CBC) and creatinine level.
    B. uric acid level and erythrocyte sedimentation rate (ESR).
    C. rheumatoid factor and red blood cell count.
    D. glucose and calcium levels.

91. Mr. Anderson's gout is probably due to:

    A. his long-term use of hydrochlorothiazide (HydroDIURIL).
    B. his history of heart failure.
    C. inactivity.
    D. a low-protein diet.

92. The goal of drug therapy during an acute episode of gout is to:

    A. relieve pain and inflammation as soon as possible.
    B. decrease uric acid blood levels.
    C. prevent infection.
    D. prevent kidney damage.

SITUATION: *Helen Adams enjoyed playing tennis three times a week at a new athletic club. She played despite pain that was increasing at the top of her right shoulder. This morning she couldn't raise her arm above her head to style her hair. She called her doctor, who explained that her symptoms are classic for a rotator cuff injury.*

    Questions 93 and 94 refer to this situation.

93. A rotator cuff is:

    A. made up of four muscles and their tendons.
    B. a ligament that connects the humerus and the scapula.
    C. a tendon that connects the deltoid muscle to the humerus.
    D. a ligament that connects the clavicle to the scapula.

94. Conservative treatment for a rotator cuff injury involves:

    A. applying ice initially, followed by heat application and rest for at least 1 week.
    B. pain medication administration and resumption of normal activities.
    C. heat application and range-of-motion exercises
    D. range-of-motion exercises and anti-inflammatory medication administration.

SITUATION: *Susan Lapin, age 34, was diagnosed with systemic lupus erythematosus. The doctor prescribes prednisone (Deltasone) to be taken every other day.*

Questions 95 and 96 refer to this situation.

95. The nurse should instruct Mrs. Lapin to take her prednisone:

    A. at bedtime.
    B. after lunch.
    C. with food before 8 a.m.
    D. 1 hour before any meal.

96. Mrs. Lapin owns a pool in her back yard. Which instruction should the nurse give her?

    A. "There are no restrictions on your activities, but plan rest periods."
    B. "Get some sun, but limit your exposure because sunburn can occur quickly."
    C. "Remember to keep your medication with you at all times."
    D. "Wear a sunscreen and avoid exposure to sunlight."

SITUATION: *Maxwell Pickney is a 48-year-old obese man who was seen for a routine checkup. His fasting blood glucose level is 135 mg/dl, so he's scheduled for a repeat test.*

Questions 97 to 100 refer to this situation.

97. Mr. Pickney asks the nurse why he has to return for another test. The nurse's best response would be:

    A. "Your fasting blood glucose level was normal, but we need a confirmation of that result."

    B. "Fasting blood glucose level tests are always repeated."

    C. "You have type 2 diabetes mellitus, so the test must be repeated."

    D. "Your fasting blood glucose level was abnormal and needs to be tested again."

98. The second fasting blood glucose level was 131 mg/dl, and Mr. Pickney was diagnosed with type 2 diabetes. When Mr. Pickney asks what caused his diabetes, the nurse should reply that type 2 diabetes is:

    A. an autoimmune disease.

    B. caused by decreased insulin levels.

    C. caused by insulin resistance.

    D. caused by eating too many sweets.

99. The initial treatment for Mr. Pickney is a meal plan change, with a goal of modest weight loss, and exercise. Modest weight loss and exercise are used to treat type 2 diabetes because each will:

    A. enhance insulin sensitivity.

    B. enhance insulin secretion.

    C. make patients feel better.

    D. prevent the progression of diabetes.

100. After a session with the dietitian, Mr. Pickney states he thinks he can change his meal plan to promote gradual weight loss. However, he expresses concern to the nurse about incorporating exercise into his busy lifestyle. The nurse should:

    A. tell him that weight loss will be sufficient.

    B. instruct him to join a local gym.

    C. instruct him to purchase a treadmill machine.

    D. help him find exercise options that fit his lifestyle.

ANSWER SHEET

	A B C D		A B C D		A B C D		A B C D
1	○ ○ ○ ○	26	○ ○ ○ ○	51	○ ○ ○ ○	76	○ ○ ○ ○
2	○ ○ ○ ○	27	○ ○ ○ ○	52	○ ○ ○ ○	77	○ ○ ○ ○
3	○ ○ ○ ○	28	○ ○ ○ ○	53	○ ○ ○ ○	78	○ ○ ○ ○
4	○ ○ ○ ○	29	○ ○ ○ ○	54	○ ○ ○ ○	79	○ ○ ○ ○
5	○ ○ ○ ○	30	○ ○ ○ ○	55	○ ○ ○ ○	80	○ ○ ○ ○
6	○ ○ ○ ○	31	○ ○ ○ ○	56	○ ○ ○ ○	81	○ ○ ○ ○
7	○ ○ ○ ○	32	○ ○ ○ ○	57	○ ○ ○ ○	82	○ ○ ○ ○
8	○ ○ ○ ○	33	○ ○ ○ ○	58	○ ○ ○ ○	83	○ ○ ○ ○
9	○ ○ ○ ○	34	○ ○ ○ ○	59	○ ○ ○ ○	84	○ ○ ○ ○
10	○ ○ ○ ○	35	○ ○ ○ ○	60	○ ○ ○ ○	85	○ ○ ○ ○
11	○ ○ ○ ○	36	○ ○ ○ ○	61	○ ○ ○ ○	86	○ ○ ○ ○
12	○ ○ ○ ○	37	○ ○ ○ ○	62	○ ○ ○ ○	87	○ ○ ○ ○
13	○ ○ ○ ○	38	○ ○ ○ ○	63	○ ○ ○ ○	88	○ ○ ○ ○
14	○ ○ ○ ○	39	○ ○ ○ ○	64	○ ○ ○ ○	89	○ ○ ○ ○
15	○ ○ ○ ○	40	○ ○ ○ ○	65	○ ○ ○ ○	90	○ ○ ○ ○
16	○ ○ ○ ○	41	○ ○ ○ ○	66	○ ○ ○ ○	91	○ ○ ○ ○
17	○ ○ ○ ○	42	○ ○ ○ ○	67	○ ○ ○ ○	92	○ ○ ○ ○
18	○ ○ ○ ○	43	○ ○ ○ ○	68	○ ○ ○ ○	93	○ ○ ○ ○
19	○ ○ ○ ○	44	○ ○ ○ ○	69	○ ○ ○ ○	94	○ ○ ○ ○
20	○ ○ ○ ○	45	○ ○ ○ ○	70	○ ○ ○ ○	95	○ ○ ○ ○
21	○ ○ ○ ○	46	○ ○ ○ ○	71	○ ○ ○ ○	96	○ ○ ○ ○
22	○ ○ ○ ○	47	○ ○ ○ ○	72	○ ○ ○ ○	97	○ ○ ○ ○
23	○ ○ ○ ○	48	○ ○ ○ ○	73	○ ○ ○ ○	98	○ ○ ○ ○
24	○ ○ ○ ○	49	○ ○ ○ ○	74	○ ○ ○ ○	99	○ ○ ○ ○
25	○ ○ ○ ○	50	○ ○ ○ ○	75	○ ○ ○ ○	100	○ ○ ○ ○

ANSWERS AND RATIONALES

1. *Correct answer:* **B**

SIADH causes antidiuretic hormone overproduction, which leads to fluid retention. Severe SIADH can cause such complications as vascular fluid overload, signaled by neck vein distention. Tetanic contractions aren't a sign of this disorder, but weight gain and fluid retention — due to oliguria — are.

> *Nursing process step:* Assessment
> *Client needs category:* Physiological integrity
> *Client needs subcategory:* Reduction of risk potential
> *Taxonomic level:* Knowledge

2. *Correct answer:* **B**

The nurse should ask the patient if she had any hemorrhaging during or after the delivery. Sheehan's syndrome, a form of hypopituitarism, is caused by anoxia from postpartal hemorrhage. The earliest signs are inability to lactate and failure to menstruate. Inability to lactate and failure to menstruate aren't normal or characteristic of gestational diabetes mellitus. Although a support group may be helpful, if the patient has hypopituitarism, this should be diagnosed and treated or she'll be infertile and experience a gradual deterioration of all functions regulated by the pituitary gland.

> *Nursing process step:* Implementation
> *Client needs category:* Physiological integrity
> *Client needs subcategory:* Reduction of risk potential
> *Taxonomic level:* Application

3. *Correct answer:* **A**

A pericardial friction rub may be present with the pericardial effusion of pericarditis. The lungs are typically clear when auscultated. Sitting up and leaning forward often relieves pericarditis pain. An S_3 indicates left-sided heart failure and isn't usually present with pericarditis.

> *Nursing process step:* Assessment
> *Client needs category:* Physiological integrity
> *Client needs subcategory:* Reduction of risk potential
> *Taxonomic level:* Knowledge

4. *Correct answer:* **C**

In an unresponsive adult, the most common cause of airway obstruction is the tongue. The rescuer should use the head-tilt, chin-lift maneuver to open the airway. If a neck injury is suspected, the jaw-thrust maneuver is recommended.

Nursing process step: Implementation
Client needs category: Physiological integrity
Client needs subcategory: Physiological adaptation
Taxonomic level: Knowledge

5. *Correct answer:* **D**

Assessing jugular vein distention should be done when the patient is in semi-Fowler's position (head of the bed elevated 30 to 45 degrees). If the patient lies flat, the veins will be more distended; if he sits upright, the veins will be flat.

Nursing process step: Assessment
Client needs category: Physiological integrity
Client needs subcategory: Reduction of risk potential
Taxonomic level: Knowledge

6. *Correct answer:* **A**

Bloody drainage on a craniotomy dressing could indicate hemorrhage and should be reported immediately to the doctor. The patient may need emergency surgery to repair the hemorrhage. A yellowish or green drainage or foul-smelling drainage should be reported but doesn't constitute a medical emergency.

Nursing process step: Implementation
Client needs category: Physiological integrity
Client needs subcategory: Reduction of risk potential
Taxonomic level: Knowledge

7. *Correct answer:* **A**

Tachycardia, hypertension, central nervous system excitation, and insomnia are adverse effects of albuterol; hypotension and lethargy aren't.

Nursing process step: Assessment
Client needs category: Physiological integrity
Client needs subcategory: Pharmacological and parenteral therapies
Taxonomic level: Application

8. *Correct answer:* **C**

TB transmission occurs when an infected person coughs or sneezes, spreading infected droplets. Many other infectious diseases can be transmitted through contact with stool, urine, or blood but not TB.

Nursing process step: Evaluation
Client needs category: Safe, effective care environment
Client needs subcategory: Management of care
Taxonomic level: Comprehension

9. *Correct answer:* **C**

Smoking should receive highest priority when trying to reduce risk factors for with respiratory complications. Losing weight and decreasing salt and caffeine intake can help to decrease risk factors for hypertension.

> *Nursing process step:* Planning
> *Client needs category:* Health promotion and maintenance
> *Client needs subcategory:* Prevention and early detection of disease
> *Taxonomic level:* Comprehension

10. *Correct answer:* **B**

Bronchoalveolar breath sounds, which are loud and coarse, are normally auscultated over the central airways. Tracheal breath sounds are normally heard over the trachea. There is no sound specifically auscultated throughout the entire lung fields. Vesicular breath sounds are heard over the peripheral lung fields.

> *Nursing process step:* Assessment
> *Client needs category:* Health promotion and maintenance
> *Client needs subcategory:* Prevention and early detection of disease
> *Taxonomic level:* Knowledge

11. *Correct answer:* **D**

The original ABG analysis reveals respiratory acidosis commonly seen with a pneumothorax. After chest tube insertion, the patient's respiratory status has improved, pH is increasing toward normal, and the $Paco_2$ is decreasing. ABG analysis in respiratory alkalosis shows an elevated pH and a low $Paco_2$. Assessment findings are more important than ABG analysis in determining if the patient requires intubation or if respiratory arrest is imminent.

> *Nursing process step:* Assessment
> *Client needs category:* Physiological integrity
> *Client needs subcategory:* Physiological adaptation
> *Taxonomic level:* Analysis

12. *Correct answer:* **B**

Inadequate hydration can cause sputum to become thick and difficult to expectorate. The patient needs to increase his oral intake of water and fruit juices. Milk products should be avoided because they may thicken sputum. I.V. fluids are necessary only if the patient's oral intake is inadequate.

> *Nursing process step:* Implementation
> *Client needs category:* Physiological integrity
> *Client needs subcategory:* Physiological adaptation
> *Taxonomic level:* Application

13. *Correct answer:* **B**

The correct ratio of compressions to ventilations when one rescuer performs CPR is 15:2.

> *Nursing process step:* Implementation
> *Client needs category:* Physiological integrity
> *Client needs subcategory:* Physiological adaptation
> *Taxonomic level:* Knowledge

14. *Correct answer:* **B**

The patient with Bell's palsy will be unable to close his eyelid on the affected side; therefore, he'll be at risk for injury to the cornea.

> *Nursing process step:* Analysis
> *Client needs category:* Physiological integrity
> *Client needs subcategory:* Reduction of risk potential
> *Taxonomic level:* Knowledge

15. *Correct answer:* **D**

The lungs and kidneys are the body's regulators of homeostasis. The lungs are responsible for removing fluid and carbon dioxide; the kidneys maintain a balance of fluid and electrolytes. The other organs play secondary roles in maintaining homeostasis.

> *Nursing process step:* Assessment
> *Client needs category:* Health promotion and maintenance
> *Client needs subcategory:* Prevention and early detection of disease
> *Taxonomic level:* Knowledge

16. *Correct answer:* **B**

The third cranial nerve (oculomotor) is responsible for pupil constriction. When there is damage to the nerve, the pupils remain dilated and don't respond to light. Glaucoma, lumbar spine injury, and Bell's palsy won't affect pupil constriction.

> *Nursing process step:* Assessment
> *Client needs category:* Physiological integrity
> *Client needs subcategory:* Physiological adaptation
> *Taxonomic level:* Application

17. *Correct answer:* **A**

Typically, a doctor will obtain four tubes of CSF. Each tube should be numbered in the order obtained to provide the most accurate fluid analysis results. No specimens should be discarded or combined.

Nursing process step: Implementation
Client needs category: Health promotion and maintenance
Client needs subcategory: Prevention and early detection of disease
Taxonomic level: Knowledge

18. *Correct answer:* **B**

Many patients have reported being able to hear when being in a comatose state. Therefore, the nurse should converse as if the patient was alert and oriented. Talking loudly is only appropriate if the patient is hard of hearing, and family members should be encouraged to talk with the patient unless contraindicated.

Nursing process step: Implementation
Client needs category: Physiological integrity
Client needs subcategory: Basic care and comfort
Taxonomic level: Application

19. *Correct answer:* **B**

Concussions are considered a minor injury with no structural signs of injury. A contusion is bruising of the brain tissue with small hemorrhages in the tissue. Coup and contrecoup are types of injuries in which the damaged area on the brain forms directly below the site of impact (coup) or at the site opposite the injury (contrecoup) due to movement of the brain within the skull.

Nursing process step: Assessment
Client needs category: Health promotion and maintenance
Client needs subcategory: Prevention and early detection of disease
Taxonomic level: Knowledge

20. *Correct answer:* **A**

Capillary refill time that's longer than 2 seconds is considered delayed and indicates decreased perfusion.

Nursing process step: Assessment
Client needs category: Health promotion and maintenance
Client needs subcategory: Prevention and early detection of disease
Taxonomic level: Comprehension

21. *Correct answer:* **A**

Increased ICP results from cerebral edema that may be caused by trauma to the head. Seizures typically don't cause significant increases in ICP. Spinal cord trauma won't affect ICP, and brain stem herniation will decrease ICP by decreasing the amount of brain contents in the skull.

Nursing process step: Assessment
Client needs category: Physiological integrity
Client needs subcategory: Physiological adaptation
Taxonomic level: Knowledge

22. *Correct answer:* C

The nurse should instruct the patient to rise slowly to a standing position to combat orthostatic hypotension. Administering I.V. fluids counteracts the effects of furosemide and may lead to fluid imbalance. Administering a vasodilator reduces the patient's blood pressure and may worsen orthostatic hypotension. Inserting an indwelling urinary catheter doesn't minimize the effects of orthostatic hypotension.

Nursing process step: Implementation
Client needs category: Physiological integrity
Client needs subcategory: Physiological adaptation
Taxonomic level: Application

23. *Correct answer:* A

Digoxin therapy is effective when the heart rate is below 100 beats/minute and above 60 beats/minute. If the patient's ECG shows supraventricular tachycardia, digoxin therapy isn't effective and another drug may be necessary to slow the patient's heart rate. Mobitz II heart block may be present if the patient is receiving too much digoxin.

Nursing process step: Evaluation
Client needs category: Physiological integrity
Client needs subcategory: Pharmacological and parenteral therapies
Taxonomic level: Analysis

24. *Correct answer:* A

A patient with retinal detachment has a painless decrease in vision and vision that is cloudy or smoky with flashing lights. The patient may also indicate that a curtain or veil is over the visual field. Intraocular pressure is normal or low. Photophobia, yellow-green halos around visual images, and blurred vision may occur with digoxin toxicity. Unilateral eye inflammation, cloudy cornea, and a moderately dilated pupil that's not reactive to light may occur with glaucoma.

Nursing process step: Assessment
Client needs category: Physiological integrity
Client needs subcategory: Reduction of risk potential
Taxonomic level: Comprehension

25. *Correct answer:* **A**

Initial treatment consists of avoiding cold, avoiding mechanical or chemical injury, and quitting smoking. Vasodilator drug therapy is generally reserved for severe cases. Hands are affected bilaterally, and amputation isn't usually done. Blood clots don't cause Raynaud's disease.

> *Nursing process step:* Implementation
> *Client needs category:* Physiological integrity
> *Client needs subcategory:* Reduction of risk potential
> *Taxonomic level:* Application

26. *Correct answer:* **D**

Unilateral hearing loss that occurs over an extended time and tinnitus are classic signs and symptoms of an acoustic neuroma. Amenorrhea, obesity, and acromegaly are signs of a pituitary tumor. Ataxia and intention tremors are seen with a cerebellar brain tumor.

> *Nursing process step:* Assessment
> *Client needs category:* Health promotion and maintenance
> *Client needs subcategory:* Prevention and early detection of disease
> *Taxonomic level:* Knowledge

27. *Correct answer:* **D**

Sucralfate should be administered on an empty stomach; therefore, it should be administered 1 hour before meals. Food in the stomach interferes with the binding of the drug to the ulcer surface.

> *Nursing process step:* Planning
> *Client needs category:* Physiological integrity
> *Client needs subcategory:* Pharmacological and parenteral therapies
> *Taxonomic level:* Knowledge

28. *Correct answer:* **B**

The nurse should encourage the patient to increase her fluid intake to approximately 3 qt (3 L)/day for 24 to 48 hours. The headache is most likely due to decreased cerebrospinal fluid (CSF) circulating around the cranium. This fluid loss allows the brain to move abnormally within the skull. The movement causes tension on the meninges and venous sinuses, causing pain. Extra oral fluid intake will increase CSF production. Lying flat may decrease pain, and raising the head of the bed may worsen the headache.

> *Nursing process step:* Implementation
> *Client needs category:* Physiological integrity
> *Client needs subcategory:* Reduction of risk potential
> *Taxonomic level:* Application

29. *Correct answer:* **C**

Because propranolol can decrease blood pressure and heart rate, the nurse should withhold the drug and notify the doctor if the patient's systolic blood pressure is less than 90 mm Hg or if the patient's pulse rate is less than 60 beats/minute.

> *Nursing process step:* Implementation
> *Client needs category:* Physiological integrity
> *Client needs subcategory:* Pharmacological and parenteral therapies
> *Taxonomic level:* Analysis

30. *Correct answer:* **A**

Vagal stimulation increases parasympathetic tone, which decreases the heart rate and may slow atrioventricular conduction.

> *Nursing process step:* Assessment
> *Client needs category:* Health promotion and maintenance
> *Client needs subcategory:* Prevention and early detection of disease
> *Taxonomic level:* Comprehension

31. *Correct answer:* **A**

The patient should be instructed to stagger antacids around other medications to avoid possible drug interactions. A patient may drink water after antacid administration, but it isn't a requirement.

> *Nursing process step:* Planning
> *Client needs category:* Physiological integrity
> *Client needs subcategory:* Pharmacological and parenteral therapies
> *Taxonomic level:* Comprehension

32. *Correct answer:* **D**

Patients who have had a total gastrectomy are at risk for developing pernicious anemia because the parietal cells in the stomach that secrete the intrinsic factor required for vitamin B_{12} absorption are no longer present. Therefore the patient will need lifelong vitamin B_{12} supplementation. Calcium, phosphorus, and vitamin D aren't helpful in preventing pernicious anemia.

> *Nursing process step:* Planning
> *Client needs category:* Physiological integrity
> *Client needs subcategory:* Pharmacological and parenteral therapies
> *Taxonomic level:* Comprehension

33. *Correct answer:* **C**

Swimming in warm water is recommended to promote comfort and flexibility. Strenuous exercise such as running and exercising in the cold may increase muscle weakness and fatigue.

Nursing process step: Planning
Client needs category: Physiological integrity
Client needs subcategory: Reduction of risk potential
Taxonomic level: Knowledge

34. *Correct answer:* **A**

Increased intraluminal pressure, transmural swelling, and inflammation can rupture the appendix and cause peritonitis. Hemorrhage and bowel obstruction aren't complications of appendicitis. Renal failure could result if the patient develops septic shock, but it's not a direct complication of appendicitis.

Nursing process step: Assessment
Client needs category: Physiological integrity
Client needs subcategory: Reduction of risk potential
Taxonomic level: Knowledge

35. *Correct answer:* **C**

The patient with angina must stop smoking. Smoking increases the blood carboxyhemoglobin level, which reduces the heart's oxygen supply, causing angina. The patient must seek immediate medical attention if chest pain doesn't subside after three nitroglycerin doses taken 10 to 15 minutes apart; serious myocardial damage or even sudden death may occur if chest pain persists for 2 hours. The patient should exercise daily to improve coronary circulation and promote weight management. The patient should eat plenty of fiber because it may decrease serum cholesterol and triglyceride levels.

Nursing process step: Planning
Client needs category: Physiological integrity
Client needs subcategory: Reduction of risk potential
Taxonomic level: Application

36. *Correct answer:* **A**

Pyridoxine commonly is administered to minimize peripheral neuropathy associated with isoniazid. Ethambutol hydrochloride is an antitubercular drug, which wouldn't be added because the patient has just begun concomitant isoniazid and rifampin therapy. Magnesium sulfate and cyanocobalamin aren't indicated for a patient taking isoniazid or rifampin; however, because the patient is probably suffering from malnutrition, cyanocobalamin may be prescribed.

Nursing process step: Implementation
Client needs category: Physiological integrity
Client needs subcategory: Pharmacological and parenteral therapy
Taxonomic level: Comprehension

37. *Correct answer:* **D**

Sudden increases in weakness with difficulty breathing and clearing secretions may be related to either a cholinergic or myasthenic crisis. An exacerbation of a myasthenic crisis from undermedication with anticholinesterase drugs or a cholinergic crisis from overmedication with these drugs may exhibit the same symptoms. General weakness isn't seen with hypertensive crisis. A hypo-osmolar state is seen in patients with Guillain-Barré syndrome, not myasthenia gravis.

> *Nursing process step:* Assessment
> *Client needs category:* Physiological integrity
> *Client needs subcategory:* Physiological adaptation
> *Taxonomic level:* Knowledge

38. *Correct answer:* **D**

When the obstruction is located high in the intestinal tract, little room exists for fluids or food. Vomiting of the gastric contents will relieve pressure and pain. The vomitus may have a fecal odor if the obstruction is low in the small bowel. Defecation may bring pain relief if the obstruction is in the lower intestinal tract. The patient typically won't have respiratory difficulty.

> *Nursing process step:* Assessment
> *Client needs category:* Physiological integrity
> *Client needs subcategory:* Reduction of risk potential
> *Taxonomic level:* Comprehension

39. *Correct answer:* **B**

When the intestinal obstruction is located high in the intestinal tract, vomitus will appear light green because it contains a small amount of bile. When the obstruction is in the lower part of the intestinal tract, the vomitus will appear dark green and have a fecal odor. Bright red–colored vomitus appears with GI bleeding.

> *Nursing process step:* Assessment
> *Client needs category:* Physiological integrity
> *Client needs subcategory:* Reduction of risk potential
> *Taxonomic level:* Knowledge

40. *Correct answer:* **A**

Liquid forms and simple compressed tablets are the only drug forms that can be administered through an NG tube. Tablets are enteric-coated to prevent stomach acids from destroying the drug; crushing the tablets would decrease their effectiveness. Time-release and controlled-delivery drugs are used to produce prolonged effects; crushing these drugs could result in overdose.

Nursing process step: Planning
Client needs category: Physiological integrity
Client needs subcategory: Pharmacological and parenteral therapies
Taxonomic level: Comprehension

41. *Correct answer:* **B**

The patient should be encouraged to avoid predisposing factors, such as stress, strenuous exercise, infection, extreme heat, surgery, and change in sleep habits.

Nursing process step: Implementation
Client needs category: Physiological integrity
Client needs subcategory: Reduction of risk potential
Taxonomic level: Application

42. *Correct answer:* **B**

Before removing the client's NG tube, the nurse should assess the patient for bowel sounds. If bowel sounds aren't present, the patient may still have a bowel obstruction or paralytic ileus, so the tube shouldn't be removed. Ability to chew, hunger, and a residual gastric volume of less than 100 ml don't determine whether an NG tube should be removed.

Nursing process step: Assessment
Client needs category: Physiological integrity
Client needs subcategory: Reduction of risk potential
Taxonomic level: Knowledge

43. *Correct answer:* **C**

Although electrolyte disturbances, respiratory arrest, and drug toxicity can cause cardiac arrest, ventricular fibrillation is the most common cause of cardiac arrest in adults.

Nursing process step: Evaluation
Client needs category: Physiological integrity
Client needs subcategory: Physiological adaptation
Taxonomic level: Application

44. *Correct answer:* **B**

Normally, the ventilation-perfusion ratio is 0.8:1. Because of gravity and pleural pressure, ventilation and perfusion are weakest at the apex and strongest at the base. Anything that interferes with ventilation, such as bronchospasm, lowers the ratio. Anything that interferes with perfusion, such as pulmonary embolism, increases the ratio. Ventilation scans are performed by having the patient inhale a radioactive substance; perfusion scans are performed by administering to the patient an I.V. injection of a radioactive substance.

Nursing process step: Evaluation
Client needs category: Health promotion and maintenance
Client needs subcategory: Prevention and early detection of disease
Taxonomic level: Analysis

45. *Correct answer:* **D**

The patient is acidotic, with a pH of 7.24. The normal $Paco_2$ and low HCO_3^- indicate a metabolic problem not compensated by the increased respiratory rate or acidosis. The patient may require mechanical ventilation because of the low Pao_2 level and known pulmonary infiltrates.

Nursing process step: Evaluation
Client needs category: Physiological integrity
Client needs subcategory: Reduction of risk potential
Taxonomic level: Analysis

46. *Correct answer:* **A**

Patients with neuropathy affecting the legs and feet will have decreased sensation and may be unaware of temperature extremes and injury. The patient should be advised to wear shoes and socks and stop smoking if possible (smoking causes vasoconstriction). Vasoconstriction will exacerbate the problem. Vitamin K intake isn't related to this problem.

Nursing process step: Planning
Client needs category: Physiological integrity
Client needs subcategory: Reduction of risk potential
Taxonomic level: Application

47. *Correct answer:* **D**

The effluent should be liquid because the water won't be removed from the stool as with an intact colon. The fecal material becomes more formed and solid as it moves through the colon.

Nursing process step: Assessment
Client needs category: Physiological integrity
Client needs subcategory: Basic care and comfort
Taxonomic level: Knowledge

48. *Correct answer:* **D**

The dietary teaching plan should include telling the patient to avoid high-fiber foods that could cause blockage. The patient should consume plenty of fluids and be encouraged to maintain a high-calorie diet that is rich in potassium.

Nursing process step: Planning
Client needs category: Physiological integrity
Client needs subcategory: Basic care and comfort
Taxonomic level: Comprehension

49. *Correct answer:* **B**

Stridor is a very loud musical sound that can be heard at a distance, usually without a stethoscope. It's caused by laryngeal spasm and mucosal swelling, which contract the vocal cords and narrow the airway. Wheeze is a continuous, high-pitched sound that has musical quality. Crackle is a short, explosive or popping sound usually heard during inspiration. Pleural friction rub is a loud, grating sound caused by inflamed or damaged pleurae.

Nursing process step: Assessment
Client needs category: Health promotion and maintenance
Client needs subcategory: Prevention and early detection of disease
Taxonomic level: Knowledge

50. *Correct answer:* **A**

Neomycin, an antibiotic, is used to decrease the bacteria in the bowel before surgery to reduce the risk of wound contamination. Antibiotics don't increase the immune system's response. Shallow breathing causes atelectasis; neomycin won't prevent it from occurring. Neomycin has no effect on bladder tone.

Nursing process step: Planning
Client needs category: Physiological integrity
Client needs subcategory: Pharmacological and parenteral therapies
Taxonomic level: Knowledge

51. *Correct answer:* **A**

Patients with hyponatremia are at high risk for seizures. Nursing interventions should be aimed at safety and protection, including using padded side rails, administering supplemental oxygen, and keeping an oral airway readily available. Peripheral edema isn't associated with SIADH. Thyrotropin is a hormone produced by the anterior pituitary gland; it has no role in SIADH. Pulmonary edema is a complication of hypernatremia and isn't commonly seen in SIADH or hyponatremia.

Nursing process step: Analysis
Client needs category: Physiological integrity
Client needs subcategory: Reduction of risk potential
Taxonomic level: Analysis

52. *Correct answer:* **A**

The patient with left-sided heart failure typically has air hunger, tachypnea, and orthopnea. Ascites, jugular vein distention, and pitting leg edema are signs of right-sided heart failure, another complication of cardiomyopathy.

> *Nursing process step:* Assessment
> *Client needs category:* Physiological integrity
> *Client needs subcategory:* Physiological adaptation
> *Taxonomic level:* Knowledge

53. *Correct answer:* **C**

Pain may be triggered by touching the face, being exposed to a cool breeze, having hair touch the face, talking, or chewing.

> *Nursing process step:* Assessment
> *Client needs category:* Physiological integrity
> *Client needs subcategory:* Reduction of risk potential
> *Taxonomic level:* Knowledge

54. *Correct answer:* **B**

Alteration in skin integrity would be the priority nursing diagnosis for daily care of the colostomy because the effluent from the colostomy can be irritating to the skin. Diarrhea isn't a concern at this point. The patient will be allowed nothing by mouth until peristalsis returns. The patient should get out of bed on the first postoperative day, so immobility shouldn't be a problem.

> *Nursing process step:* Analysis
> *Client needs category:* Physiological integrity
> *Client needs subcategory:* Reduction of risk potential
> *Taxonomic level:* Analysis

55. *Correct answer:* **D**

Although microorganisms that cause sepsis syndrome can enter through the skin, GI tract, or respiratory tract, the most common portal of entry is the urinary tract via urinary catheters, suprapubic tubes, and cystoscopic examination.

> *Nursing process step:* Assessment
> *Client needs category:* Safe, effective care environment
> *Client needs subcategory:* Safety and infection control
> *Taxonomic level:* Knowledge

56. *Correct answer:* **B**

Daily weight measurement is the most accurate means of monitoring hydration status at home. The patient should be encouraged to increase dietary intake of both sodium and potassium, particularly if diuretics are prescribed. Pulse checks and urine specific gravity measurements are unnecessary in a patient with chronic SIADH.

> *Nursing process step:* Evaluation
> *Client needs category:* Physiological integrity
> *Client needs subcategory:* Reduction of risk potential
> *Taxonomic level:* Analysis

57. *Correct answer:* **A**

A chest X-ray discloses the position of the chest tube to determine the procedure's effectiveness. The X-ray isn't done to advance the tube, although the doctor may decide to adjust the tube after reviewing the X-ray. Tomography — used to study cavities, neoplasms, and lung densities — visualizes a single layer of the lungs. An ultrasound or echogram records sound waves that penetrate the lungs.

> *Nursing process step:* Evaluation
> *Client needs category:* Physiological integrity
> *Client needs subcategory:* Physiological adaptation
> *Taxonomic level:* Application

58. *Correct answer:* **A**

Otorrhea and rhinorrhea are classic signs of a basilar skull fracture. Injury to the dura commonly occurs with this fracture, resulting in cerebrospinal fluid (CSF) leaking through the ears and nose. Any fluid suspected of being CSF should be checked for glucose or have a halo test done.

> *Nursing process step:* Assessment
> *Client needs category:* Physiological integrity
> *Client needs subcategory:* Physiological adaptation
> *Taxonomic level:* Knowledge

59. *Correct answer:* **B**

Prosopagnosia, the inability to recognize oneself and significant others, may be alleviated if the patient is frequently exposed to photographs of himself and his significant others.

> *Nursing process step:* Planning
> *Client needs category:* Psychosocial integrity
> *Client needs subcategory:* Coping and adaptation
> *Taxonomic level:* Application

60. *Correct answer:* **A**

The purpose of a CPM machine is to facilitate joint mobility. The degree of flexion will be increased daily to help the patient regain normal range of motion. It's the nurse's responsibility to monitor the degree of flexion according to the doctor's or therapist's order and to ensure the knee is placed directly over the knee gatch of the machine. Although ambulating with assistance and crutches or a walker may be allowed postoperatively, bed rest isn't usually necessary. Active range of motion isn't necessary when CPM is being used. Massaging an immobile extremity is contraindicated due to the risk of mobilizing a blood clot.

> *Nursing process step:* Planning
> *Client needs category:* Physiological integrity
> *Client needs subcategory:* Reduction of risk potential
> *Taxonomic level:* Application

61. *Correct answer:* B

Osteoclasts break down the matrix of bone and bring about resorption of the mineral contents. Inhibiting osteoclast activity slows the demineralization of bone. Osteoblasts synthesize collagen and enhance the mineralization of bone. Nonhormonal drugs have no effect on estrogen or vitamin D, both of which are important for maintaining bone mass.

> *Nursing process step:* Not applicable
> *Client needs category:* Physiological integrity
> *Client needs subcategory:* Pharmacological and parenteral therapies
> *Taxonomic level:* Application

62. *Correct answer:* C

Cardiac tamponade is associated with decreased cardiac output, resulting in decreased blood pressure. Removing a small amount of blood may improve cardiac output and blood pressure. Pericardial blood doesn't clot rapidly because it's defibrinated by cardiac motion within the cardiac sac. If blood clots rapidly, the needle may have entered the heart. Patients with cardiac tamponade may have muffled heart sounds. If pericardiocentesis is effective, heart sounds become normal.

> *Nursing process step:* Evaluation
> *Client needs category:* Physiological integrity
> *Client needs subcategory:* Physiological adaptation
> *Taxonomic level:* Analysis

63. *Correct answer:* B

The effects of rest and activity on pain is one of the significant differences between rheumatoid arthritis and osteoarthritis. A patient with rheumatoid arthritis experiences morning joint stiffness; a patient with osteoarthritis experiences more pain as the day progresses and may function better after a night of rest.

> *Nursing process step:* Assessment
> *Client needs category:* Physiological integrity
> *Client needs subcategory:* Reduction of risk potential
> *Taxonomic level:* Knowledge

64. *Correct answer:* C

Minimal I.V. fluids are provided to reduce cerebral edema. The head of the bed should be at 30 degrees to facilitate venous return, thus decreasing intracranial pressure. Neurologic assessment should be performed every 1 to 2 hours. A pillow may be used to promote comfort.

> *Nursing process step:* Implementation
> *Client needs category:* Physiological integrity
> *Client needs subcategory:* Reduction of risk potential
> *Taxonomic level:* Application

65. *Correct answer:* B

S_1 is best heard at the apex of the heart. The second heart sound (S_2) is best heard over the base of the heart at the end of ventricular systole. The low-pitched, rumbling, crescendo-decrescendo murmur common with mitral stenosis can be auscultated in the mitral area. The low, rumbling, crescendo-decrescendo murmur found in tricuspid stenosis can be auscultated in the tricuspid area of the heart.

> *Nursing process step:* Assessment
> *Client needs category:* Health promotion and maintenance
> *Client needs subcategory:* Prevention and early detection of disease
> *Taxonomic level:* Comprehension

66. *Correct answer:* C

Fluid restriction is essential in treating chronic SIADH. Fluids typically are restricted to 27 to 34 oz (800 to 1,000 ml)/day. If diuretics are prescribed, sodium and potassium supplements may be needed. A hypertonic sodium chloride I.V. solution might be used in the acute phase of treatment if the patient is severely hyponatremic.

> *Nursing process step:* Implementation
> *Client needs category:* Physiological integrity
> *Client needs subcategory:* Reduction of risk potential
> *Taxonomic level:* Application

67. *Correct answer:* C

The best possible Glasgow Coma Scale score is 15; the lowest, 3. A score of 8 or less indicates coma. When associated with a new head injury, it indicates a serious traumatic injury, and the airway may be compromised and need intubation.

> *Nursing process step:* Assessment
> *Client needs category:* Physiological integrity
> *Client needs subcategory:* Reduction of risk potential
> *Taxonomic level:* Application

68. *Correct answer:* **B**

Promethazine requires cautious use in a patient with hepatic or cardiovascular disease, respiratory or seizure disorder, glaucoma, and prostatic hyperplasia.

> *Nursing process step:* Implementation
> *Client needs category:* Physiological integrity
> *Client needs subcategory:* Pharmacological and parenteral therapies
> *Taxonomic level:* Application

69. *Correct answer:* **A**

During therapy with any cephalosporin, the patient should ingest yogurt or buttermilk, which replenishes normal GI flora, to prevent intestinal superinfection.

> *Nursing process step:* Planning
> *Client needs category:* Physiological integrity
> *Client needs subcategory:* Basic care and comfort
> *Taxonomic level:* Application

70. *Correct answer:* **B**

Vancomycin is contraindicated in a pregnant patient or one with known hypersensitivity or a hearing loss.

> *Nursing process step:* Planning
> *Client needs category:* Physiological integrity
> *Client needs subcategory:* Pharmacological and parenteral therapies
> *Taxonomic level:* Comprehension

71. *Correct answer:* **D**

Angina is caused by altered tissue perfusion to the myocardium, which results in ischemia. Treatment is aimed at reversing ischemia. Pain and anxiety should also be addressed, but they don't take priority over altered tissue perfusion. Cardiac output may or may not be affected with angina.

> *Nursing process step:* Analysis
> *Client needs category:* Physiological integrity
> *Client needs subcategory:* Reduction of risk potential
> *Taxonomic level:* Analysis

72. *Correct answer:* **D**

The primary mode of transmission for hepatitis A is through fecal contamination of food or water. Hepatitis A is also commonly transmitted through sexual contact with people previously infected with hepatitis A. Blood is the primary mode of transmission for hepatitis B and C.

Nursing process step: Assessment
Client needs category: Safe, effective care environment
Client needs subcategory: Safety and infection control
Taxonomic level: Comprehension

73. *Correct answer:* **B**

A barky cough usually occurs with croup, with the coughing frequency increasing at night. Crackles are popping noises usually heard during inhalation. They indicate that fluid, pus, or mucus is in the smaller airways. When heard, the nurse should instruct the patient to cough and breathe deeply; the nurse should then auscultate again. The sounds may have cleared. Wheezing is a high-pitched musical sound. It can be heard during inhalation and exhalation and usually accompanies an asthma attack or bronchospasm.

Nursing process step: Assessment
Client needs category: Physiological integrity
Client needs subcategory: Reduction of risk potential
Taxonomic level: Application

74. *Correct answer:* **A**

The patient should be monitored closely and given low-flow oxygen to decrease chances of depressing the respiratory drive. Increasing fluids to liquefy secretions, humidifying the air, and performing postural drainage are also important for a patient with acute bronchitis.

Nursing process step: Implementation
Client needs category: Physiological integrity
Client needs subcategory: Reduction of risk potential
Taxonomic level: Analysis

75. *Correct answer:* **C**

A urine output of 30 ml/hour or more indicates that the patient has received adequate volume replacement and that renal perfusion is normal. Any volume less than 30 ml/hour indicates the need for more fluids.

Nursing process step: Evaluation
Client needs category: Physiological integrity
Client needs subcategory: Reduction of risk potential
Taxonomic level: Analysis

76. *Correct answer:* **B**

The priority in the initial treatment of patients in anaphylactic shock is maintaining airway patency. Anaphylactic shock is associated with the sudden onset of severe respiratory distress. Bronchospasm and laryngeal edema may lead to airway obstruction. I.V. access should be initiated to administer antihistamines and other drugs. Infusing a bolus of crystalloids isn't necessary because the hypotension in this type of shock is caused by vasodilation, not hypovolemia. Therefore, the patient's blood pressure would remain low even after the fluid bolus.

Nursing process step: Implementation
Client needs category: Physiological integrity
Client needs subcategory: Physiological adaptation
Taxonomic level: Application

77. *Correct answer:* C

Lyme disease is a tick-borne disease that progresses through distinctly separate stages. In the first stage, the disease presents with red-ringed, circular skin lesions called erythema chronicum migrans. At the same time the lesions appear, the patient generally experiences headache, stiff neck, fever, and malaise. During the second stage, cardiomegaly, neuritis, and myopericarditis may appear. The final stage includes arthritic pain, chronic synovitis, lack of coordination, facial palsy, paralysis, and dementia.

Nursing process step: Assessment
Client needs category: Health promotion and maintenance
Client needs subcategory: Prevention and early detection of disease
Taxonomic level: Comprehension

78. *Correct answer:* B

The presence of an increased number of epithelial cells, especially when they exceed the number of WBCs, indicates a contaminated specimen. Proper cleaning and retrieval of the specimen may not have taken place. The presence of bacteria, WBCs, and pus suggests spyelonephritis or a urinary tract infection.

Nursing process step: Planning
Client needs category: Safe effective care environment
Client needs subcategory: Safety and infection control
Taxonomic level: Analysis

79. *Correct answer:* C

Pyelonephritis is diagnosed by the presence of leukocytosis, hematuria, pyuria, and bacteriuria. The patient presents with fever, chills, and flank pain. Because there is often a septic picture, the white blood cell count is more likely to be elevated, not low. Ketonuria indicates a diabetic state.

Nursing process step: Assessment
Client needs category: Physiological integrity
Client needs subcategory: Reduction of risk potential
Taxonomic level: Comprehension

80. *Correct answer:* **B**

Hydration and analgesia are the priority interventions for the patient with a kidney stone. I.V. fluids are given to hydrate the patient and help flush out the stone. Fluids at a keep-vein-open rate would be inadequate for this patient. An indwelling urinary catheter and an NG tube usually aren't necessary.

Nursing process step: Planning
Client needs category: Physiological integrity
Client needs subcategory: Reduction of risk potential
Taxonomic level: Application

81. *Correct answer:* **C**

Didanosine should be administered on an empty stomach regardless of the dosage form used. Administering the drug with meals can decrease the drug's absorption by 50%. The powdered form should be mixed in 4 oz (120 ml) of water. Don't use fruit juice or other beverages that may be acidic; they decrease the drug's effectiveness. Specific positioning isn't necessary after taking didanosine.

Nursing process step: Implementation
Client needs category: Physiological integrity
Client needs subcategory: Pharmacological and parenteral therapies
Taxonomic level: Knowledge

82. *Correct answer:* **B**

Candida albicans is treated with nystatin (Mycostatin) and doesn't require treatment for sexual partners. *Neisseria gonorrhoeae, Trichomonas vaginalis,* and *Chlamydia trachomatis* are sexually transmitted diseases that require that partners be treated.

Nursing process step: Planning
Client needs category: Safe, effective care environment
Client needs subcategory: Safety and infection control
Taxonomic level: Comprehension

83. *Correct answer:* **A**

Patients who have undergone gastrectomy surgery are at risk for pernicious anemia because they're unable to absorb vitamin B_{12} due to a lack of intrinsic factor secreted in the stomach. I.V. drug users aren't at risk for pernicious anemia. Patients with colostomies have an intact stomach, so they don't lack intrinsic factor and therefore aren't at risk for pernicious anemia. Alcoholics are prone to folic acid deficiency.

Nursing process step: Assessment
Client needs category: Physiological integrity
Client needs subcategory: Reduction of risk potential
Taxonomic level: Application

84. *Correct answer:* **B**

Patients who require valve replacement must take warfarin (Coumadin) postoperatively to prevent clot formation. The patient won't need an iron supplement, and she shouldn't take aspirin while taking warfarin because of its anticoagulant effect.

> *Nursing process step:* Evaluation
> *Client needs category:* Physiological integrity
> *Client needs subcategory:* Reduction of risk potential
> *Taxonomic level:* Application

85. *Correct answer:* **D**

The symptoms specific to epidural opioids are itching, nausea, vomiting, and urine retention. Opioid narcotics given by any route can cause excessive sedation, respiratory depression, hypotension, and confusion. Inadequate pain relief usually is associated with inappropriate doses for the individual patient.

> *Nursing process step:* Assessment
> *Client needs category:* Physiological integrity
> *Client needs subcategory:* Pharmacological and parenteral therapies
> *Taxonomic level:* Knowledge

86. *Correct answer:* **A**

The CPM machine flexes and extends the knee through controlled range of motion, lessening postoperative stiffness. The motion may increase the amount of blood evacuated from the joint. In some patients, it increases pain. The patient receives anticoagulants to reduce the risk of clot formation.

> *Nursing process step:* Evaluation
> *Client needs category:* Physiological integrity
> *Client needs subcategory:* Reduction of risk potential
> *Taxonomic level:* Knowledge

87. *Correct answer:* **B**

After joint replacement surgery, prophylactic use of antibiotics is recommended before dental procedures and any time transient bacteremia is expected. This is necessary to prevent the prosthesis from becoming infected. Infection of the prosthesis could result in the need to remove it. Taking her temperature won't prevent infection. When the surgical wound is healed, there is no need to avoid swimming.

> *Nursing process step:* Planning
> *Client needs category:* Physiological integrity
> *Client needs subcategory:* Reduction of risk potential
> *Taxonomic level:* Knowledge

88. *Correct answer:* **B**

The primary treatment for compartment syndrome is to relieve the source of the pressure. The cast would be removed or split to relieve the external pressure. If symptoms persist, a fasciotomy would be considered, to relieve the internal pressure. Limb elevation above the heart would decrease arterial perfusion and make the problem worse. Vasodilators don't increase tissue perfusion in compartment syndrome.

> *Nursing process step:* Implementation
> *Client needs category:* Physiological integrity
> *Client needs subcategory:* Physiological adaptation
> *Taxonomic level:* Application

89. *Correct answer:* **C**

During fasciotomy the fascia is opened along the length of the muscle compartment and the skin is left open to prevent further compression from swelling. Sterile dressings are applied but without applying pressure. The wound is watched closely, and usually the compartment can be closed in 3 to 5 days. When the wound is closed, it may be sutured or secured with tape. A skin graft may be needed to complete closure at a later date.

> *Nursing process step:* Implementation
> *Client needs category:* Physiological integrity
> *Client needs subcategory:* Reduction of risk potential
> *Taxonomic level:* Comprehension

90. *Correct answer:* **B**

Serum uric acid levels will be elevated during all stages of gout. During acute episodes the ESR is elevated. White blood cell count is also elevated during acute episodes, but the results of the CBC, rheumatoid factor, and creatinine, glucose, and calcium levels don't help diagnose gout.

> *Nursing process step:* Assessment
> *Client needs category:* Physiological integrity
> *Client needs subcategory:* Reduction of risk potential
> *Taxonomic level:* Knowledge

91. *Correct answer:* **A**

Prolonged use of hydrochlorothiazide can cause hyperuricemia. As uric acid accumulates in the blood, urate crystals are deposited in the joints, promoting an inflammatory response. Reducing protein in the diet usually isn't helpful in treating gout. Heart failure and inactivity aren't associated with gout.

Nursing process step: Assessment
Client needs category: Physiological integrity
Client needs subcategory: Pharmacological and parenteral therapies
Taxonomic level: Application

92. *Correct answer:* **A**

Treatment for an acute episode of gout is aimed at reducing pain and inflammation as soon as possible, usually with anti-inflammatory drugs. After the acute episode has subsided, other drugs may be given to increase uric acid excretion or decrease its synthesis.

Nursing process step: Evaluation
Client needs category: Physiological integrity
Client needs subcategory: Pharmacological and parenteral therapies
Taxonomic level: Knowledge

93. *Correct answer:* **A**

The rotator cuff is made up of four muscles and their tendons, which provide stability to the ball-and-socket shoulder joint. These muscles are the supraspinatus, subscapularis, infraspinatus, and teres minor.

Nursing process step: Assessment
Client needs category: Physiological integrity
Client needs subcategory: Reduction of risk potential
Taxonomic level: Comprehension

94. *Correct answer:* **A**

Application of ice followed by heat and rest for 1 week should bring about improvement in partial tears or inflammation of the rotator cuff. Anti-inflammatory medications may also be used. If symptoms improve, rehabilitation to strengthen the rotator cuff can begin. If there is no improvement, studies such as magnetic resonance imaging may be done to determine if there is a complete tear. A complete tear usually requires surgical repair.

Nursing process step: Implementation
Client needs category: Physiological integrity
Client needs subcategory: Reduction of risk potential
Taxonomic level: Knowledge

95. *Correct answer:* **C**

Taking prednisone (or any glucocorticoid) in the early morning rather than at bedtime helps the patient maintain the normal pattern of cortisol production by the adrenal glands. This production peaks during the early morning; because cortisol production depends on the body's cortisol level, taking prednisone in the early morning suppresses the patient's endogenous cortisol production. Taking prednisone with food reduces gastric irritation; taking the drug before or after a meal or snack would be less effective.

Nursing process step: Implementation
Client needs category: Physiological integrity
Client needs subcategory: Pharmacological and parenteral therapies
Taxonomic level: Application

96. *Correct answer:* **D**

Because exposure to ultraviolet light can activate systemic lupus erythematosus, the patient should avoid direct exposure to sunlight and wear sunscreen and protective clothing to filter out reflected rays. Giving the patient no restrictions or telling her she can sunbathe for a limited time may lead to dangerous exposure to ultraviolet light. The patient shouldn't keep her medication outside near the pool; it could get wet.

Nursing process step: Implementation
Client needs category: Physiological integrity
Client needs subcategory: Reduction of risk potential
Taxonomic level: Application

97. *Correct answer:* **D**

Type 2 diabetes is diagnosed with two fasting blood glucose levels ≥126 mg/dl or a casual plasma glucose level ≥200 mg/dl and symptoms. Because his first fasting blood glucose level was >126 mg/dl, it must be repeated to make the diagnosis of type 2 diabetes.

Nursing process step: Implementation
Client needs category: Health promotion and maintenance
Client needs subcategory: Prevention and early detection of disease
Taxonomic level: Application

98. *Correct answer:* **C**

The pathophysiology of type 2 diabetes involves insulin resistance, impaired insulin secretion, and inappropriate hepatic glucose production. Type 2 diabetes isn't an autoimmune disease. Although type 2 diabetes is characterized by elevated insulin levels, because of insulin resistance, that insulin isn't effective. Eating sweets doesn't cause diabetes. However, it may contribute to the development of diabetes if eating sweets causes obesity.

Nursing process step: Implementation
Client needs category: Physiological integrity
Client needs subcategory: Reduction of risk potential
Taxonomic level: Knowledge

99. *Correct answer:* **A**

Modest weight loss (5% to 10% of body weight) and exercise both decrease insulin resistance, which improves insulin sensitivity. These management modalities don't enhance insulin secretion, but the insulin that's secreted is more effective. Although modest weight loss and exercise generally help patients feel better, this isn't the major reason these modalities are prescribed. The natural history of type 2 diabetes is a gradual inability of the pancreas to maintain the required insulin secretion. Therefore, it's unlikely that modest weight loss and exercise will prevent the progression of diabetes for the rest of the patient's life, although they will delay the progression as long as the patient maintains euglycemia.

> *Nursing process step:* Implementation
> *Client needs category:* Physiological integrity
> *Client needs subcategory:* Basic care and comfort
> *Taxonomic level:* Application

100. *Correct answer:* **D**

In making lifestyle changes, helping patients to problem solve and come up with options and solutions that appeal to them is more effective than a prescriptive approach. Although weight loss is effective, it's more successful when accompanied by an exercise program, and exercise is most effective in decreasing insulin resistance.

> *Nursing process step:* Implementation
> *Client needs category:* Physiological integrity
> *Client needs subcategory:* Reduction of risk potential
> *Taxonomic level:* Application

SELECTED REFERENCES

Assessment Made Incredibly Easy. Springhouse, Pa.: Springhouse Corp., 1998.

Baere, P. G., and Myers, J. L. *Principles and Practice of Adult Health Nursing: Learning Guide*, 3rd ed. St. Louis: Mosby–Year Book, Inc., 1997.

Berger, K. *Fundamentals of Nursing*, 2nd ed. Stamford, Conn.: Appleton & Lange, 1998.

Black, J., and Matassarin-Jacobs, E. *Medical-Surgical Nursing: Clinical Management for Continuity of Care*, 5th ed. Philadelphia: W.B. Saunders Co., 1997.

Bloom, B.S., et al. *Taxonomy of Educational Objectives: The Classification of Educational Goals, Handbook 1*. New York: David McKay, 1956.

Cleveland, L., et al. *Nursing Pharmacology and Clinical Management*. Philadelphia: Lippincott, Williams & Wilkins, 1998.

deWit, S. *Essentials of Medical-Surgical Nursing*, 4th ed. Philadelphia: W.B. Saunders Co., 1998.

Handbook of Medical-Surgical Nursing, 2nd ed. Springhouse, Pa.: Springhouse Corp., 1998.

Luckmann, J. *Saunders Manual of Nursing Care*. Philadelphia: W.B. Saunders Co., 1997.

Mastering Medical-Surgical Nursing. Springhouse, Pa.: Springhouse Corp., 1997.

Medical-Surgical Nursing, 3rd ed. Springhouse Notes Series. Springhouse, Pa.: Springhouse Corp., 1997.

Monahan, F., and Neighbors, M. *Medical-Surgical Nursing Foundations for Clinical Practice*, 2nd ed. Philadelphia: W.B. Saunders Co., 1998.

National Council Detailed Test Plan for the NCLEX-RN Examination. Chicago: National Council of State Boards of Nursing, Inc., 1997.

Polaski, A., and Tatro, S. *Luckmann's Core Principles and Practice of Medical-Surgical Nursing*. Philadelphia: W.B. Saunders Co., 1996.

Smeltzer, S., and Bare, B. *Brunner and Suddarth's Textbook of Medical-Surgical Nursing*, 8th ed. Philadelphia: Lippincott, Williams & Wilkins, 1996.

INDEX

A

ABG. *See* Arterial blood gas.
Acetaminophen (Tylenol), 243, 244, 260
Acoustic neuroma, symptoms of, 281, 303
Acquired immunodeficiency syndrome, 244, 245, 261
Acromegaly, 216, 235, 236
Acute myeloblastic leukemia, 248, 265
Addisonian crisis, 214, 233
Adenoma, pituitary, 213, 216
  high corticotropin levels and, 232
  preoperative teaching for patient with, 236
Adrenal insufficiency, 214, 233, 234
Adult respiratory distress syndrome, 9, 10
  mechanical ventilation for, 27
  trauma and, 26
AIDS. *See* Acquired immunodeficiency syndrome.
Airway clearance, ineffective, tracheostomy and, 11, 29
Airway obstruction, cardiopulmonary resuscitation and, 277, 297
Albuterol (Proventil), 278, 298
Alcoholism, chronic, 150, 167
Allopurinol (Zyloprim), 248, 265
Alpha-interferon therapy, 244, 260
ALS. *See* Amyotrophic lateral sclerosis.
Aluminum hydroxide, 147, 163
Alveolocapillary membrane damage, 10, 27
Alzheimer's disease, 85, 103
Amantadine (Symadine), 84, 103
American Cancer Society, 226
Amyotrophic lateral sclerosis, 74, 91
Anaphylactic shock, maintaining airway patency and, 290, 315, 316
Anemia, 252, 253, 291
  aplastic, 270, 271
  pernicious, 271, 272, 282, 304, 317
Aneurysm, cerebral. *See* Cerebral aneurysm.
Anger, tachycardia and, 37, 53
Angina, nursing diagnosis for patient with, 289, 314
Angioplasty, percutaneous transluminal coronary, 46, 64

Angiotensin-converting enzyme inhibitors, for hypertension, 38, 54
Antacids, 282, 304
Antibiotics, 43, 107, 292
  diarrhea and, 123
  prophylactic use of, 61, 318
Anticoagulant, 14, 46
  administering, during percutaneous transluminal coronary angioplasty, 64
  interaction with guaifenesin, 33
Antihypertensive drugs, 47, 65
Anuria, 141, 155
Aortic aneurysm, thoracic, 43, 60
Aortic dissection, 43, 60
Aphasia, global, 72, 89
Appendectomy, 111, 128
Appendicitis, 110, 283
  knowledge deficit and, 127, 128
  peritonitis and, 305
  signs of, 127
ARDS. *See* Adult respiratory distress syndrome.
Arrhythmias
  atrial, 24
  cardiac, 25
Arterial blood gas, 4, 10, 11, 279
  chest tube insertion and, 299
  metabolic acidosis and, 28
  respiratory acidosis and, 19
  respiratory alkalosis and, 28, 29
Arterial occlusive disease, 48, 67, 254, 273
Arterial pulse, 36, 52
Arthrocentesis, 243, 259
Arthroscopy, 184, 185
  decreased sensation and, 201
  treating joint conditions with, 200
Aseptic necrosis, 181, 196
Aspiration, risk for, bronchoscopy and, 7, 24
Aspirin
  enteric-coated, 243, 259
  idiopathic thrombocytopenic purpura and, 245, 262
  postoperative bleeding and, 39, 56

U

Ulcerative colitis, 114, 132
Urinary catheter, 141, 144, 286
  aspirating urine and, 156
  maintaining drainage system's patency and,
    160
  sepsis syndrome and, 310
Urine output, 147, 217, 290
  diabetes insipidus and, 237
  fluid intake and, 164, 315
Urine pH, normal, 142, 157
Urine retention, 106, 122

V

Vagal stimulation, 282, 304
Vagotomy, 109, 125
Valsalva's maneuver, 32
Vasoconstriction, 76, 94
Vaso-occlusive crisis, 251, 252
  fluid intake and, 269
  mesenteric infarction and, 270
  priapism and, 270
Vasopressin (Pitressin), 208, 225
Vasospasm, 73, 75, 90, 93
Vecuronium bromide, 4, 20
Ventilation-perfusion ratio, 284, 307
Ventricular fibrillation, 40, 55, 57, 284, 307
Venturi mask, 23
Vincristine (Oncovin), 255, 274
Vitamin B_{12}, 253, 254, 282
  neurologic dysfunction and, 272
  pernicious anemia and, 272, 304
Vitamin D, decreased activation of, renal
    failure and, 143, 159
Vomiting, increased intracranial pressure
    and, 71, 87

WXY

Warfarin (Coumadin)
  for preventing clot formation, 291, 318
  variable dose response of, 183, 199

Z

Zidovudine (AZT)
  anemia caused by, 245, 261
  interaction with acetaminophen, 243, 244,
    260